THE H.E.R.B.A.L. GUIDE Dietary Supplement Resources for the Clinician

ROBERT ALAN BONAKDAR, MD, FAAFP

Director of Pain Management
Scripps Center for Integrative Medicine
La Jolla, California

Co-Director
Natural Supplements: An Evidence-Based Update Conference

Assistant Clinical Professor
Department of Family and Preventative Medicine (Voluntary)
University of California, San Diego School of Medicine
San Diego, California

Wolters Kluwer | Lippincott Williams & Wilkins
Health

Philadelphia • Baltimore • New York • London
Buenos Aires • Hong Kong • Sydney • Tokyo

Acquisitions Editor: Sonya Seigafuse
Product Manager: Kerry Barrett
Vendor Manager: Bridgett Dougherty
Senior Manufacturing Manager: Benjamin Rivera
Marketing Manager: Kim Schonberger
Creative Director: Doug Smock
Production Service: Aptara

530 Walnut Street
Philadelphia, PA 19106 USA
LWW.com

Printed in China

Library of Congress Cataloging-in-Publication Data

The H.E.R.B.A.L. guide : dietary supplement resources for the clinician / Robert Alan Bonakdar.
p. ; cm.
Includes bibliographical references and index.
ISBN 978-0-7817-8268-5 (alk. paper)
1. Dietary supplements—Handbooks, manuals, etc. 2. Materia medica, Vegetable—Handbooks, manuals, etc. 3. Herbs—Therapeutic use—Handbooks, manuals, etc. I. Title. II. Title: Herbal guide.
[DNLM: 1. Dietary Supplements. 2. Complementary Therapies. 3. Industry. 4. Phytotherapy. QU 145.5 B697h 2010]
RM258.5.B66 2010
615′.321—dc22

2009045889

To purchase additional copies of this book, call our customer service department at (800) 638-3030 or fax orders to (301) 223-2320. International customers should call (301) 223-2300.

Visit Lippincott Williams & Wilkins on the Internet: at LWW.com. Lippincott Williams & Wilkins customer service representatives are available from 8:30 am to 6 pm, EST.

10 9 8 7 6 5 4 3 2 1

RRS0912

To my wife, Jennifer, and the entire Bonakdar and Prine family for your never-ending love and support.

CONTRIBUTORS

Sue Akeroyd, PhC, MPS, MRPharmS (Medicines)
Regulatory Consultant
Victoria, Australia

Randall S. Alberte, PhD
Chief Scientific Officer
HerbalScience Group LLC.
Naples, FL

Sloan Ayers
HerbalScience Group LLC
Naples, Florida

Marilyn Barrett, PhD
Pharmacognosy Consulting
Mill Valley, CA

Stephanie Bethune, ND
Stonington Natural Health Center
Stonington, CT

Joseph M. Betz, PhD
Director, Dietary Supplement Methods and Reference Materials Program
Office of Dietary Supplements
National Institute of Health
Bethesda, MD

Mark Blumenthal
Founder and Executive Director
American Botanic Council
Editor, HerbalGram & HerbClip
Austin, TX

Robert Alan Bonakdar, MD, FAAFP
Director of Pain Management
Scripps Center for Integrative Medicine
Assistant Clinical Professor
Department of Family and Preventative Medicine (Voluntary)
University of California, San Diego, School of Medicine
La Jolla, CA

Ryan Bradley, ND, MPH
Research Assistant Professor-Bastyr University
Director-Diabetes & Cardiovascular Wellness Program-Bastyr Center for Natural Health

Thomas Brendler
Founder, PlantaPhile®
Berlin, Germany

Tod Cooperman, MD
President
ConsumerLab.com
White Plains, New York

Rebecca B. Costello, PhD, FACN
Office of Dietary Supplements
National Institutes of Health
Bethesda, MD

Amanda McQuade Crawford, Dip Phyto, MNIMH, RH (AHG), MNZAMH
Consultant Medical Herbalist
Los Angeles, CA

Annette Dickinson, PhD
President, Dickinson Consulting, LLC
St. Paul, MN

Tieraona Low Dog, MD
Fellowship Director
Arizona Center for Integrative Medicine
Clinical Associate Professor of Medicine
University of Arizona Health Sciences Center
Tucson, AZ

Julian Duval
President/CEO
San Diego Botanic Gardens
(formerly known as Quail Botanical Gardens)
Encinitas, CA

Daniel Fabricant, PhD
Vice President, Scientific and Regulatory Affairs Natural Products Association
Washington, DC

Ryan C. Fink
HerbalScience Group LLC
Naples, FL

Paula Gardiner, MD, MPH
Assistant Professor
Department of Family Medicine
Boston University Medical School
Boston, MA

Cathy-Ann Garvey, RD
Scripps Center for Integrative Medicine
La Jolla, CA

Robert T. Gow
HerbalScience Group LLC
Naples, FL

Justine Greene, MD, MSTOM
San Diego, CA

Philip J. Gregory, PharmD
Editor, Natural Medicines Comprehensive Database
Assistant Professor, Pharmacy Practice
Center for Drug Information & Evidence-Based Practice
Creighton University

Mary L. Hardy, MD
Medical Director. The Simms/Mann Integrative Oncology Program
University of California, Los Angeles
Los Angeles, California
Co-Director of the Integrative Medicine and Wellness Program
Venice Family Clinic
Venice, California

David Kiefer, MD
Clinical Assistant Professor of Medicine, Program in Integrative Medicine
University of Arizona
Adjunct Faculty, Bastyr University

Dan Li
HerbalScience Singapore Ptd Ltd

Matthew McMichael
HerbalScience Group LLC
Naples, FL

Cydney E. McQueen, PharmD
Clinical Associate Professor, Pharmacy Practice and Administration
UMKC School of Pharmacy
Kansas City, MO

Simon Y. Mills, MA, MCPP, FNIMH
Managing Director, Sustaincare Community Interest Company
Principal Investigator, UK Department of Health Project: Integrated Self Care in Family Practice
Secretary, European Scientific Cooperative on Phytotherapy (ESCOP)
Fellow, Prince's Foundation of Integrated Health
Specialist Advisor, House of Lords Select Committee on Complementary and Alternative Medicine
Past President, British Herbal Medicine Association, National Institute of Medical Herbalists, College of Practitioners of Phytotherapy

Margie Moore, RN, LAc
Scripps Center for Integrative Medicine
La Jolla, CA

Wadie Najm I., MD, MEd
Clinical Professor
Department of Family Medicine & Geriatrics
University of California, Irvine
Orange, CA

Rajul Patel, PharmD, PhD
Assistant Professor, Pharmacy Practice
Thomas J. Long School of Pharmacy and Health Sciences
University of the Pacific
Stockton, CA

Laura N. Provan, MA
Director, Corporate Communications
U. S. Pharmacopeia
Rockville, MD

David Rakel, MD
Director, University of Wisconsin Integrative Medicine
Department of Family Medicine
University of Wisconsin School of Medicine and Public Health
Madison, WI

Celtina K. Reinert, PharmD
Integrative Pharmacist
Sastun Center of Integrative Health Care
Overland Park, KS

Bill Roschek, Jr, PhD
HerbalScience Group LLC
Naples, FL

Carolyn Sabatini
Director, Government and Corporate Relations
Pharmavite LLC

Andrew Shao, PhD
Vice President, Scientific & Regulatory Affairs
Council for Responsible Nutrition
Washington, DC

Victor S. Sierpina, MD, ABFP, ABHM
WD and Laura Nell Nicholson Family Professor of Integrative Medicine
Professor, Family Medicine
University of Texas Distinguished Teaching Professor
University of Texas Medical Branch
Galveston, Texas

William J. Skinner, RPh, Esq
Editor, Natural Medicine Law
Newsletter Muscatatuck Publishers, Inc.
Boynton Beach, FL

Robert D. Smith
HerbalScience Group LLC
Naples, FL

V. Srini Srinivasan, PhD
Vice President, USP Certification Programs
International Sites Support
United States Pharmacopeia

George Sypert
HerbalScience Group LLC
Naples, FL

Joel B. Taller
Gowling Lafleur Henderson LLP
Ottawa, Canada

Michael Traub, ND, DHANP, FABNO
North Hawaii Community Hospital
Medical Director, Lokahi Health Center
Kailua Kona, HI

Julia Whelan, MS, AHIP
Reference and Education Services Librarian
Countway Library of Medicine, Harvard Medical School
Boston, MA

FOREWORD

Journey into the Jungle

Since becoming fascinated with plants at the age of 5, I have made my way through the beautiful jungles of green plants and related dietary supplements. I have gone through working at greenhouses, botanic gardens, earning an advanced degree in botany, and a full career with the United States Department of Agriculture (USDA). I have visited several rain forests and jungles, especially in Latin America, studying useful plants and the people who use them. A fascinating and rewarding journey! I have come to appreciate the intricate and delicate balance that plants and derived nutritional supplements have with their environment. At the same time it is clear that plants markedly influence other organisms, including, of course, people and the whole Gaian planet. We are indelibly indebted to the plants and the nutrients they contain. Skilled clinicians are needed to disseminate the field and laboratory research on these nutrients to patients in need of education and intervention. These competing priorities and levels of evidence create a real jungle which The H.E.R.B.A.L. Guide tries to decipher in a very practical way.

I have had the pleasure of working with the editor of The H.E.R.B.A.L. Guide, Dr. Robert Bonakdar, over the last several years as faculty of the conference he founded and co-directs: Natural Supplements: An Evidence-Based Update. And the more evidence we gather, the more we see that natural medicines and supplements can be very competitive with synthetic pharmaceuticals. During our interactions at the conferences and more often on tours at the Quail Botanical Gardens (now the San Diego Botanic Garden) he has shared with me his ambitious but simple premise: Herbal and dietary supplements deserve to be discussed and managed by clinicians. There are many learning curves to be encountered in the nutritional jungle where many challenges exist. Fortunately for this journey Dr. Bonakdar has enlisted expert "field-guides" who are ready to decipher the intricacies of regulation, safety, efficacy, education, and clinical management to guide readers to their healthier destination.

He has assembled contributions from many noted authors, many of whom I have known as friends for years, including Marilyn Barrett, Joe Betz, Mark Blumenthal, Rebecca Costello, Amanda McQuade Crawford, Annette Dickinson, Paula Gardiner, Mary Hardy, David Keifer, Tieraona Low Dog, Wadie Najm, David Rakel, Victor Sierpina, and Michael Traub. He has also attempted to categorize the hurdles of the jungle that may trip up the clinician, making the hurdles surmountable. So, whether you are on your first guided trip through the jungle or a seasoned expert, take heart: the goal is in the journey. There are no easy answers out there, especially at first. Many plants, formulas, tincture, bottles, studies, and patient inquiries will seem confusing at first. However, on closer inspection with the magnifying glass that these chapters provide, you will begin to separate the seed from the chaff, both of which may contain bioactive ingredients! Indeed, the deeper we delve into these plant species, the more we see that most contain thousands of phytochemicals, almost all of which are biologically active and pleiotropic and antagonistic, additive, and/or synergic. There is a veritable chaotic jungle of interacting biologically active phytochemicals of some 300,000 species of higher plants inside each individual. One clearly needs skillful guidance.

On my first grazing trips at age 5, I was led by a neighbor in suburban Birmingham, Alabama, a wise old widower full of wood lore, who patiently taught me chestnuts and watercress. I still have these two nutritious food plants here in my Green Pharmacy Garden. Admittedly, it is the hardier Chinese chestnut I grow today. Since moving north from Alabama, I have visited more than 50 countries, inquiring about useful plants, foods, and medicines. And I have spent an aggregate of more than 6 years in Latin American travels. And in my 80th year on this planet, I even told the *Wall Street Journal*, "don't go on your first grazing trip alone." Grazing is our term among those of us who like to forage for wild foods, among them the many nutritious weeds. Don't venture into the jungle alone! Go with a good local guide. And the world and literature of nutritional supplements is a veritable jungle. Recently, I have expressed the considered opinion that the whole food is often better than the nutritional supplements. But few Americans are lucky enough to have a 6-acre garden with more than 300 useful plant species that they recognize. And almost all Americans are deficient in several vitamins, minerals, amino acids, carbohydrates, and so forth. Americans on the run do not always have the time, patience, and knowledge to go grazing. They must weave their way through the supplemental jungle if they are to correct these deficiencies, many of which deficiencies have serious consequences for their health.

Throughout my career, in interactions with many cultures using botanic medicines, I have waited for the time that the cultural respect and understanding in the United States paralleled that seen in other cultures. I have waited for a time when patients can go to a trusted provider to discuss the topic and get advice, encouragement, and guidance. It is my feeling that The H.E.R.B.A.L. Guide will positively influence the clinician–patient dialogue and the interdisciplinary partnership needed to advance this cause. With knowledge of the terrain The H.E.R.B.A.L. Guide provides many learned friends to guide you on your way. The first dietary supplement journey is a jungle. Dr. Bonakdar and The H.E.R.B.A.L. Guide provide clinicians with the practical tools they need for a successful journey. In the end, The H.E.R.B.A.L. Guide has helped provide both an introduction into the complexity of the jungle and the tools to adapt, appreciate, and learn from it.

To your health! My best to you on your journey!

Jim Duke, PhD
(Author of *The Green Pharmacy*, Rodale Press)

PREFACE

Why a clinical guide?

Some years ago, as a resident in family medicine I had the humbling experience of taking care of a gentleman hospitalized with complications related to his advanced prostate cancer. He had attempted multiple previous conventional therapies and during this admission due to increasing symptoms was noted to be taking a number of "supplements." As the intern (lowest seniority on the care team) and having some interest in complementary and alternative medicine (CAM), I was charged with the duty of going into his room to direct him to discontinue his supplements.

The request was odd on many levels. The resident was unsure of why he was asking me to do this, only that it would make his job easier. Moreover, there was no discussion of what the supplements may be doing for him. In fact, there had been no clear discussion of what he was taking, at what dose, and for how long. As the directive rolled off his tongue, we both looked at each other somewhat confused both at the request and how I would deal with it. Luckily, residency prepares you for many uncomfortable situations.

I walked into his dark room, now filled with two men very tired. I was exhausted by a night of multiple admissions and Bill sat there, gaunt, unshaven, and hollow from dealing with an advancing cancer and severe obstructive urinary symptoms. I was not sure of the best approach in this situation but decided to simply ask him about his condition and what brought him to this point. The ensuing conversation, late in the evening, interrupted by my pager and news of other admissions, was both informative and transformative for both of us.

He readily let me know how bad his cancer was getting: fatigue, wasting, increasing urinary symptoms, as well as the associated fear and depression. He told me of the increasing disassociation he was experiencing from the medical support system as his cancer was advancing. He mentioned that the alienation was even more so as he mentioned the use of CAM with his providers, something he had done less and less of to save himself the trouble.

He elaborated that he began the use of saw palmetto among other supplements as a means of improving his urinary flow, which had gotten progressively worse even with the best of treatments attempted. He noted that although small, the gains with his supplements were noticeable and represented a rare improvement as compared to the numerous procedures and chemotherapies he had attempted, which he perceived had brought him little relief, often at a high cost.

As we talked I could see his shoulders and guardedness relaxing, with mine following soon after. He brought out his bag of supplements, the same bag that had alerted the hospital staff that he needed "to be talked to." As I sat there, I felt somewhat lost in time, partially because I was a fatigued intern late in the shift, but more importantly because I had connected with a patient in need at a deeper level than possible during my typical clinical encounters. This need transcended his condition but was one which I felt was all too common in our patients: *a desperate need to discuss and reintegrate the fragmented pieces of their healthcare choices (in this case dietary supplements) with the members of his healthcare team.*

The members of his team, including myself, whom he had repeatedly entrusted to provide the most invasive and high-risk treatments, appeared to care the least about the CAM care he was pursuing or the fear, despair, and hopelessness he was feeling. In an instant I felt shameful of the system that allowed the members of care team, which most needed to know EVERYTHING he was utilizing, thinking, and considering, to fall into an easy place of ignorance. The lack of genuine interest in what he was taking as well as lack of disclosure and discussion created a scenario in which the best possible care was not possible. For many reasons and likely previous uncomfortable interactions in this area, we did not want to know, he did not want to tell, and we went on with the hypocrisy of comprehensive care.

The propagation of this system caused disrespect to all parties: the patient, the clinician, and the supplement representative of a healing choice. This contrasted significantly with how I had encountered herbal supplements during a Richter Fellowship I had completed in Southeast Asia. I had witnessed the respect, continuity of knowledge, and ongoing discussion implicit in use of herbal medicine. Here the scenario was one of a disrespected supplement that had been relegated to some secretly horded bottles, too precious to give up and too laborious to discuss. The physician has become disrespected as someone not knowledgeable, helpful, or worth consulting on the matter. In the end the integrative relationship was neither respected nor possible, having been relegated to a convenient discussion of the risks and benefits of the next procedure.

As Bill and I continued to entrust, I heard the story of his supplements, recorded them for the medical chart, counseled him the little that I could about his supplements (especially in regard to his upcoming procedure), and discussed a number of strategies that he should consider and discuss with his health care providers. During this interaction, I felt more like a physician than I had at nearly any time in my training. I was listening, educating, and mostly just allowing the fragmentation to mend. We both felt like stranded buoys in a lonely ocean that had found comfort in the conversation. We both realized that neither of us had all the answers regarding his supplements. Indeed, I would say that that is how most scenarios go in this area. But simply having the conversation with full disclosure, empathy, and humility allowed better communication and hopefully better care.

Subsequent to the admission I placed a list of all supplements in the medical chart and when the resident asked me whether the situation had been dealt with I said yes, knowing that his definition and mine were vastly different. Bill went on to have a procedure for urinary obstruction, which helped restore function, and was discharged not long after that. I remember that at his discharge after morning rounds he was shaven, more lively, and a different man than at admission. As he was leaving, he showed me his medication list that was now meshed and organized with his supplement list, ready to be used for his future clinical visits.

Bill was also leaving with another tool. He told me on his way out that he had hope that he could openly discuss his supplements, receive nonjudgmental discussion, and that someday "everything would be out of the bag and on the table." I smiled, shook his hand, and thanked him for the conversation.

After the experience I contacted our hospital's Pharmacy and Therapeutics Committee (which handles the policy surrounding medications in the hospital) and found that no real policy existed regarding dietary supplements. Mainly, the tactic was to have patients stop them immediately. I also found in surveying my fellow residents and attendings that they routinely did not ask, discuss, or record supplement use. The small amount of literature I could find on the subject corroborated this sad situation. With the patient experience and information I gathered, I was convinced that a better model for dealing with dietary supplements existed. Frankly, any system was more helpful than what was in place.

Disheartened and motivated by the situation I began developing and identifying currently available materials for clinical discussion and counseling surrounding supplements. This included a form for recording dietary supplements in a manner parallel to prescription medication, resources for clinician–patient dialogue of dietary supplements, and the H.E.R.B.A.L. mnemonic for capturing the key steps involved in the dialogue. I began lecturing on evidence-based use and discussion of dietary supplements to clinicians, most notably at the American Academy of Family Physicians and the Society for Teachers of Family Medicine and founded the annual conference at Scripps Clinic entitled, *Natural Supplements: An Evidence Based Update*. The clinical guide appeared to be a natural progression of these efforts to capture the needed resources as well as presenting supplement use in the context of condition management, as often it arises in the clinical visit.

In the end as much as I would like to say I created the clinical guide to help my fellow clinicians or patients like Bill who will hopefully benefit, I must admit that the motivation was selfish. I envisioned and edited this book because of the feeling I had when I was asked to enter Bill's room that night as an intern. It created a feeling of discomfort, emptiness, and embarrassment that I wish to never again experience as a clinician. I cannot claim the guide will make all such scenarios obsolete, but I hope that as clinicians enter the room and talk with patients who are using supplements they will have a vastly different experience. Instead of missed opportunities, I hope they experience what I have come to enjoy more often, an opportunity to be the integrative clinician we all wish to be, partnering with our patients in improving and empowering health through open discussion, resources, and advocacy.

Yours in Health,

Robert Bonakdar, MD, FAAFP

ACKNOWLEDGMENTS

This book would not have been possible without the support and encouragement of numerous people. My acknowledgment:

- To the clinicians who have given of their expertise and who engage their patients in a discussion of dietary supplement as a part of whole person care.
- To the researchers and experts whose contributions were essential for providing a more complete understanding of the field.
- Natural Medicines Comprehensive Database, especially Jeff M. Jellin, PharmD, and Philip J. Gregory, PharmD, for their incredible support throughout my education as well as in creating this book.
- The Staff of the Scripps Center for Integrative Medicine, most notably Mimi, Rauni, Raneth, Cathy, Margie, and Darlene, as well as my clinical partner who keeps me sane, David Leopold, MD.
- To all the patients who have taught me.
- To all the clinicians who have thought me how to learn.
- To the former Sharp Family Practice Residency Program, the hardest working group of residents, faculty, and staff dedicated to bringing health care to patients in San Diego.
- To Michael Hart, MD, former Residency Director of the Sharp program, who wholeheartedly encouraged and supported the creation and presentation of the H.E.R.B.A.L. mnemonic. Dr. Hart, we miss you and your encouragement to appreciate life and all that is around us lives on.
- To the expert herbalists, most notably Mark Blumenthal and Jim Duke, PhD, who have painstakingly attempted to keep what is sacred in plants alive.
- To the faculty and staff of the Scripps conference *Natural Supplements: An Evidence-Based Update*, especially Julie Simper. I would not have been in a position to create this book without the knowledge and expertise I gained from you at the conference.
- To the staff of the San Diego Botanic Garden (Formerly Quail Botanical Garden) (especially, Julian Duval), for helping me better understand and get in touch with plant medicine—thank you for creating a space where this is possible.
- To Sonya Seigafuse and Kerry Barrett of Lippincott Williams & Wilkins for believing in the importance of this topic as well as their patience in making it a reality.
- And most importantly, to my entire family for their patience and support throughout the process and for always believing in me.

CONTENTS

**All chapters have been written by Robert Alan Bonakdar unless otherwise noted*

I The H.E.R.B.A.L. Mnemonic

II Understanding Dietary Supplements

V Efficacy

VI Clinical Management

VII Resources and Education

VIII Case Studies

IX Quick Reference Guide

I

The H.E.R.B.A.L. Mnemonic

CHAPTER 1

The H.E.R.B.A.L. Mnemonic—Introduction and Overview

Robert Alan Bonakdar

As the preface points out, the mnemonic came out of a frustration in the typically patient encounter with less than optimal discussion and management of dietary supplements. Even with current efforts, multiple surveys point out that physicians do not ask and patients do not disclose supplement use, especially in certain demographics. This was most notably reported in a National Center for Complementary and Alternative Medicine (NCCAM)/AARP survey, which demonstrated that 77% of patients failed to inform their clinician regarding the use of complementary and alternative medicine or dietary supplements. In this same population, 74% and 59% of patients were taking one or more prescription or over-the-counter medications, respectively (1).

Clearly, there is a need to take the discussion to a higher level, both in how often it is brought up and what is done with the information exchanged. First, asking about supplement use in an open, nonjudgmental manner is key in encouraging true disclosure and discussion. If the patient feels that the clinician is truly interested in this piece of information, disclosure will be more likely and complete. Second, providing the clinician with resources and education has been found to be a predictor for increasing comfort and confidence in pursuing the discussion. Hearing the patient out entails going beyond simply the supplement list. It is also about the details of use including motivation for use, the brand, dose, length, and perceived outcome of treatment.

The H.E.R.B.A.L. mnemonic was developed to capture and reinforce the key steps in a discussion on dietary supplements. The steps have gone through several modifications since it was first developed in training and presented at the Society for Teachers of Family Medicine and the American Academy of Family Physicians Annual Scientific Assembly. What has been most striking since I have introduced the mnemonic is how overwhelmed clinicians feel with the prospect of discussing supplements and how underwhelmed they are with resources available to help them with this task.

Thus, the H.E.R.B.A.L. mnemonic stands as a starting point to systematically place the pieces of the dietary supplement puzzle together. Because discussion often begins with education and resources, the goal of the mnemonic and the book is to provide both a framework for the discussion and a foundation of knowledge and resources to facilitate the discussion. Each section of the H.E.R.B.A.L. mnemonic is elaborated upon to allow the clinician to understand the step's importance in the context of patient care. Supporting resources and handouts are listed in the appendix which is available online for download. In time I hope that you come to appreciate the window into the patient that dietary supplement discussion allows and that this guide will help make the most of the opportunity.

Reference

1. National Center for Complementary and Alternative Medicine (NCCAM)/AARP survey. Complementary and alternative medicine: what people 50 and older are using and discussing with their physicians. http://www.aarp.org/aarp/presscenter/pressrelease/articles/medicine_use.html. Published January 2007. Accessed March 3, 2009.

CHAPTER 2

Hear the Patient Out

Robert Alan Bonakdar

RESPECT AND COMFORT

The most important step in fully hearing patients out is making them feel respected, comfortable, and valued in having the dietary supplement discussion. Surveys point out that lack of disclosure by patients can be partially linked to clinician's previous dismissive or negative interaction involving dietary supplements. There are many steps that you and your clinic can initiate that will encourage the discussion as a partnership exercise. Steps that help engender this are having background literature in the clinic that supports the discussion as well as staff who can help initiate the discussion in a open nonjudgmental manner.

FULL DISCLOSURE AND DISCUSSION = FULL CARE

Another common misconception held by patients is that clinicians do not need to know about supplements use. In one survey, 30% of respondents stated that they did not discuss complementary and alternative medicine because they "**Didn't know they should**" (1). In another survey, 61% stated "**It wasn't important for my doctor to know**" (2). This stems from several likely factors including that patients may view supplements as not requiring discussion for various reasons. In addition, they may view some clinicians as not able to help them with questions they have in this area. Moreover, the more interaction patients have where supplements are not discussed (as compared to other care options), the more likely they are to have reinforcement that non-discussion is typical.

To change this trend, it is important to let patient know in as many ways as possible the importance of disclosure and discussion. In general, this can be done with wording on handouts and "medication lists" which ask patients to list all supplements being used (see chapter 11), in addition to prescription and over-the-counter medication. Moreover, handouts and statements from providers emphasize that clinicians have the best chance of helping patients in their care efforts if they are aware of all treatments being pursued, including dietary supplements. Educating patient as noted below on the ways dietary supplement can impact care can also be a powerful shift for some patients.

ASKING THE BIG QUESTION

Asking about supplement use in an open, nonjudgmental manner is essential in encouraging true disclosure and discussion. Several studies have noted that when patients are directly questioned about use of CAM including DS, the disclosure rate can be two or more times highter than that seen from a questionnaire alone (3,4). If the patient feels that the clinician is truly interested in this piece of information, disclosure will be more likely and complete. Hearing the patient out entails going beyond simply the supplement list. It is also about delving into the details behind supplement use. These details include the motivation for use, the brand, dose, length of treatment, overseeing clinician, potential benefit, and side effects and level of satisfaction with treatment.

When hearing the patient out, it is common to have the patient tell you about strong motivating factors that led the patient to dietary supplements. These may include previous positive experience, discussion with other clinicians, or suggestion by non–health care providers or media. It is also important to note that the supplements are often a sign of attempts to improve general wellness as well as to fortify their attempts at dealing with a chronic condition. In all cases, it is important to note the motivations and their importance to the patient. It is then often an excellent opportunity to understand their motivation for optimizing health and transition both to supplement choices which may be appropriate and other care choices which will help them attain their goals (i.e., diet, exercise, stress management).

References

1. National Center for Complementary and Alternative Medicine (NCCAM)/AARP survey. Complementary and alternative medicine: what people 50 and older are using and discussing with their physicians. http://www.aarp.org/research/health/prevention/cam_2007.html. Published January 2007. Accessed March 3, 2009.
2. Eisenberg DM. Perceptions about complementary therapies relative to conventional therapies among adults who use both: results from a national survey. *Ann Int Med* 2001;135(5): 344–351.
3. Jones HA, Metz JM, Devine P, et al. Rates of unconventional medical therapy use in patients with prostate cancer: standard history versus directed questions. *Urology* 2002; 59(2):272–276.
4. Metz JM, Jones H, Devine P, et al. Cancer patients use unconventional medical therapies far more frequently than standard history and physical examination suggest. *Cancer J* 2001;7(2):149–154.

CHAPTER 3

Educating the Patient: What's Your Source of Information and Supplement?

Robert Alan Bonakdar

DIETARY SUPPLEMENT AS A LIFESTYLE CHOICE

Before discussing education regarding dietary supplements, a helpful transition point that took me some time to absorb is the fact that dietary supplements are lifestyle choices more than pills. In the typical scenario, it is helpful to think of prescription medications as directives that are provided to the patient by the clinician and dietary supplements (DS) as lifestyle choices which are typically initiated by the patient based on a number of factors including personality, peer group, educational levels, etc. A patient usually has a lot more invested in the DS than the prescription medication and just as the clinician must invest time and resources in understanding and modifying other lifestyle choices such as diet and exercise, the same is true of DS. In this regard, it is quite helpful to view the DS dialogue in most cases not only as a directive to start a new agent but also as a lifestyle discussion which will require a sensitivity to the background of the situation and the patient with appropriate counseling to arrive at common ground.

EDUCATION—THE CLINICIAN PROVIDING A ROADMAP

It is also important to view the education as a two-way process in which the patient often alerts the clinician to supplements she/he is considering or utilizing which may be completely unfamiliar. It is common and understandable that the clinician may feel intimidated regarding his/her specific knowledge base. However, in most cases it is neither expected nor possible for the clinician to be a supplement encyclopedia for the more than 60,000 supplements estimated on the market. Surveys have pointed out that patients are seeking guidance from a trusted source more than absolute knowledge when discussing supplements. As Verhoed and colleagues point out in a survey of cancer patients' needs and expectations regarding discussion of DS, the clinician is more expected to provide a road map than be an encyclopedia:

> *Patients expected their physicians to be supportive, caring, kind and to show an interest in them. They also expected their physicians to be accepting and nonjudgmental regarding complementary therapy use and to reinforce a sense of hope.* (1)

THE DETAILS ARE ESSENTIAL

The road map includes making sure the patient is clear on the broad definition of DS so that you are both discussing the whole of what the patient may be utilizing in this area. The clinician should use this opportunity to inform patients, if they are not already aware, that DS vary widely with what and how DS are taken often predicting benefit. It is vitally important for the clinician and patient to know the details of the supplement including brand, dose, formulation, and preparation. This attention to detail becomes most relevant and helpful when reevaluating the supplement at follow-up and needing to make important decisions regarding whether to continue and if so, potential changes in dose, brand, or preparation to optimize results.

One example of this comes from a previous meta-analysis of glucosamine for osteoarthritis of the knee which found that one type of glucosamine was responsible for the majority of the evidence for benefit:

> *Collectively, the 16 identified RCTs provided evidence that glucosamine is both effective and safe in OA. Most of the trials reviewed only evaluated the Rotta preparation of glucosamine sulfate. It is not known whether different glucosamine preparations prepared by different manufacturers are equally effective in the therapy of OA.* (2)

In clinical experience, many patients assume that one brand of a certain supplement is similar to others and if one brand does not work then neither will others. After learning the details of what they are taking, a good percentage of patients who are taking supplements for an appropriate indication get improved results when they are educated and transitioned to a more evidence-based DS in the same class.

In addition to education on the source of the supplement, it is important to balance the source of information. Because most patients receive their information on DS from sources other than a clinician (family, friends, Internet, media), it is often helpful to understand their views and if appropriate, attempt to balance the patient's current understanding regarding supplements. This can often be the most difficult part of the discussion, especially if the patient has very polarizing and unwavering views on supplements. However, having talked with many patients who may otherwise be viewed initially as dogmatic either in their beliefs or the information they provide on supplements, several strategies have been helpful to keep in mind.

REMEMBER THE MESSAGE *BEHIND* THE BOTTLE

First, it is important to keep in mind the basic fact that most patients are simply attempting to utilize strategies to improve their health. Although the DS bottle may be the first and most convenient strategy for patients, it does not mean that it is the *only* approach they are open to, especially if they know the full menu of options. I have found that in many cases the supplement bottle is the easiest thing to grab (both figuratively and literally) for patients to signal they want to take a more proactive approach to their health. (more on in Chapter 13 The Dietary Supplement User). One example of bringing the discussion to this level may be, **"I see that you are trying many approaches to improve your cholesterol. That is great. Let's talk about the pros/cons of some options to come up with the best ones for you."** In this way, the patients does not fear that you are immediately for or against any therapy, but that your are working with them to come up with the best option, whether or not that includes the DS they brought into the clinic.

BUILDING TRUST THROUGH EDUCATION

The next step is building trust and partnership which may take some time. As patients come to know you and your clinic as a resource in helping them optimize and streamline their care, several key things may happen. First, the discussion of DS will be more fluid. Instead of the patient worrying about the reaction they will receive, they will be anticipating the discussion. Second, the trust built by saying "I don't know (the specifics of) that supplement and need to get back to you," will begin to mean that they will get useful feedback and resources regarding this option. This is no different than a situation in which another new therapy is mentioned and the clinician needs to do research before providing recommendation.

EDUCATION AND THE ONGOING LEARNING PROCESS

Last, the education step is not only about building trust by providing input on specific treatment options but also about providing new tools for searching. As I continue to discuss supplements with patients, we try to find a common set of resources so that our discussions can be more productive and individualized. What may start out as a 50-page printout from a site with multiple testimonials may progress to a short review of a supplement that the patient accesses on a trusted and agreed-upon resource which can help focus the discuss for his/her individual needs. At this level the patient becomes the ultimate educator of the clinician by providing relevant, up-to-date information that can be a source of lively discuss regarding treatment options. What was "Hey, Doc I found this internet ad for an arthritis cure—what do you think" is transformed to "Hey, Doctor B, this article talks about a specific type of glucosamine for lessening the need for knee replacement—what do you think?"

The educational transition does not come immediately in most cases and is similar to other areas of counseling such as dietary or exercise changes. However, most patients who are looking for guidance in this often-confusing area will come to trust and depend on your valuable input. For the few who do not, you have at least done your job in providing balanced feedback and resources which will hopefully have an important impact on the patient's future health. In both scenarios, as discussed next, it is vitally important to document your discussion, educational steps, and recommendations for future reference.

References

1. Verhoed M, White MA, Doll R. Cancer patients' expectations of the role of family physicians in communication about complementary therapies. *Cancer Prev Control* 1999;3(3): 181–187.
2. Towheed TE, Anastassiades TP, Shea B, et al. Glucosamine therapy for treating osteoarthritis. *Cochrane Database Syst Rev* 2001;(1):CD002946.

CHAPTER 4

Record

Robert Alan Bonakdar

IF IT'S NOT RECORDED—YOU MUST HAVE TALKED ABOUT SUPPLEMENTS . . .

One of the most often overlooked areas in the dietary supplements (DS) dialogue is documentation. A survey of DS use by Cohen and colleagues (1) in patients older than 65 years of age found that even though 63% were utilizing some type of DS, only 35% of all supplements were documented in the medical charts. This is likely due to clinicians consciously or subconsciously not viewing the discussion the same as one regarding prescription medications. This is a pervasive misconception that needs to be reversed for many reasons. From a starting point of time invested, if a clinician is going through the steps of discussing an active biological ingredient which can have a positive or negative impact on health (similar to a prescription medication) then it is worthy of including in the medical chart.

RECORD TO CLARIFY

Second, a number of potential problems can arise from nondocumentation. These include the potential for unintended redundancy and interaction in therapies. At the least this can cause confusion as to the cause of clinical change (i.e., change in blood sugar) and at the far extreme a potential negative scenario. The need for documentation is especially true for patients who are using polypharmacy and for clinics that share a medical chart and depend on the documentation of colleagues to have the full story. Simply put, the lack of documentation takes away most of the benefit gained by initiating the discussion as the information gained does not become a documented springboard for future discussion.

SUPPLEMENT STOCKPILING—WHAT AM I TAKING THIS FOR?

Third, an immediate benefit of documentation includes a thorough understanding for the patient and clinician of the indications and appropriateness for what is being taken. When the clinician performs this so-called *therapeutic inventory* there are cases of unintentional *supplement stockpiling*. This occurs when one DS is initiated with or without input and is then added to by future DS without a full discussion or understanding of how the previous meshes with the current. Because these decisions are often made without an advocate involved, it is often easier to add-on than to strategically review, compare, and focus therapy. As one extreme example points out, I have had several patients whose DS, once sorted and ingredients compared to one another, were at significantly higher than recommended doses for vitamin A—without their knowledge. Simply putting all the details on paper can at times be a helpful and therapeutic exercise for the patient and clinician to update and focus therapy with additional resources provided in the online Appendix.

RECORDING THE DETAILS

Once documentation is initiated, the details are just as important to record. We would not see a heart patient and feel satisfied at simply noting "Taking an anti-hypertensive and statin." However, we often feel complete having placed only "Ginkgo" or "Glucosamine" in the chart. This is even more pertinent in the field of DS where there are a multitude of potential choices within a specific supplement. Thus, it is important to record not only the supplement name used but also the brand, dose, preparation, formulation, and other details as relevant. This attention to detail is not only helpful in informing all clinicians about current DS therapy and minimizing potential reactions and interactions but also to direct care toward the most helpful agents. As noted in the education section, once the patient and the clinician are aware that the specifics matter and may predict clinician improvement, it is then important to record these details and allow future decisions to be based on this background. This will be pointed out in several of the patient cases presented in section 8.

REGULAR REVIEW AND UPDATING

Once you, your staff, and the patient have teamed up to create a current dietary supplement list with the pertinent details, it is vital to view the list as dynamic. Thus, even more so than prescription and over-the-counter medications, supplements and their details tend to shift between visits. At follow-up, make a point to ask not only whether the supplement previously recorded is helpful, and thus potentially worthwhile in continuing, but also whether the brand or dose has shifted. Because the patient is in control of the purchase, dose and brand, changes are not uncommon and reviewing these regularly will help the clinician have all the facts when providing guidance on ongoing therapy.

If certain patients have an especially extensive supplement and medication list, it will likely be helpful for your staff to remind them to update the details, either online or through a list they bring in to the office to expedite the discussion. Several resources to help facilitate recording and discussion are listed in the online Appendix.

Reference

1. Cohen RJ, Ek K, Pan CX. Complementary and alternative medicine (CAM) use by older adults: a comparison of self-report and physician chart documentation. *J Gerontol A Biol Sci Med Sci* 2002;57(4):M223–M227.

CHAPTER 5

Be Aware of Reactions/Interactions

Robert Alan Bonakdar

PRACTICING THE ART OF MEDICINE

It is not uncommon for clinicians to be reminded of a potential reaction or interactions involving dietary supplements (DS) through a case study or report. Unfortunately, they are just that, potential and case studies, some well done and some not. This leaves the clinician in a difficult situation regarding the use of DS, especially with other agents such as the over-the-counter and prescription medications. Because the amount of information available on the reaction potential of some supplements, especially how they coexist with other substances, is evolving, the clinician is often unsure of how relevant the information is for his/her patient. We have very few trials that demonstrate a likely interaction (St. John's Wort with indinavir) or noninteraction (Panax ginseng and warfarin in ischemic stroke patients) in a controlled setting (1,2).

In most scenarios, the clinician is truly practicing the art of medicine where she/he has some guidance from the literature and an individual patient requires advice on how to proceed. Fortunately, several resources are available to enable the clinician to triage scenarios involving DS. First, the excellent chapters in section 4 provide guidance as to the most likely reactions and interactions. In addition, several recent articles have allowed clinician to know the likelihood of interaction based on the patient's clinical scenario as noted below.

PRIORITIZING THE MOST LIKELY

Researchers at the Mayo clinic performed a cross-sectional, point-of-care survey combined with chart reviews to determine patterns and severity of potential interactions. The researchers found that no patients were harmed seriously because of interactions and that 94% of the potential clinically significant interactions were found with four common classes of prescription medications (antithrombotic medications, sedatives, antidepressant agents, and antidiabetic agents). In addition, 68% of the potential clinically significant interactions were related to five common natural products (garlic, valerian, kava, ginkgo, and St John's Wort). In conclusion, the authors noted:

> A small number of prescription medications and dietary supplements accounted for most of the interactions. The actual potential for harm was low .... *This information likely will help educate patients and physicians about these potential interactions*. (3)

Articles like these help both clinicians and patients focus on the most likely scenarios that demand the most discussion and monitoring. In addition, as some supplements are being used in new combinations with other supplements, over the counter (OTC) and prescriptions medications, it is always pertinent to keep supplement in mind when a new reaction has occurred, positive or negative. This may be a change in a laboratory value such as the international normalizing ratio (INR) or blood sugar or an a new symptom or sign such as unexplained rash. After the typical culprits have been ruled out, it is important to have a complete and up-to-date list of supplements to confirm that this is not a likely cause or contributing agent. If the potential is there, a number of resources for monitoring and reporting appropriately are listed in section 4.

References

1. Piscitelli SC, Burstein AH, Chaitt D, Alfaro RM, Falloon J. Indinavir concentrations and St John's wort. *Lancet* 2000;355(9203):547–548.
2. Lee SH, Ahn YM, Ahn SY, Doo HK, Lee BC. Interaction between warfarin and Panax ginseng in ischemic stroke patients. *J Altern Complement Med* 2008;14(6):715–721.
3. Sood A, Sood R, Brinker FJ, et al. Potential for interactions between dietary supplements and prescription medications. *Am J Med* 2008;121(3):207–211.

CHAPTER 6

Agree to Discuss

Robert Alan Bonakdar

HELPING YOUR PATIENT HELP YOU

As soon as your patient has left the clinical encounter the most important part of your educational efforts will be initiated. Clinicians may rely on the fact that medications require prescription before initiation and thus inherently provide an opportunity for input and oversight. Conversely, because most supplements are considered or initiated before clinical input, it is crucial that patients realize that you, your staff, and your recommended resources are available in a more proactive manner. It is much more efficient for a supplement to be reviewed and initial recommendation provided prior to the follow-up at which point the clinician often picks up newly initiated supplements in "mid-stream."

Although it is impossible to have input on every supplement decision that a patient makes, it is important for patients to know that you look forward to the opportunity of hearing from them about new supplements they are considering. You may even have a set of resources, such as the ones reviewed in chapter 42 that you recommend they utilize before initiation. In addition, let them know that they can contact your office regarding any questions in this area and that you and your staff will be available to give timely feedback to help them make balanced and informed decisions.

SETTING UP A SYSTEM

Although this may seem like additional work at no benefit, fielding a call such as "Doctor B, I am considering supplement x for my cholesterol, what do you think?" can be triaged quite effectively. Using nursing input the patient's chart can be reviewed for relevant medical conditions, other supplements, and medication and this can be quickly cross-referenced with the intended supplement based on it safety/ efficacy profile. If the supplement is not a good choice, a call back from your office with the rationale can help educate the patient. If the supplement is a good idea you can help the patients by giving them suggestions on dosing and brands which can best help them derive the benefits for which they are looking. Once any changes have been made, a follow-up appointment is recommended to discuss effects of the new regimen.

AVOIDING THE SUPPLEMENT STARE SYNDROME

The benefit of this agreement is best termed avoiding the "*Supplement Stare Syndrome.*" I often ask my patients whether they have an easy time making decisions when at the supplement aisle. They often mention that it is quite an ordeal going through the numerous and often-confusing choices in a particular section. What if you could help your patients decide if they needed to go to a certain aisle and if so what is the most beneficial dose, brand, and formulation they should look for? I cannot tell you how many patients have thanked me for providing input into this frustrating scenario and the time it has saved them in their supplement decision-making process. Having the patients prepared with a handout with the details is the key to expediting the process and ensuring that they actually initiate the therapy you had discussed. The effort placed in providing the details is saved many times over because the patient and clinician are on the same page. This is in contrast to a supplement purchased without input after dealing with the supplement stare syndrome. The supplement finally obtained may be inconsistent with current evidence for benefit based on sub-optimal dosage, use, formulation, brand or other factors. It is much more productive reviewing a therapeutic supplement trial for benefit when the choice initiated was one that had a strong potential of benefit.

AN ONGOING RELATIONSHIP

Once patients come to know that you are available and that your advice is timely and helpful, you will be one step ahead of the follow-up visit at which point you will, in a more in-depth and face-to-face manner, review their supplement choices and move ahead to assessment. A typical scenario might be, "I see you called our office about 8 weeks ago to ask us about specific supplements for your knee arthritis. Were you able to start the ones we recommended and if so, what have you noticed?" This is much more productive conversation than starting at step 1 with a number of supplement choices that you would have wished to have provided input on before initiation. Make sure you thank them for keeping your office in the loop for this important decision and in most cases you will be thanked for decreasing the Supplement Stare Syndrome.

CHAPTER 7

Learn

Robert Alan Bonakdar

MAKING CONNECTIONS

One of the biggest challenges regarding supplements is that they appear to represent a new area of required learning for the busy clinician. This can be daunting but with the right resources not very much different than becoming familiar with newly approved medications, procedures, or diagnostic tests. In addition, the science of dietary supplements, especially herbal medicine, provides a greater understanding and deeper respect both for the plants and currently available therapeutics.

STAYING AHEAD OF THE CURVE

As the use of dietary supplements increases, there will be greater and greater expectation for clinicians to be a resource point for patients and to recognize the role of dietary supplements in various clinical scenarios. In some cases, dietary supplements have been incorporated as components of (re)certification examinations. In addition, increasing numbers of US training programs expect their graduates to have core competencies in the area of dietary supplements. This is similar to several European countries, including Germany, where the licensing examination for physicians includes a section on herbal medicine (1).

It is prudent for the busy clinician to get familiar with various learning resources in this area (as reviewed in chapter 42). Among these resources are books, Internet, and PDA-based resources which will allow learning that is most accessible to the clinician. Several of these resources also have patient handout options so that the information can be easily shared in a manner that parallels what the clinician' is learning.

KNOWING WHO IS ON YOUR TEAM

Last, in addition to using referenced sources, it is prudent to become familiar with colleagues and experts who have a special interest in this area (see section 6). In many case, the specific patient scenario that you are dealing with may not be one that is published or clear-cut. Moreover, the evidence-based supplement you read about in Europe may not be what is on the shelf in your city. However, there are likely experienced clinicians and experts whom you can consult to help you guide care with practical knowledge. Because dietary supplements take on many forms and traditions, it is important for you to view the education and counseling as "taking a village."

It is impractical for one clinician to gain knowledge about all potential dietary supplements and their clinical use. However, it is possible to create a team of clinicians in your area with interested physicians, nurses, pharmacists, dieticians, naturopaths, traditional herbalist, and others who will be able to provide valuable input in specific cases. With this type of backing, as well accessible resources for learning and education, the task of managing dietary supplements can transition from a chore to an engaging clinical interaction.

Reference

1. Schilcher H. The significance of phytotherapy in Europe—an interdisciplinary and comparative survey. *Acta Hort (ISHS)* 1993;332:55–62. http://www.actahort.org/books/332/332_9.htm. Accessed March 1, 2009.

CHAPTER 8

Frequently Asked Questions—A Road Map to Supplement Answers

Robert Alan Bonakdar

As I planned the sections in this book I tried to remember the many questions I have had (and continue to have) on this topic. I also noted the frustration and confusion clinicians have shared with me when describing their experiences with the topic. These moments typically bring up pertinent questions which are searching for answers. For some readers these questions may be in the area of regulation, for others it may be more about dosing or charting. As you look at the sections below, please review the questions and see which section has the most pertinent questions whose answers may help your practice or scenario. In many cases that is the section to start with and return to others as questions arise. In this way, the guide will provide the most appropriate road map on your dietary supplement journey.

- SECTION I: THE H.E.R.B.A.L. MNEMONIC
  - Why should I bring up the topic?
  - How should I approach the topic with my patients?
  - What steps are needed to appropriately manage supplements?
  - Is there a simple way to capture the necessary information regarding dietary supplements?
- SECTION II: UNDERSTANDING DIETARY SUPPLEMENTS
  - Why are dietary supplements so popular and how do they fit in with complementary and alternative medicine?
  - What exactly is a dietary supplement?
  - How do I read a dietary supplement label and how is it different from other labels?
  - Who in my practice is most likely to use supplements?
  - How is dietary supplement viewed legally?
- SECTION III: REGULATION
  - Are supplements regulated and if so who does this differ from over the counter (OTC)/prescription medications?
  - What is DSHEA?
  - How do I find a well-regulated supplement?
  - What are health claims?
  - How are supplements regulated around the world?
  - What is the role of industry and organizations in regulation and oversight?
  - What is the role of third party review/testing?

- SECTION IV: REACTIONS AND INTERACTIONS
  - What are the most common reactions I have to consider clinically?
  - How likely are interactions and what are most likely scenarios?
  - What do I do if I am aware of a potential reaction/interaction—how do I report it?
- SECTION V: EFFICACY
  - Where do herbal supplements come from and does this matter?
  - What does it mean to be standardized and how is this done?
  - How do I know if a supplement trial is well done when I read it?
  - Does the formulation used in trials really make a difference?
  - Where can I find research-tested brands?
  - Where can I find reviews of the trials?
  - Where are dietary supplements trials being done?
- SECTION VI: CLINICAL MANAGEMENT
  - How should herbs be managed?
  - How can a team approach be utilized for managements?
  - Who can help co-manage supplements?
    - What are the roles of the herbalist pharmacist, physician, dietician, nurse, naturopath, and Traditional Chinese medicine (TCM) practitioner?
- SECTION VII: RESOURCES AND EDUCATION
  - Are there any evidence-based resources available for dietary supplements?
  - Are there any points of care resources available for dietary supplements?
  - Where can I find free supplement handouts?
  - Where can I find continuing medical education (CME) in this area?
  - Are there any resources to help me teach others in this area?
- SECTION VIII: DIETARY SUPPLEMENT CASE STUDIES
  - How can I incorporate these supplements in a real-world setting for my patient with "Condition X" including the brand and dose?
  - How do you strategize the various supplements you can use for "Condition X"?
- SECTION IX: QUICK REFERENCE GUIDE
  - How do I get started with potential recommendations?
  - I need supplement answers fast for the patient in room 3 what is my go to recommendation, if any, source before they leave the clinic?
- SECTION X: ONLINE APPENDIX
  - Are there any handouts to educate my patients on dietary supplement use and discussion?
  - Are there any intake forms to help record and manage supplement use?

CHAPTER 9

A Pathway for Dietary Supplement Management

Robert Alan Bonakdar

The following pathway attempts to summarize the typical flow of discussion surrounding dietary supplements (DS) as well as the components of the H.E.R.B.A.L. mnemonic and book that may be supportive. Typically, the patient brings up a particular dietary supplement (DS) or condition for which supplement(s) may be a potential, "I'm thinking of taking 'DS' for my condition." Similarly, the clinician may be looking for additional options in a clinical scenario and wonder whether there are any DS which fit the need. This springs into the review and discussion of safety and efficacy that must take into account the unique patient scenario (medical history, allergies, medi-cations, other supplements). Subsequently, the clinician and patients must be savvy in connecting the available clinical evidence with actual products available. This is often the most complex aspect of the search as the formula desired from the available evidence may be different from what is actually available based on many factors. Thus, the clinician and the patient must often use available resources to come up with the best-case scenario of a well-regulated supplement, which most consistently approaches what they are hoping to introduce.

Next, the clinician and the patient approach the scenario of clinical management that should parallel as much as possible other treatments in the clinic. This would include appropriate charting regarding administration (brand, dose, frequency, etc.), counseling regarding utilization including compliance, and scheduled follow-up to evaluate response. In most cases, the follow-up is essential to discuss continuation as previous versus a change in the administration of the DS (typically the dose or formulation) or initiation of an alternate or additional supplement based on timing of the follow-up.

In each step, the clinician is pointed toward sections of the book or resources in the online Appendix, which may help answer the questions at hand. Based on regular use, it is hoped that the pathway helps both streamline and support the typical DS scenario so that both the clinician and the patient find the discussion helpful and timely.

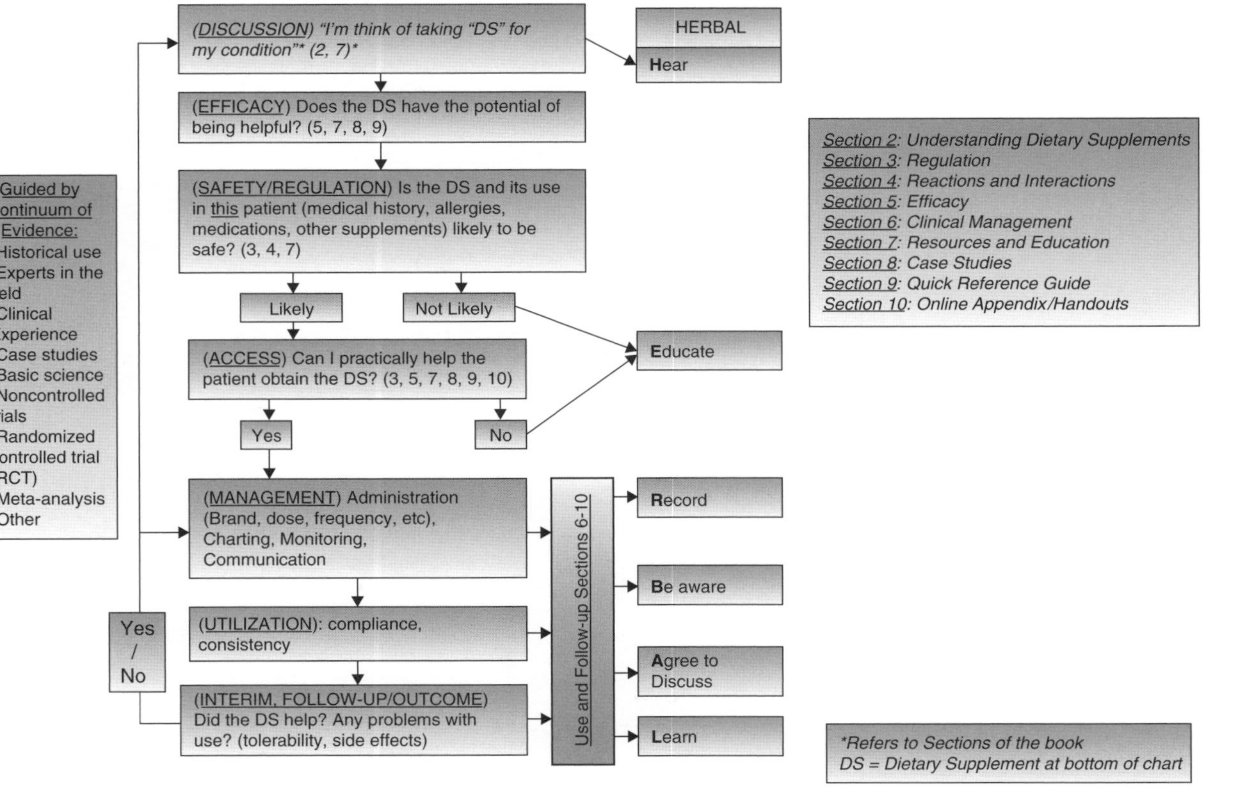
Guided by Continuum of Evidence:
•Historical use
•Experts in the field
•Clinical Experience
•Case studies
•Basic science
•Noncontrolled trials
•Randomized controlled trial (RCT)
•Meta-analysis
•Other
(DISCUSSION) "I'm think of taking "DS" for my condition"* (2, 7)*
HERBAL
Hear
(EFFICACY) Does the DS have the potential of being helpful? (5, 7, 8, 9)
(SAFETY/REGULATION) Is the DS and its use in this patient (medical history, allergies, medications, other supplements) likely to be safe? (3, 4, 7)
Likely
Not Likely
Educate
(ACCESS) Can I practically help the patient obtain the DS? (3, 5, 7, 8, 9, 10)
Yes
No
(MANAGEMENT) Administration (Brand, dose, frequency, etc), Charting, Monitoring, Communication
(UTILIZATION): compliance, consistency
(INTERIM, FOLLOW-UP/OUTCOME) Did the DS help? Any problems with use? (tolerability, side effects)
Yes / No
Use and Follow-up Sections 6-10
Record
Be aware
Agree to Discuss
Learn
Section 2: Understanding Dietary Supplements
Section 3: Regulation
Section 4: Reactions and Interactions
Section 5: Efficacy
Section 6: Clinical Management
Section 7: Resources and Education
Section 8: Case Studies
Section 9: Quick Reference Guide
Section 10: Online Appendix/Handouts
*Refers to Sections of the book
DS = Dietary Supplement at bottom of chart

Figure 9.1 • A pathway for dietary supplement (DS) management.

II

Understanding Dietary Supplements

CHAPTER 10

Dietary Supplements in the Context of CAM: Prevalence and Discussion

Robert Alan Bonakdar

Any discussion of dietary supplements is not complete without a review of complementary and alternative medicine (CAM) and integrative medicine. Although dietary supplements represent the most common type of CAM, they typically coexist with a number of other health care choices. A brief overview of these therapies provides context for the discussion of dietary supplements and the other CAM options which many patients use concomitantly. More specific information on dietary supplement utilization is provided in chapter 13.

Summary Points

- CAM represents a diverse set of therapies which are increasing in overall use
- CAM is used commonly to treat specific conditions such as pain
- CAM use is more common in certain socioeconomic groups
- Dietary supplements are the most common type of CAM therapy utilized
- Dietary supplements typically shift in popularity and sales based on a number of factors
- Patients and clinicians often do not discuss use of dietary supplements

The following discussion is provided from materials and research conducted by the National Center for Complementary and Alternative Medicine (NCCAM), a component of the National Institutes of Health. These include the following sites and reports which the reader is recommended to review in full:

1. *What Is CAM? Accessed at http://nccam.nih.gov/health/whatiscam/overview.htm on May 29, 2009*
2. *The Use of Complementary and Alternative Medicine in the United States. Accessed at http://nccam.nih.gov/news/camstats/2007/camsurvey_fs1.htm* (1).
3. *Complementary and Alternative Medicine: What People 50 and Older Are Using and Discussing with Their Physicians. The 2006 NIH/AARP report accessed at http://assets.aarp.org/rgcenter/health/cam_2007.pdf.*

DEFINITIONS

- **Complementary medicine** is used **together with** conventional medicine. An example of a complementary therapy is using aromatherapy to help lessen a patient's discomfort following surgery.

- **Alternative medicine** is used **in place of** conventional medicine. An example of an alternative therapy is using a special diet to treat cancer instead of undergoing surgery, radiation, or chemotherapy that has been recommended by a conventional physician.
- **Integrative** medicine combines treatments from conventional medicine and CAM for which there is evidence of safety and effectiveness.

CATEGORIES

NCCAM groups CAM practices into four domains, recognizing that there can be some overlap. In addition, NCCAM studies CAM whole medical systems, which cut across all domains. A brief overview of these categories as provided by NCCAM as well as a more complete list of CAM therapies from the 2007 National Health Interview Survey (NHIS) is noted in Table 10.1.

Whole Medical Systems

Whole medical systems are built upon complete systems of theory and practice. Often, these systems have evolved apart from and earlier than the conventional

TABLE 10.1 Complementary and Alternative Medicine Therapies Included in the 2007

National Health Interview Survey (NHIS)[a]	
Acupuncture*	Movement therapies
Ayurveda*	Alexander technique
Biofeedback*	Feldenkreis
Chelation therapy*	Pilates
Chiropractic or osteopathic manipulation*	Trager psychophysical integration
Deep breathing exercises	Natural products (nonvitamin and nonmineral, such as herbs and other products from plants, enzymes, etc.)
Diet-based therapies	Naturopathy*
Atkins diet	Progressive relaxation
Macrobiotic diet	Qi gong
Ornish diet	Tai chi
Pritikin diet	Traditional healers*
South beach diet	Botanica
Vegetarian diet	Curandero
Zone diet	Espiritista
Energy healing therapy/Reiki*	Hierbero or Yerbera
Guided imagery	Native American healer/Medicine man
Homeopathic treatment	Shaman
Hypnosis*	Sobador
Massage*	Yoga
Meditation	

[a]An asterisk (*) indicates a practitioner-based therapy.

medical approach used in the United States. Examples of whole medical systems that have developed in Western cultures include homeopathic medicine and naturopathic medicine. Examples of systems that have developed in non-Western cultures include traditional Chinese medicine and Ayurveda.

Mind–Body Medicine

Mind–body medicine uses a variety of techniques designed to enhance the mind's capacity to affect bodily function and symptoms. Some techniques that were considered CAM in the past have become mainstream (e.g., patient support groups and cognitive-behavioral therapy). Other mind–body techniques are still considered CAM, including meditation, prayer, mental healing, and therapies that use creative outlets such as art, music, or dance.

Biologically Based Practices

Biologically based practices in CAM use substances found in nature, such as herbs, foods, and vitamins. Some examples include dietary supplements, herbal products, and the use of other so-called natural but as yet scientifically unproven therapies (e.g., using shark cartilage to treat cancer).

Manipulative and Body-Based Practices

Manipulative and body-based practices in CAM are based on manipulation and/or movement of one or more parts of the body. Some examples include chiropractic or osteopathic manipulation, and massage.

Energy Medicine

Energy therapies involve the use of energy fields. They are of two types:

- **Biofield therapies** are intended to affect energy fields that purportedly surround and penetrate the human body. The existence of such fields has not yet been scientifically proven. Some forms of energy therapy manipulate biofields by applying pressure and/or manipulating the body by placing the hands in, or through, these fields. Examples include qi gong, Reiki, and therapeutic touch.
- **Bioelectromagnetic-based therapies** involve the unconventional use of electromagnetic fields, such as pulsed fields, magnetic fields, or alternating-current or direct-current fields.

USE OF COMPLEMENTARY AND ALTERNATIVE MEDICINE AND SUPPLEMENTS

The NHIS survey on **The Use of Complementary and Alternative Medicine in the United States** was based on interviews of more than 23,000 adults and 9,000 children. This was a follow-up to a similar survey conducted in 2002 (2).

Overall use of CAM appears to be approximately 38% of US adults and approximately 12% of children as noted in Figure 10.1. This represents an increase from 2002.

As noted earlier, the most common CAM therapy in this category is dietary supplements as used by 17.7%. Other common therapies are noted in Figure 10.2.

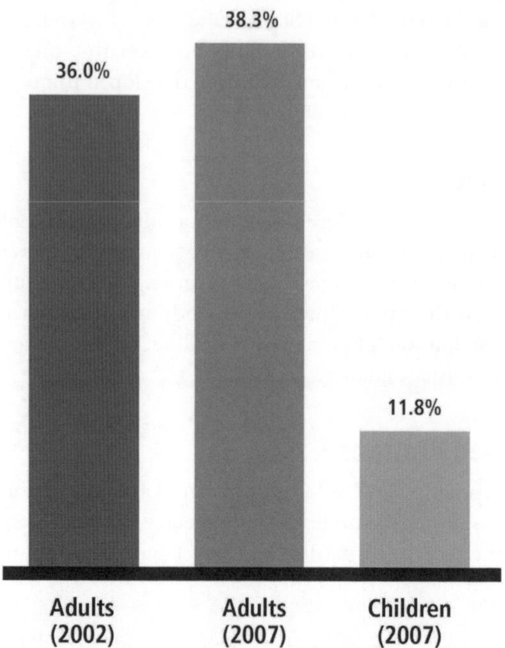

Figure 10.1 • CAM Use by US Adults and Children. Percentage of US adults in 2002 versus 2007 and children in 2007 who used complementary and alternative medicine (CAM) in the past 12 months. The figures show that CAM use among adults has remained relatively steady from 2002 to 2007. (From Barnes PM, Bloom B, Nahin R. *Complementary and Alternative Medicine Use Among Adults and Children: United States, 2007*. CDC National Health Statistics Report #12. December 10, 2008. Courtesy of National Center for Complementary and Alternative Medicine, NIH, DHHS.)

Within dietary supplements, the most common supplements include fish oil/omega 3, glucosamine, echinacea, flaxseed, ginseng, ginkgo, garlic, and coenzyme Q10. This contrasts with the finding of the 2002 survey which showed the most popular supplement as echinacea, ginseng, ginkgo, and garlic supplements with other supplements in the top 10 including St. John's Wort, peppermint, ginger, and soy. These top supplements are noted in Figure 10.3. The difference in survey results is common for a number of reasons which are important for the clinician to keep in mind including:

1. *Difference in survey methods*. In this specific case, the 2002 survey asked about use in the last 12 months and the 2007 survey asked about use in the last 30 days which can garner different answers.
2. *New research* which may increase or decrease the popularity of specific supplements
3. *Shift in advertising* promoting certain dietary supplements
4. *Recalls or warnings* regarding the safety or interaction of certain supplements
5. *New guidelines* which may include specific dietary supplements (i.e. Plant Sterols as part of the Treatment of High Cholesterol (Adult Treatment Panel (ATP III))
6. *Change in other options* available including new prescription or non-CAM therapies on the market
7. *Cost and availability* of specific supplements
8. *Change in level of discussion* of specific supplements based on factors above

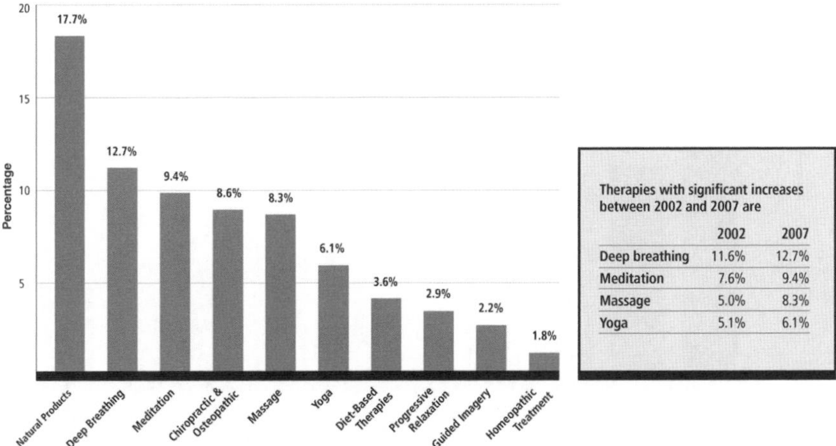

Figure 10.2 • Ten Most Common CAM Therapies Among Adults—2007. Percentage of adults in 2007 who used the 10 most common complementary and alternative medicine (CAM) therapies. The most commonly used CAM therapy among adults in 2007 was nonvitamin, nonmineral natural products. Box shows therapies with significant increases in use between 2002 and 2007: deep breathing, meditation, massage, and yoga. (From Barnes PM, Bloom B, Nahin R. *Complementary and Alternative Medicine Use Among Adults and Children: United States, 2007*. CDC National Health Statistics Report #12. December 10, 2008. Courtesy of National Center for Complementary and Alternative Medicine, NIH, DHHS.)

COMPLEMENTARY AND ALTERNATIVE MEDICINE USE BASED ON CONDITIONS

Typically, Americans use CAM to treat a particular condition as opposed to prevention or wellness. The most common condition is pain which was more specifically and commonly back pain or problems, neck pain or problems, joint pain and arthritis. Nonpain conditions including colds, anxiety and insomnia, or high cholesterol were also common reasons for CAM use (Fig. 10.4).

COMPLEMENTARY AND ALTERNATIVE MEDICINE USE BASED ON DEMOGRAPHICS

Typically, CAM use appears to be more common in the following category of patients and consumers:

- Women
- Certain ethnic/racial groups including Native American/Eskimos and whites (Fig. 10.5)
- Those aged 30 to 69 (Fig. 10.6)
- Those with higher levels of education
- Those who were more affluent
- Those living in the West

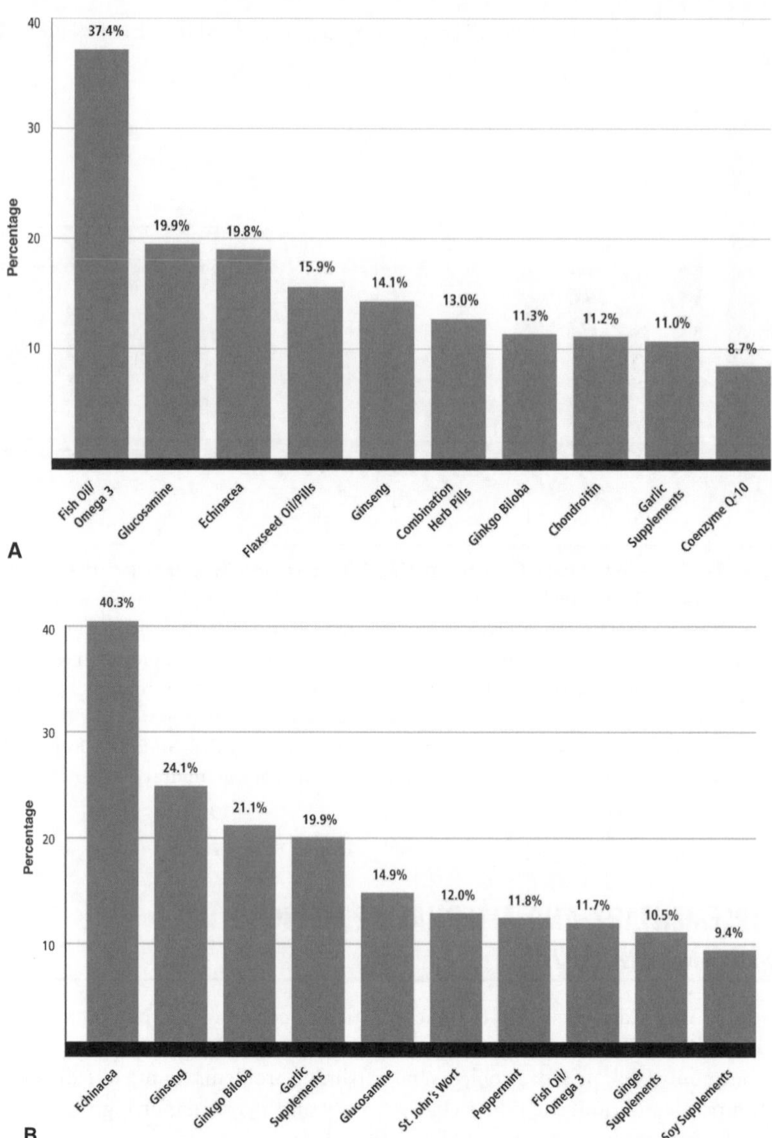

Figure 10.3 • Ten Most Common Natural Products Among Adults—for 2007 (A) and 2002 (B)[*]. Among adults who used nonvitamin, nonmineral natural products in the last year—percentages for the top 10 natural products used in last 30 days among adults in 2007 and percentages for the top 10 natural products used in the last 12 months for 2002. In 2007, the most popular natural products were fish oils/omega 3, glucosamine, echinacea, and flaxseed. In 2002, the most popular natural products were echinacea, ginseng, ginkgo, and garlic supplements.

[*]Percentages for specific natural products for 2002 and 2007 cannot be directly compared because the 2002 survey asked about use in the last 12 months whereas the 2007 survey asked about use in the last 30 days. (Part A from Barnes PM, Bloom B, Nahin R. *Complementary and Alternative Medicine Use Among Adults and Children: United States, 2007*. CDC National Health Statistics Report #12. December 10, 2008. Courtesy of National Center for Complementary and Alternative Medicine, NIH, DHHS, and Part B from Barnes P, Powell-Griner E, McFann K, Nahir R. *Complementary and Alternative Medicine Use Among Adults: United States, 2002*. CDC Advance Data Report #343. May 2004.)

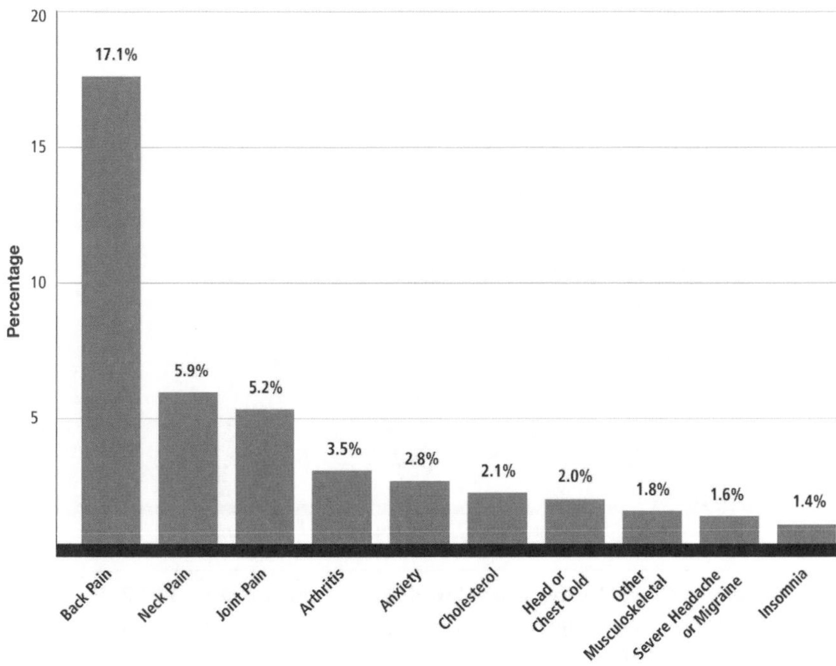

Figure 10.4 • Diseases/Conditions for Which CAM Is Most Frequently Used Among Adults—2007. Percentage of adults in 2007 who used complementary and alternative medicine (CAM) during the last 12 months by specific disease and condition. In 2007, problems such as back/neck, and joint pain and arthritis were some of the most common reasons for CAM use. (From Barnes PM, Bloom B, Nahin R. *Complementary and Alternative Medicine Use Among Adults and Children: United States, 2007*. CDC National Health Statistics Report #12. December 10, 2008. Courtesy of National Center for Complementary and Alternative Medicine, NIH, DHHS.)

DISCUSSION IS SUBOPTIMAL

The low level of clinician–patient discussion is best exemplified by findings of the 2006 National Institutes of Health/American Association of Retired Persons report, **Complementary and Alternative Medicine:** *What People 50 and Older Are Using and Discussing with Their Physicians* (3). Among other findings, this survey of 1,559 people noted a significant lack of discussion. Overall 77% did not talk about CAM use with their physicians with reasons given for nondiscussion including:

1. Physicians never asked (42%)
2. Patients did not know that they should talk with their physicians (30%).
3. Lack of time (19%).
4. Do not think physician knows the topic (17%)
5. Physician would have been dismissive or told you not to do it (12%)

Those who did speak to their physicians were more likely to be women and those with higher income and education. The discussions that did take place typically focused on efficacy, safety, and potential interactions. These discussions are especially important as nearly ¾ of this population took one or more prescription medications with 20% taking more than five and 59% taking over-the-counter medications.

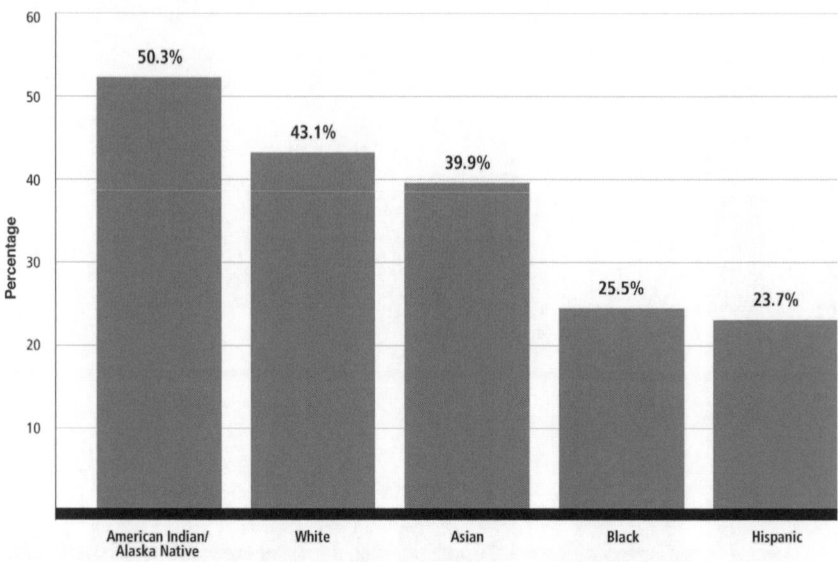

Figure 10.5 • CAM Use by Race/Ethnicity Among Adults—2007. Percentage of adults in 2007 who used complementary and alternative medicine (CAM) during the past 12 months, by race/ethnicity. CAM use is greater among American Indians/Alaska Natives, whites, and Asians than among blacks and Hispanics. (From Barnes PM, Bloom B, Nahin R. *Complementary and Alternative Medicine Use Among Adults and Children: United States, 2007.* CDC National Health Statistics Report #12. December 10, 2008. Courtesy of National Center for Complementary and Alternative Medicine, NIH, DHHS.)

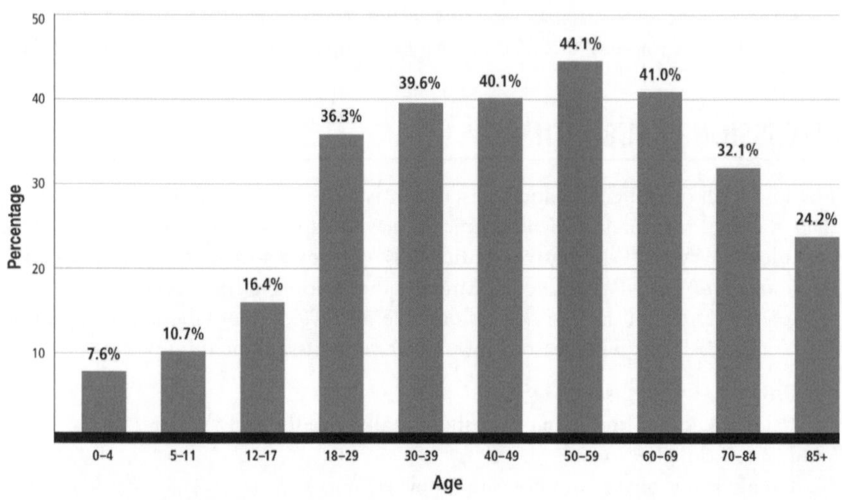

Figure 10.6 • CAM Use by Age—2007. Percentage of persons in 2007 who used complementary and alternative medicine (CAM) during the past 12 months, by age. CAM use is greatest among those aged 30 to 69. (From Barnes PM, Bloom B, Nahin R. *Complementary and Alternative Medicine Use Among Adults and Children: United States, 2007.* CDC National Health Statistics Report #12. December 10, 2008. Courtesy of National Center for Complementary and Alternative Medicine, NIH, DHHS.)

SUMMARY

As patients increase their use of dietary supplements it is important for clinicians to realize that these choices are typically made within the larger context of CAM that involves a large number of therapies and systems of healing. Thus, as clinicians increase their discussion of dietary supplements it is imperative to also ask about sources of information, use, and other providers so supplements can best be understood in the context of the larger integrative care model. By beginning to view dietary supplement more as a lifestyle choice that is linked to other health care options, clinicians have the greatest chance of understanding, motivating, and counseling patients.

References

1. Barnes PM, Bloom B, Nahin R. *Complementary and Alternative Medicine Use Among Adults and Children: United States, 2007*. CDC National Health Statistics Report #12. December 2008.
2. Barnes P, Powell-Griner E, McFann K, Nahin R. *Complementary and Alternative Medicine Use Among Adults: United States, 2002.* CDC Advance Data Report #343. May 27, 2004.
3. Complementary and alternative medicine: what people 50 and older are using and discussing with their physicians. The 2006 NIH/AARP report. http://assets.aarp.org/rgcenter/health/cam_2007.pdf.

CHAPTER 11

What Is a Dietary Supplement? (It's More Than That Multivitamin Pill)

Robert Alan Bonakdar

There are many ways to approach the definitions for a dietary supplement based on whom you are asking. Some of the more common views, including regulatory, legal, insurance-related, functional, and practical, are briefly reviewed below. The goal of this review is to demonstrate that dietary supplements can be viewed very differently from various perspectives and that these definitions are part of an evolving continuum. It is important for the clinician to keep these various definitions in mind as patients may have very traditional or emerging understanding of dietary supplementation. Moreover, the way clinicians ask about dietary supplements will help patients best describe their dietary supplement habits, be it a traditional multivitamin pill or less traditional functional foods.

REGULATORY

An important definition to start with is the official one provided by Congress in the Dietary Supplement Health and Education Act (DSHEA) of 1994 and covered in detail by Dr. Dickinson in chapter 16. Importantly, DSHEA placed dietary supplements in a special category under the umbrella of "foods," not drugs, and requires that every supplement be labeled as such. More specifically, dietary supplements were defined as products:

- Taken by mouth in various forms, including:
  - Tablets
  - Capsules
  - Soft gels
  - Gel caps
  - Liquids
  - Powders
- Containing a "dietary ingredient" intended to supplement the diet, including one or more of the following:
  - Vitamins
  - Minerals
  - Herbs or other botanics
  - Amino acids
  - Substances such as enzymes, organ tissues, and metabolites.

- Found in various forms including:
  - Extracts, concentrates, etc.
  - Other forms, such as a bar, may require labeling that the product represents a conventional food or a sole item of a meal or diet (1).

LEGAL AND INSURANCE DEFINITION

As William Skinner writes in chapter 14 the legal definition can vary widely by state. These legal variations include who may "prescribe" a dietary supplement as well as what may be considered for insurance coverage. As one example, New York public health law defines prescription and some nonprescription drugs including supplements similarly including the possibility of insurance coverage. Specifically, "... Any drug that does not require a prescription under such act, but which would otherwise meet the criteria under this article for inclusion on the preferred drug list ... shall be considered to be a prescription drug for purposes of this article ..." With this law in place, certain clinically tested dietary supplements have a history of coverage in a manner similar to prescription medications.

This type of law does not exist in most states, so insurance carriers typically decide how a supplement is viewed in regard to coverage. In most cases, insurers will cover only certain Food and Drug Administration–approved prescription drugs. As dietary supplements are defined by DSHEA within the category of food, this typically will make dietary supplements noncovered entities. However, certain natural products may have coverage based on how they are approved or prescribed as several examples point out. First, certain natural products, such as niacin and fish oils, exist both as dietary supplements and as prescriptions medications that received Food and Drug Administration approval for specific indication (i.e., hypertriglyceridemia). Moreover, dietary supplements may exist as medical foods that can only be acquired by prescription from a qualified health care provider (i.e., (genistein, zinc and cholecalciferol) Fosteum). Last, dietary supplements may petition for and receive a qualified health claim (see as reviewed in chapter 17).

As these examples point out, the same substance, based on how it is researched, submitted, approved, packaged, and taken, can be regulated and covered in vastly different ways. It is important for the practitioner to keep this in mind as this may determine access, affordability, compliance, and legitimacy in various environments.

PRACTICAL DEFINITIONS TO CONSIDER

"Everything You Consume"

The clinician needs to place the regulatory and legal definitions in the context of practical patient understanding and utilization of dietary supplements. Examples of this include patients who have very focused or expanded views of dietary supplementation.

FUNCTIONAL FOODS

Functional foods are typically fortified with increased levels of vitamins, minerals, fiber, protein, and/or dietary supplements such as herbal extracts, probiotics, plant sterols, omega-3 fatty acids, or soy just to name a few. These added ingredient may end up in final products ranging from omega-3 fatty acid fortified cereals to probiotic yogurts drinks, cholesterol-lowering spreads, vitamin-fortified breads, and herbal extract infused energy drinks. In recent years, the number of functional foods on the market has grown dramatically to the point that the traditional means by which a consumer acquired required and supplemental nutrients may no longer be pills or capsules. From the standpoint of the clinician, the form of the supplement should not be the main issue, but more importantly what the supplement provides and the rationale behind its use.

This trend is especially important for clinicians to keep in mind as the way questions are posed pick up or miss to patients may miss important avenues for dietary supplementation. As an example, asking, "do you take any vitamins or mineral supplement?" may not register as any of the fortified foods a patient may be utilizing for various reasons. This may underestimate supplements which the patient is actually obtaining in noncapsule form and decrease the opportunity for charting, discussion and counseling.

In this scenario it is important for the clinician to expand the definition of dietary supplements to less traditionally recognized forms. This can be accomplished by educating the patient on the broad definition of supplements and by asking and recording if they are utilizing any of these forms (see Appendix for supplement intake forms). Not only will this facilitate the job of the clinician in understanding what patients are truly utilizing but also in many cases it will help patients erase artificial barriers on what should or should not be discussed.

"Beyond Taken by Mouth"

Although the DSHEA only views supplements as those taken orally, many patients and consumers are using "supplements" in other forms. A few examples of these include transdermal (herbal hormonal and analgesic creams, ointments, and patches); injectable (vitamin B_{12}, homeopathics, steroid precursors); intravenous (glutathione, chelation); and inhaled (intranasal aromatherapy). To some patients these non-oral forms may be the major "supplement" to their diet and lifestyle but are not mentioned because they do not occur in the traditional oral supplementation form.

In this scenario the clinician needs to broaden the definition by asking about non-oral intake that is not officially considered "dietary supplements" but which may influence care. The term "natural supplements" may be useful in the above examples as it may key in on substances and therapies beyond official "dietary supplements." This discussion may also bring up other clinicians who are coordinating these therapies who are important to keep in mind when formulating or changing care options.

Although there are many definitions applied to dietary supplements, the most important one for the clinician to keep in mind includes a combination of the above. In essence, by starting with basic legal and regulatory definitions and then broadening to capture the potential unique natural supplement use of each patient, the clinician is most practically able to gain full disclosure. And as discussed elsewhere in the book, full disclosure paralleled with open, nonjudgmental discussion has the greatest potential of allowing full care.

Reference

1. U. S. Food and Drug Administration Center for Food Safety and Applied Nutrition. Overview of dietary supplements. http://www.cfsan.fda.gov/~dms/ds-oview.html#what. Accessed March 16, 2009.

CHAPTER 12

Understanding Dietary Supplement Labels and Dosing

David Kiefer

Chapter ID: Suzanne is 51 years old and completely perplexed about the meaning on the packaging for several products she recently purchased to help her through menopause. She wants to take calcium; each tablet of her calcium supplement contains 500 mg of calcium carbonate. She asks you how many to take daily. Moreover, she purchased black cohosh, 350 mg per capsule, and it is recommended to ingest three capsules daily for the relief of symptoms of menopause. Do you counsel her that this dosage is too much? Not enough? What should she look for on a label that would indicate a quality black cohosh product?

BACKGROUND

There are an estimated 30,000 supplements for sale in the United States currently (ref). As a result of the Dietary Supplement Health and Education Act (DSHEA) of 1994 (see chapter 16), these supplements are treated technically as foods, and as such are monitored after they reach the shelves of grocery stores, pharmacies, and health food stores. This postmarketing surveillance is in stark contrast to the regulatory climate of pharmaceuticals in the United States that have to undergo several phases of testing *prior* to be allowed for public sale. As a result of this, regulations have been established about what is allowed on dietary supplement labels; knowledge of this will help health care practitioners to better counsel patients and ensure that they are purchasing quality and effective products.

This chapter will

- review what is allowed and not allowed on a dietary supplement label,
- describe what should be on an herbal medicine label for the different formulations (dried herb, tincture, extract, etc.),
- delineate characteristics of a good versus a bad dietary supplement label, and
- list the third-party evaluation groups.

EDUCATING THE PATIENT

There are three main types of statements that are allowable on dietary supplements (see Table 12.1), the details of which are overseen by the U.S. Food and Drug Administration Center for Food Safety and Nutrition (www.cfsan.fda.gov/~dms/hclaims.html),

TABLE 12.1 Categories of Label Claims

Claim Category	What It Does Do	What It Does Not Do
Structure/function	Comments on how a particular product promotes wellness related to a structural part or function of the body	Provide information relevant to the diagnosis, prevention, treatment, or cure of any specific disease
Nutrient Content	Describes the amount of a substance in a product	Apply to those nutrients for which a daily value has *not* been established
Health Claim	Makes a connection between a substance and the reduced risk of a disease or health-related condition	There are still limits about the phrasing of these claims depending on the type of approval received.

though the Federal Trade Commission may become involved if issues surrounding advertising develop. One of the allowable statements on a label is called a structure/function claim, a phrase that comments on how a particular product promotes wellness related to a structural part or function of the body. This statement cannot mention anything related to the diagnosis, prevention, treatment, or cure of any specific disease and has to carry a disclaimer on the label to that effect. Examples of this kind of phrasing include how a certain supplement builds strong bones, maintains cell integrity, promotes liver function, supports heart health, or maintains bowel regularity.

Nutrient Content claims use terms such as high, low, free, more, reduced, and lite to describe the amount of a compound in a product. These claims may also include percentage claims if no daily value percentage exists. The Food and Drug Administration's Food Labeling Guide (www.cfsan.fda.gov/~dms/flg-toc.html) lists what nutrients and their content claims are allowable.

Health Claims are the most stringent and evidence-based phrases allowable on a dietary supplement label. A petition is made through one of three methods of scientific review (NLEA Authorized Health Claim, a Health Claim Based on Authoritative Statements, and Qualified Health Claims) that differ primarily in the strength of the evidence for the claim and the source of the claim (scientific literature, scientific body, governmental organization, etc.). Once approved, a statement can be placed on the label. An example of an Approved Health Claim, based on significant scientific agreement, is "Healthful diets with adequate folate may reduce a woman's risk of having a child with a brain or spinal cord defect," whereas a Qualified Health Claim, based on some preliminary evidence, is "Supportive but not conclusive research shows that consumption of EPA and DHA omega-3 fatty acids may reduce the risk of coronary heart disease. One serving of [Name of the food] provides [ ] gram of EPA and DHA omega-3 fatty acids."

Other requirements from the Food and Drug Administration include a descriptive name (including a statement that it is a "supplement"); the name and place of business of the manufacturer, packer, or distributor; contact information for reporting adverse effects; net contents of the product; and a "Supplement Facts"

TABLE 12.2 General Needs for Herbal Medicine Labeling

Characteristic	Example
Latin scientific name (*Genus species*)	*Echinacea purpurea*
Plant part being used	Root bark powder
Recommend dose	30–60 drops of tincture three times daily
Special characteristics depending on herbal medicine form	See Table 12.3

panel which lists a serving size, a complete list of ingredients, and the percent daily value of relevant ingredients. Reviewing a particular label for these characteristics can help health care providers, patients, and consumers begin to get an idea about the quality of a dietary supplement.

Beyond these generalities, determining what should be on a supplement label depends on the specific dietary supplement involved. Health care providers can help patients effectively use dietary supplements by first being up-to-date on the evidence basis for various nutrients for a given demographic. Calcium intake recommendations are a good example. Recommendations from scientific research are based on a patient's gender, age, and risk factors, and are usually stated in elemental calcium. Furthermore, some nuances from the medical literature are surfacing and would be available to health care practitioners doing a basic search on medical databases; for example, one might find that no more than 500 mg of elemental calcium should be taken in any one dose, and that generally calcium carbonate is reasonably absorbed when taken with meals (taking advantage of stomach acid) except in low acid environments when preliminary data indicate that calcium citrate may be slightly better absorbed. Putting this all together, a health care provider will want to tailor calcium product recommendations based on each patient and mention paying attention to the form, dose, and elemental calcium amounts listed on the label (as opposed to total calcium compound [i.e., calcium carbonate, calcium citrate, etc.)]. This approach can be applied to any other specific dietary supplement.

Specifics to Herbal Medicines

Herbal medicines are another example of a type of dietary supplement that have characteristics to be aware of when reading dietary supplement labels. There are general herbal medicine label needs (i.e., all labels for an herbal medicine should have these characteristics; Table 12.2), and, as mentioned above for dietary supplements as a whole, some labeling needs will differ for each plant. In general, all herbal medicine labels should specifically mention the Latin scientific name for a plant, including the *Genus* and *species*, or any variety or *subspecies*. No longer is "echinacea" sufficient for health care providers or patients/consumers to adequately critique an herbal medicine product containing that plant. Instead, current taxonomy dictates that a product specifically lists which of the three main echinacea species are being included: *Echinacea purpurea*, *Echinacea pallida*, *Echinacea pallida* var. *angustifolia*. Furthermore, every herbal medicine label should have the plant part being used; this would correlate with the physiological condition being treated.

TABLE 12.3 Herbal Medicine Labeling for Two Common Herbal Medicine Forms

Form	Important Label Characteristics	Example
Tinctures	• Strength/ratio (expressed as kilogram of herb to liters of solvent, or ounce to ounce): most are 1:2–1:5 • Percentage alcohol or glycerin (the most common solvents)	*Panax ginseng*: 1:2 dry root to extract ratio, 23%–29% grain alcohol
Standardized extracts	• Marker compound(s) • Percentage standardization	*Ginkgo biloba*: 50:1 standardized extract containing 6% terpene lactones and 24% flavonolglycosides

One example of why this is important is stinging nettle (*Urtica dioica*); the *root* is used for benign prostatic hypertrophy, but the *leaf* is used as an anti-inflammatory for conditions like arthritis and allergic rhinitis. Some labeling characteristics appear depending on what herbal medicine form the product is (Table 12.3). For example, some plants are more often used in raw form, such as an infusion made from peppermint (*Mentha* × *piperita*) leaves, whereas in other cases, a standardized extract is used, such as with butterbur (*Petasites hybridus*) for migraine or allergic rhinitis treatment. Although there is some variety in approach among herbal medicine experts, as health care providers explore clinical herbal medicine some patterns in herbal medicine form begin to surface which then translate into what should be on a given herbal medicine label. Literature is beginning to list the standardized extracts used in research trials (1); some health care providers are focusing their herbal medicine practice on these studied and proven forms (see chapter 31).

Third-Party Evaluation Organizations

There are four main groups involved with the evaluation and rating of dietary supplements (2, 3) (Table 12.4). These groups range from nonprofit groups providing information to consumers (NSF International) to industry and trade organizations that provide certification of quality to member businesses (Natural Products Association; ConsumerLab). ConsumerLab has voluntary (businesses apply for certification and are then tested) and nonvoluntary (products are chosen from retail shelves for testing) programs, in addition to providing some information free of charge for consumers on its Web site. The U.S. Pharmacopeia will test products and ingredients for identification, strength, purity, and quality, in addition to providing basic education tools online for consumers, patients, and health care practitioners.

LEARN

Health care practitioners should make a habit of regularly checking the Web site for the Food and Drug Administration (4) for updates to approved health claims and

TABLE 12.4 Third-Party Evaluation Groups

Organization	Details	Web Site
ConsumerLab	• Voluntary and nonvoluntary industry programs • Membership provides full access to product testing results; some limited information free of charge on Web site	www.consumerlab.com
Natural Products Association TruLabel	• An industry and trade group, primarily advocating on the legislative level • Random testing program through TruLabel; 17,000 product labels listed • Good Manufacturing Practices (GMP) certification	www.naturalproductsassoc.org
NSF International	• A nonprofit organization providing information for consumers and certification for industry groups • GMP auditing • Product testing to American National Standards Institute parameters	www.nsf.org
U.S. Pharmacopeia	• Product testing and certification program • GMP audit • Manufacturing documentation review	www.uspverified.org

labeling changes. In addition to the references listed for this chapter, several helpful tools for ongoing learning include the following:

1. U.S. Pharmacopeia Web site (www.uspverified.org) for resources on dietary supplement labeling including a video "Choosing a Dietary Supplement" (5)
2. The Dietary Supplements Labels Database (http://dietarysupplements.nlm.nih.gov) through the National Library of Medicine. The database includes information from the labels of more than 2,000 brands of dietary supplements.
3. Natural Medicines Comprehensive Database (www.Naturaldatabase.com). This subscription-funded site provides label information for more than 26,000 products.

SUMMARY

There is very specific information that should be contained on a dietary supplement label with respect to ingredients, health information, and dosing. There are generalities that health care practitioners and consumers should be aware of, in addition to unique aspects relevant to particular classes of products, such as herbal medicines. Being aware of these characteristics will help patients achieve the most out of their dietary supplement use by making sure that only products of the highest quality and most in line with scientific evidence are being prescribed and purchased.

References

1. Blumenthal M, ed. *The ABC Clinical Guide to Herbs*. Austin, TX: American Botanical Council; 2003.
2. Whybark MK. Third party evaluation programs for the quality of dietary supplements. *HerbalGram* 2004;64:30–33.
3. Blumenthal M. *Identifying High Quality Herbal dietary Supplements: A Discussion of Issues About Quality and Clinical Reliability*. American Botanical Council. Scripps Conference on Dietary Supplements; 2006.
4. U.S. Food and Drug Administration and Center for Food Safety and Nutrition. Dietary supplements. www.cfsan.fda.gov/~dms/supplmnt.html. Accessed December 12, 2007.
5. U.S. Pharmacopeia. www.usp.org/USPVerified/. Accessed December 12, 2007.

CHAPTER 13

The Dietary Supplement User: Predictors and Implications for the Clinician

Robert Alan Bonakdar

The Dietary Supplement (DS) User: Key Points

- DS use ranges from 18% to 73% of the population based on survey methodology. In general, DS use is increasing and is conservatively noted in at least one third to more than one half of the US population.
- DS use may improve, but does not guarantee, adequate nutrient intake, especially in populations at risk for deficiency such as the elderly.
- A change in health status (recent medical diagnosis, quitting smoking) is associated with initiation or shift in DS use. Use appeared highest in subjects with conditions that have poorer prognosis or less available medical options.
- DS users are not likely to openly discuss the topic until brought up by a clinician.
- DS nonusers may be members of specific populations most likely to require focused supplementation based on nutrient deficiency.

INTRODUCTION

Dietary supplements (DS), based on various definitions, are currently utilized by one third to more than half of all adults in the United States. As many DS users do not disclose use with their clinicians, it is important for the clinician to initiate discussion regarding interest in and utilization of DS. This chapter discusses important demographics, predictors, and health-related behaviors of the DS user that are helpful for the clinician to keep in mind. These predictors can have implications for strategizing discussion when interacting with and providing guidance to patients who are DS users and nonusers.

PREVALENCE OF USE

The percentage of the population utilizing DS varies on the basis of several key factors including the population examined as well as survey methodology including qualifying definitions for DS and level of use. For example, the Tomorrow Project Survey noted an extensive DS use of 69.8 % (1). This survey was a general population telephone survey of approximately 12,000 men and women (aged 35 to 69 years) in which DS use was defined as any type of seven discrete supplement categories including multivitamins utilized at least weekly in the year prior. In contrast, the personal interviews of more than 31,044 subjects older than age 18 years performed by Centers for Disease Control and Prevention/ National Institutes of Health surveyed all complementary and alternative medicine modalities utilized. Although natural products were the most commonly utilized complementary and alternative medicine approach (excluded prayer), use was noted at a lower level of 18.9% (2). Other surveys tend to demonstrate higher levels of use. In the National Health and Nutrition Examination Survey IV (NHANES), use of any dietary supplement in the last month was 52%, demonstrating a steady increase from NHANES I, II, & III surveys with 23%, 35%, and 40% use, respectively (3). In other surveys demonstrating increasing use, the Hawaii–Los Angeles Multiethnic Cohort survey of adults without chronic disease, 48% of men and 56% of women reported use of multivitamin supplements at least weekly over the past year and the US Food and Drug Administration Health and Diet telephone survey noted a 73% prevalence rate for DS use in adults in the previous 12 months (4, 5).

DEMOGRAPHICS OF THE DIETARY SUPPLEMENTS USER

Several demographic factors tend to consistently predict DS use in previous surveys as summarized in Table 13.1 (6–11). In general, use is higher in women than men with a previous survey demonstrating 2.2 times higher DS use in women (95% CI, 1.4 to 3.3) (12). Ethnicity also predicts use with non-Hispanic whites demonstrating greater use than non-Hispanic blacks or Mexican Americans. Surveys note that DS users, on average, are older, married, and have a higher level of education and income. As recent research has attempted to link DS use with specific health outcomes, it is imperative that these demographic factors are taken into consideration when making potential associations.

TABLE 13.1 Predictors of Dietary Supplements Use

Female
Married
Non-Hispanic white
Residence in metropolitan area
Higher level of education
Higher income
Health status, behaviors, and beliefs:
Lower body mass index
Higher level of physical activity
Vegetarian diet
Higher fruit, vegetable, and fiber intake
Lower fat intake
Consumption of wine but not beer or hard liquor (distilled spirits)
Former or never smoker
Belief that DS will prevent illness and promote health

HEALTH STATUS, BEHAVIOR, AND BELIEFS OF THE DIETARY SUPPLEMENTS USER

The health status and behavior of the DS user also deserve attention. In general, those who exhibit healthier lifestyles demonstrate higher DS use. This is defined in various surveys as having a higher level of physical activity; lower body mass index, lower alcohol intake (specifically beer and hard liquor), and being a nonsmoker. Specific beliefs in the role of DS use in disease and health are also apparent. For example, DS users believe more strongly that use will prevent illness and promote health (13).

Attitudes regarding the importance of following a healthful diet are also predictive of DS use. This attitude is demonstrated with DS users more likely to follow a vegetarian diet and/or having preexisting higher fruit, vegetable, fiber intake and lower dietary fat intake. These dietary habits appear to place the DS user at a slightly (2% to 8%) higher likelihood of meeting nutrient adequacy when compared with nonusers. Conversely, DS nonusers are more likely to be in subpopulation that may receive less adequate nutrient intake from foods and benefit from DS as noted below in discussion of adults over 50.

Several important points regarding DS in the context of dietary intake should be kept in mind. In some cases the DS user, especially if already reaching adequacy for diet nutrients, may be at potential risk for exceeding the tolerable upper intake level for nutrients such as vitamin A, iron, and zinc. Conversely, as noted in a survey of adults older than age 50, supplementation may improve but does not guarantee, adequate nutrient intake (6). In this survey, although a significantly smaller percentage of DS users had dietary intake below the estimated average requirement (EAR) compared with nonusers, less than 50% of the DS users and nonusers met the EAR for folate, vitamin E, and magnesium from food sources alone. With use of DS, however, more than 80% met the EAR for nutrients including vitamins A, B_6, B_{12}, C, and E; folate; iron; and zinc.

Next, the above dietary trends appear to be most consistent for DS users with more specialized supplement choices (14). One example comes from the North Carolina Strategies to Improve Diet, Exercise, and Screening study in which participants' use of five different DS categories were evaluated in relation to fruit and vegetable consumption. Those subjects using a multivitamin/multimineral along with a single supplement or any nonvitamin/nonmineral products (such as an herbal DS) were likely to be consuming more vegetables and higher-quality fruits and vegetables than did DS nonusers. Subjects with more basic DS use (daily multivitamin only) had dietary patterns that were more similar to those of DS nonusers.

The above dietary patterns in relation to DS use provide several key points for the clinician. First, DS may improve, but do not guarantee acceptable nutrient status, especially in certain populations. Second, patients who are already making healthy dietary choices are more likely to utilize DS, especially specialized DS. In this scenario the clinician questioning a patient may use answers about multivitamin use or specialized DS to postulate dietary patterns and the need for DS, especially in relation to meeting recommended dietary intake. This is especially important in populations, such as the elderly, who are more likely not to meet adequate intake and may benefit from focused supplementation in conjunction with dietary counseling. A summary of key demographics and predictors of DS use is provided in Table 13.1.

SPECIAL POPULATIONS

Pediatric

The use of DS in the pediatric population exhibits patterns, which deserve special attention. In a number of surveys approximately 50% of preschoolers utilize a multivitamin DS (15). In a survey of 8,285 preschool children, 54.4% of 3-year-olds were given some type of vitamin and mineral DS. Children who received DS had parents whose demographics were similar to the typical adult DS user noted above, namely, these parents were older, well-educated, non-Hispanic whites with higher household incomes. Children who were first born and whose mothers reported their children as having issues with poor appetite, eating problems, or food allergy were more likely to receive DS. In addition, children who had a medical diagnosis or who had received nutritional counseling from a health care provider were also more likely to use DS, regardless of the clinical setting. Unfortunately, in some groups, including children participating in an Aid to Families with Dependent Children program, DS use was noted to be quite low (16). Thus, unless there is specific health care practitioner's advice to do so, the authors summarize: "...groups at risk for nonuse are likely the same groups whose circumstances may predispose a need for supplementation."

As noted above, the use of DS in children appears to be linked to medical diagnosis. In a survey of 505 chronically ill children with a variety of conditions, 62% of the population was utilizing DS, with the highest percentage noted in subjects with cancer (17). Use appeared highest in subjects with conditions associated with less available medical options or those with poorer prognosis.

Adolescents and Young Adults

In the adolescent and young-adult population somewhat different predictive factors were noted as compared to adults. Approximately 25.7% of 14 to 18 year olds and 20% of 18 to 30 year olds were using DS with current or previous smoking, moderate/heavy alcohol use, and higher physical activity levels noted as predictive factors (18, 19). Importantly, only a quarter of DS users were discussing use with a health care professional even though prescription medication was utilized in more than 50% of the subjects and was a predictive factor for DS use. In this population DS use has also been associated with performance and appearance enhancement (20, 21). In a study of female college students, the most important predictor of the use of multivitamin supplements was the belief that use would help them look and feel good (22, 23).

Other Populations

The use of DS in other specific population including women who are pregnant or lactating, is reviewed elsewhere in the book.

A SHIFT IN HEALTH

Medical Conditions and Change in Health

The use of DS in populations with specific medical diagnoses has been evaluated in a number of surveys. With some exception, studies demonstrate higher DS use in those with a diagnosis versus healthy controls (24). This shift appears to correlate with other lifestyle strategies employed in this population aimed at improving health outcomes (25). The best example of this may be in cancer in which 64% to 81% of survivors reported using vitamin or mineral supplements (26). Moreover, 14% to 48% of those with cancer noted that they initiated or increased DS use after diagnosis (26).

In other chronic conditions besides cancer, DS use tends to be more specialized (27). The California Health Interview evaluated DS use in those with and without cancer and among those with and without other chronic conditions. Both those with cancer or a chronic condition had higher use than individuals without a diagnosis but differed in their choice of DS. A cancer diagnosis is associated with vitamin use, but not other nonvitamin DS. Conversely, those living with other chronic conditions had higher use of all nonvitamin DS, except multivitamins. The authors postulate that nonvitamin DS use among cancer survivors may be initiated for the treatment of other chronic conditions or comorbidities.

IMPLICATION FOR THE HEALTH CARE PROFESSIONAL

The clinician should routinely consider a number of factors that predict DS use when encountering patients. Foremost is the fact that most patients considering or utilizing DS do not openly discuss this with a health care professional. This issue is discussed in detail elsewhere, (chapter 10) but should prompt an open, nonjudgmental discussion by the clinician with strategies to optimize use in the setting of safety and efficacy (chapter 44). In addition to inquiring about the use of DS in all patients at their initial encounter, clinicians should be aware of populations most likely to benefit from DS discussion based on predictors noted in Table 13.1. In these specific populations, the use of DS should be more regularly reviewed and may represent an ideal opportunity for DS and lifestyle counseling. Several examples of populations that should be specifically highlighted during the clinical encounter are noted below:

- **Patients with a new medical diagnosis.** Patients should be asked whether they are considering or have started a new DS based on the diagnosis, and if so, their goals for doing do. Discussion can often lead to review of DS in the context of other options for management of the condition or comorbidities (i.e., cancer-related fatigue or neuropathy).
- **Patients on specific prescription medications.** Patients taking specific prescription medications that may put them at increased risk of interaction should be asked about use of specific DS (i.e., St. John's Wort and cyclosporine). This topic is further discussed in chapter 26.
- **Patients at risk for suboptimal dietary intake.** Certain populations whose dietary pattern, socioeconomical status, or clinical state places them at higher risk of not meeting requirements for certain nutrients should be counseled on dietary and DS interventions. Examples in this scenario are numerous but include children with elevated body mass index and iron deficiency (28); breast-fed infants with vitamin D deficiency (29); patients on home enteral feedings with trace element deficiency (30); elderly nursing home patients with deficiencies including zinc, selenium, vitamins B_{12}, B_1, B_6, and D (31).
- **Patients at risk of excessive or inappropriate use.** Patients who are likely to meet dietary guidelines through their diet alone and who are currently using DS in a

manner that may create acute or chronic toxicity should be counseled. Examples include long-term high-dose use of certain supplements such as vitamin A (32) or inappropriate use of ergogenic/performance enhancement supplements such as stimulants, steroids, and steroid precursors.

CONCLUSION

As use of DS continues to increase, clinician–patient discussion regarding this topic continues to be suboptimal. In this scenario, the clinician should be aware of both widespread use and particular demographics that may predict DS use. With this information the clinician may be better prepared to initiate focused discussion on the safety and efficacy of DS as noted above. This discussion can be helpful in improving patient–clinician partnership by understanding the motivations and circumstances that may prompt DS. Furthermore, this discussion may improve review of appropriate clinical strategies, including and beyond DS, which can optimize nutrient intake and disease management.

References

1. Robson PJ, Siou GL, Ullman R, Bryant HE. Sociodemographic, health and lifestyle characteristics reported by discrete groups of adult dietary supplement users in Alberta, Canada: findings from The Tomorrow Project. *Public Health Nutr* 2008;11(12):1238–1247.
2. Barnes PM, Powell-Griner E, McFann K, Nahin RL. Complementary and alternative medicine use among adults: United States, 2002. *Adv Data* 2004;(343):1–19.
3. Rock CL. Multivitamin-multimineral supplements: who uses them? *Am J Clin Nutr* 2007;85(1):277S–279S.
4. Murphy SP, White KK, Park SY, Sharma S. Multivitamin-multimineral supplements' effect on total nutrient intake. *Am J Clin Nutr* 2007;85(1):280S–284S.
5. Timbo BB, Ross MP, McCarthy PV, Lin CT. Dietary supplements in a national survey: prevalence of use and reports of adverse events. *J Am Diet Assoc* 2006;106(12):1966–1974.
6. Sebastian RS, Cleveland LE, Goldman JD, Moshfegh AJ. Older adults who use vitamin/mineral supplements differ from nonusers in nutrient intake adequacy and dietary attitudes. *J Am Diet Assoc* 2007;107(8):1322–1332.
7. Foote JA, Murphy SP, Wilkens LR, Hankin JH, Henderson BE, Kolonel LN. Factors associated with dietary supplement use among healthy adults of five ethnicities. *Am J Epidemiol* 2003;157:888–897.
8. Archer SL, Stamler J, Moag-Stahlberg A, et al. Association of dietary supplement use with specific micronutrient intakes among middle-aged American men and women: the INTERMAP Study. *J Am Diet Assoc* 2005;105:1106–1114.
9. Reedy J, Haines PS, Campbell MK. Differences in fruit and vegetable intake among categories of dietary supplement users. *J Am Diet Assoc* 2005;105:1749–1756.
10. Jasti S, Siega-Riz AM, Bentley ME. Dietary supplement use in the context of health disparities: cultural, ethnic and demographic determinants of use. *J Nutr* 2003;133(suppl):2010S–2013S.
11. Stang J, Story MT, Harnack L, Newmark-Sztainer D. Relationships between vitamin and mineral supplement use, dietary intake, and dietary adequacy among adolescents. *J Am Diet Assoc* 2000;100:905–910.
12. Hedderson MM, Patterson RE, Neuhouser ML, et al. Sex differences in motives for use of complementary and alternative medicine among cancer patients. *Altern Ther Health Med* 2004;10(5):58–64.

13. Conner M, Kirk SF, Cade JE, Barrett JH. Why do women use dietary supplements? The use of the theory of planned behaviour to explore beliefs about their use. *Soc Sci Med* 2001;52(4):621–633.
14. Reedy J, Haines PS, Campbell MK. Differences in fruit and vegetable intake among categories of dietary supplement users. *J Am Diet Assoc* 2005;105(11):1749–1756.
15. Yu SM, Kogan MD, Gergen P. Vitamin-mineral supplement use among preschool children in the United States. Pediatrics [serial online]. 1997;100(5):e4. http://pediatrics.aappublications.org/content/vol100/issue5/index.shtml. Accessed October 27, 2006.
16. Sharpe TR, Smith MC. Use of vitamin–mineral supplements by AFDC children. *Public Health Rep* 1985;100:321–324.
17. Ball SD, Kertesz D, Moyer-Mileur LJ. Dietary supplement use is prevalent among children with a chronic illness. *J Am Diet Assoc* 2005;105(1):78–84.
18. Picciano M, Dwyer J, Radimer K. Dietary supplement use among infants, children, and adolescents in the United States, 1999–2002. *Arch Pediatr Adolesc Med* 2007;161(10):978–985.
19. Gardiner P, Kemper KJ, Legedza A, Phillips RS. Factors associated with herb and dietary supplement use by young adults in the United States. *BMC Complement Altern Med* 2007;7:39.
20. Jenkinson DM, Harbert AJ. Supplements and sports. *Am Fam Physician* 2008;78(9): 1039–1046.
21. Calfee R, Fadale P. Popular ergogenic drugs and supplements in young athletes. *Pediatrics* 2006;117(3):e577–589.
22. Pawlak RD, Brown D, Meyer MK, et al. Theory of planned behavior and multivitamin supplement use in Caucasian college females. *J Prim Prev* 2008;29(1):57–71.
23. Dwyer JT, Garceau AO, Evans M, et al. Do adolescent vitamin-mineral supplement users have better nutrient intakes than nonusers? Observations from the CATCH tracking study. *J Am Diet Assoc* 2001;101:1340–1346.
24. McDavid K, Breslow RA, Radimer K. Vitamin/mineral supplementation among cancer survivors: 1987 and 1992 National Health Interview Surveys. *Nutr Cancer* 2001;41:29–32.
25. Patterson RE, Neuhouser ML, Hedderson MM, Schwartz SM, Standish LJ, Bowen PJ. Changes in diet, physical activity, and supplement use among adults diagnosed with cancer. *J Am Diet Assoc* 2003;103:323–328.
26. Velicer CM, Ulrich CM. Vitamin and mineral supplement use among US adults after cancer diagnosis: a systematic review. *J Clin Oncol* 2008;26(4):665–673.
27. Miller MF, Bellizzi KM, Sufian M, Ambs AH, Goldstein MS, Ballard-Barbash R. Dietary supplement use in individuals living with cancer and other chronic conditions: a population-based study. *J Am Diet Assoc* 2008;108(3):483–494.
28. Nead KG, Halterman JS, Kaczorowski JM, Auinger P, Weitzman M. Overweight children and adolescents: a risk group for iron deficiency. *Pediatrics* 2004;114(1):104–108.
29. Wagner CL, Greer FR; American Academy of Pediatrics Section on Breastfeeding; American Academy of Pediatrics Committee on Nutrition. Prevention of rickets and vitamin D deficiency in infants, children, and adolescents. *Pediatrics* 2008;122(5):1142–1152.
30. Oliver A, Allen KR, Taylor J. Trace element concentrations in patients on home enteral feeding: two cases of severe copper deficiency. *Ann Clin Biochem* 2005;42(Pt 2):136–140.
31. Seiler WO. Clinical pictures of malnutrition in ill elderly subjects. *Nutrition* 2001;17(6): 496–498.
32. Sheth A, Khurana R, Khurana V. Potential liver damage associated with over-the-counter vitamin supplements. *J Am Diet Assoc* 2008;108(9):1536–1537.

CHAPTER 14

Dietary Supplements and Prescribing—A Legal Perspective

William J. Skinner[1]

This chapter gives an overview of some important legal issues regarding prescribing or recommending vitamins, minerals, and other dietary supplements.

RECOMMENDING OR PRESCRIBING DIETARY SUPPLEMENTS

Recommending and prescribing dietary supplements follows the usual examination of the patient, taking a history, and deciding on a theory of treatment, while making a record of subjective, objective, assessment and plan (SOAP), the same as you would for prescription medication. Indeed, if you prescribe it, the dietary supplement "becomes" prescription medication. But the dietary supplement may not be paid for by certain insurance or public assistance plans, and they may not be filled by a pharmacist, or recorded in a medication record in the same manner as prescription drugs.

WHAT ARE DIETARY SUPPLEMENTS?

First, a baseline is needed as to what this chapter is calling "dietary supplements." The statutory definition (1) in the Dietary Supplement Health and Education Act of 1994 defines them as vitamins, minerals, herbs or other botanics, amino acids, dietary substances for use by man to supplement the diet by increasing the total daily intake, or concentrates, metabolites, constituents, extracts, or combinations of these.

Dietary supplements represent a wide range of substances that must be ingested or swallowed but not rubbed on, not gargled, and not used as conventional food or drink. By legal definition dietary supplements are supposed to supplement the diet, pure and simple.

However, dietary supplements are generally not mentioned by state law except in statutes that are restrictive in who can use or prescribe them, or that require certain

[1]William J. Skinner is a registered pharmacist since 1960. He has practiced law since 1965 in the field of food and drug law, health law, congressional relations, advertising, intellectual property, and trials including medical and dental malpractice. He has been the publisher and editor of Natural Medicine Law™ Newsletter since 1997, which can be reviewed and searched at www.natmedlaw.com/. All laws, regulations, and case citations can be provided by author on request at editor@natmedlaw.com.

labeling or forbid the sale of certain ingredients.[2] You must become aware of these kinds of exceptions or peculiar twists in the law wherever you practice and prescribe.

WHAT DOES IT MEAN TO PRESCRIBE OR RECOMMEND?

The second baseline we need to consider is what it means to recommend or prescribe. Here we have to go to state and federal law, maybe common law (law made by courts usually based on precedent when no statutory law is or was available). We go to the statutes because there are many laws on the books pertaining to the use of various substances which may include dietary supplements. Where you practice is the most important because you do not want to prescribe or recommend something that is forbidden to be prescribed or recommended in your state unless certain conditions are followed.

Prescribing presupposes a license that includes the privilege to prescribe or recommend products for treatment. Unlicensed persons can get into more trouble than prescribing may be worth. For example, less than 10 years ago a naturopathic physician in New Jersey had an undercover investigator sign a statement that he was advised he was not a medical physician and that the patient should see a medical physician before implementing the naturopath's recommendations. Subsequently, the naturopath recommended certain over-the-counter dietary products, The New Jersey attorney general later charged the naturopath with the unlicensed practice of medicine in violation of the Medical Practices Act, N.J.S.A. 45:9-18 and 22. The Division of Consumer Affairs filed a criminal complaint 2 days later charging the naturopath with the unauthorized practice of medicine based on the same conduct.

The attorney general sought an injunction resulting in certain restrictions and an agreement to pay $5,000 in civil penalties and $3,554.07 in investigative costs, plus interest. A week later the Essex County prosecutor took the criminal case to the grand jury where the investigator was called as the only witness. An indictment was returned charging the naturopath with practicing medicine without a license. Before the trial the naturopath filed a motion to dismiss the indictment as it was a violation of the Double Jeopardy Clause and that the investigator's conduct before the grand jury misled the grand jury in failing to disclose the disclaimer signed by the naturopath. The trial court agreed in part and dismissed the criminal indictment on double jeopardy grounds, but the Appellate Division reversed finding no bar on double jeopardy grounds but dismissed the indictment because of the investigator's misconduct.

Subsequently, the Supreme Court of the United States did not take this case on a petition for certiorari. This means usually that four out of nine Justices did not find

---

[2]California Health and Safety Code Section 110423-110423.8 restricts the sale and prescription of epinephrine group alkaloids and steroid hormone precursors; and California Health and Safety Code Section 110423.101 says some of these restrictions do not apply to (a) a California licensed health care practitioner who is practicing within his or her scope of practice and who prescribes or dispenses, or both, dietary supplement products containing ephedrine group alkaloids in the course of the treatment of a patient under the direct care of that licensed health care practitioner, except that a licensed health care practitioner shall not prescribe or dispense dietary supplements containing ephedrine group alkaloids for purposes of weight loss, body building, or athletic performance enhancement. Indiana Code IC 16-42-23-4 states that amygdalin use is not endorsed, but the chapter does not prevent a physician from prescribing amygdalin (laetrile) as a dietary supplement to a patient not suffering from a known malignancy, disease, illness, or physical condition upon execution of the written informed request.

any merit in the appeal. Thus, one can conclude, in a practical sense, that a license is necessary under most state laws if you are engaging in the practice of medicine or holding yourself out as a medical physician and recommending dietary supplements. Prescribing or recommending products for a fee is not a good idea if you are not licensed.

But keep in mind that there are professions other than medicine in which the sale of dietary supplements is a part of the expectations of the license. So, naturopathic physicians in some states are allowed to prescribe and sell dietary supplements. States may permit pharmacists, grocers, door-to-door sales people, and others to sell dietary supplements.

DIFFERENCES IN STATE LAW ON PRESCRIBING

To give readers some idea of the differences in state law definitions of prescribing, take a look at California, Texas, Indiana, and New York. California Health and Safety Code defines who may write or issue a prescription. In addition to physicians, this list includes practitioners including nurse midwives, naturopathic physicians, and optometrists, who are not always in other state laws. Texas Health & Safety Code, defines "prescription" to mean "an order from a practitioner, or an agent of the practitioner designated in writing as authorized to communicate prescriptions (licensed midwife, registered nurse, or physician assistant)." Indiana Code defines "Prescribe" as "to direct, order, or designate the use of or manner of using a drug, medicine, or treatment by spoken or written words or other means" and defines "Prescription" as " . . . a written order to or for an ultimate user for a drug or device."

Interestingly, New York's Public Health Law § 270 (13) defines prescription and nonprescription drugs as "a drug ... for which a prescription is required under the federal food, drug, and cosmetic act. Any drug that does not require a prescription under such act, but which would otherwise meet the criteria under this article for inclusion on the preferred drug list may be added to the preferred drug list under this article; and, if so included, shall be considered to be a prescription drug for purposes of this article; provided that it shall be eligible for reimbursement under a state public health plan when ordered by a prescriber authorized to prescribe under the state public health plan and the prescription is subject to the applicable provisions of this article." Thus, this New York statute allows for certain substances, including dietary supplements to be placed on the "preferred drug list" and to have them considered for coverage and reimbursement similar to prescription agents.

You can see that states differ on definitions and what may be included. Therefore, it is paramount that you know the law where you are licensed to recommend or prescribe dietary supplements.

ISSUES TO BE AWARE OF WHEN CONSIDERING OR NOT RECOMMENDING DIETARY SUPPLEMENTS FOR PREVENTION AND MANAGEMENT

To be competent to prescribe or recommend, you must be acquainted with the practice guidelines and subspecialty recommendation (when available) as well as scientific literature, including the recent clinical studies that attempt to determine the effects of dietary supplements in various diseases and conditions. The American Society of Anesthesiologists was one of the first to adopt some practice guidelines regarding the use of herbs before surgery. The organization developed a brochure explaining about 15 herbs that should be discontinued before surgery, but this same brochure describes vitamins and dietary supplements as something to speak to your physician about before anesthesiology (2). Other organizations that have published guidelines include the American Dietetic Association and the Society for Endocrinology. The clinicians should be aware of practice guidelines in this area published by their specialty organizations or governing bodies.

When definitive practice guidelines are not available the clinician must attempt to synthesize available knowledge from various sources. Some basic ways to do this are to keep up with the National Institutes of Health/Office of Dietary Supplements studies and reports, the Institute of Medicine/National Research Council Food and Nutrition Board decisions about vitamins and minerals, the reports of the Food and Drug Administration, and additional resources listed in chapter 42.

One additional difficulty encountered by the clinician utilizing dietary supplements is the wide variation in formulations utilized in clinical trials and those available on the market which are dissimilar to those clinically tested. The clinician should attempt to follow research-tested formulations whenever available. These recommendations are exemplified by commentary made in a recent glucosamine sulfate study in *Rheumatology*, June 2007 (3):

> Glucosamine Sulfate (GS) has shown positive effects on symptomatic and structural outcomes of knee OA. These results should not be extrapolated to other glucosamine salts [hydrochloride or preparations (over-the-counter or food supplements)] in which no warranty exists about content, pharmacokinetics and pharmacodynamics of the tablets.

DIETARY SUPPLEMENT—DRUG INTERACTIONS

Another factor in prescribing and recommending dietary supplements is interactions. Some of these will be found under "Drug–Drug" interactions in the medical literature. One common example is calcium supplementation for osteoporosis. You can learn in the 2004 *Surgeon General's Report on Bone Health and Osteoporosis* (4) about the need for calcium in various age levels, what the importance of vitamin D and the dose for various age levels is in relation to calcium. However, it is important to also be aware that calcium can cause gastric irritation when combined with products like aspirin, erythromycin, and bisacodyl. Calcium can also reduce the bioavailablity of levothyroxine, ciproflaxin, phenytoin, and digoxin and limit the absorption of iron, thiamin, zinc, and B_{12} (5). Dietary supplement interaction and resources are covered in chapter 26.

PROFESSIONAL LIABILITY INSURANCE AND PRESCRIBING

Your professional liability insurance may define what you are allowed to recommend or prescribe and there are cases in which experts differ about what is allowable under policy language. So, where tea tree oil was injected to remove a wart and complications occurred, a court ruled this was a homeopathic remedy that was excluded from insurance coverage (6). Actually, tea tree oil is not a homeopathic remedy in the opinion of most experts, but the evidence before the court, in this case, including expert witness testimony said that tea tree oil was a homeopathic remedy; therefore, the court was led to make a decision saying the physician's insurance did not cover the damages done by the use of the substance.

The mention of professional liability insurance raises the possibility of prescribers being sued. Professional negligence occurs when a prescriber is prescribing or recommending something that is not within the recognized "standard of care" or conventional protocols of treatment. Standard of care proof in a court room trial requires at a minimum that an expert, qualified by education, training, and experience, and accepted by the trial judge, give testimony that what the defendant in the case has done is not within the standard of care and that those actions were the proximate cause of damages to the patient. Many states have laws and even court rules that define the level of specificity for "standard of care," "expert witness qualifications," "causation," and other legal terms in medical malpractice cases. A prescriber must be aware that going too far from "normal" is inviting scrutiny of those practices, especially when patient injuries occur.

Some states also want to make sure that prescribers are following appropriate protocols for handling patients when using alternative and complementary medicine. The Texas Medical Board has adopted standards which include practice guidelines (7). These standards define alternative and complementary medicine, conventional medicine, and reasonable potential for therapeutic gain, plus set forth standards for patient assessment, disclosure, treatment plans, periodic treatment review, adequate medical records, demonstration of therapeutic validity, and clinical investigations.

CONSUMER PROTECTION

In the fall of 2006, Congress passed the Dietary Supplement and Nonprescription Drug Consumer Protection Act, Public Law No: 109-462, approved December 22, 2006. This new law requires:

> . . . a manufacturer, packer, or distributor whose name appears on the label of a nonprescription drug or dietary supplement marketed in the United States to: (1) submit to the Secretary of Health and Human Services within 15 business days any report of a serious adverse event associated with use of such drug or supplement in the United States; (2) submit within 15 business days any related medical information that is received within one year of the initial report; (3) maintain records related to each report for six years; and (4) permit inspection of such records. Allows a retailer whose name appears on the label as a distributor to authorize the manufacturer or packer to submit the required reports so long as the retailer directs all reported adverse events to such manufacturer or packer.
>
> Requires the Secretary to develop systems to ensure that duplicate reports of a serious adverse event are consolidated.
>
> Allows the Secretary to establish an exemption from such reporting that would have no adverse effect on public health.

Considers a serious adverse event report to be: (1) a safety report that may be accompanied by a statement, which shall be included in any public disclosure of the report, that denies that the report or the records constitute an admission that the product involved caused or contributed to the adverse event; and (2) a record about an individual and a medical or similar file the disclosure of which violates the Freedom of Information Act unless all personally identifiable information is redacted.

Provides that the submission of any adverse event report shall not be construed as an admission that the drug or supplement involved caused or contributed to the adverse event.

Prohibits any state or local government from establishing or continuing any requirements related to a mandatory system for adverse event reports for nonprescription drugs or dietary supplements that are not identical to the requirements of this Act.

Prohibits the responsible person from: (1) refusing to permit access to any required record; or (2) failing to establish or maintain any record, or make any report, required under this Act.

Deems a nonprescription drug or dietary supplement that is marketed in the United States to be misbranded unless its label includes a domestic address or phone number for the reporting of a serious adverse event.

Prohibits the falsification of a serious adverse event report.

Prohibits the importation of a drug or supplement subject to this Act if the Secretary has credible information indicating that the responsible person has not complied with the requirements of this Act or has not allowed access to its records (8).

Prescribers are going to be involved in reporting these adverse reports as much as they are involved in reporting prescription drug reports. Prescribers will be a major source of reports to manufacturers, distributors, and other sellers along with injured patients, pharmacists who hear from patients, and others about the adverse events.

Prescribers will have more difficulty attributing adverse events with products containing multiple ingredients such as botanics. The typical Chinese or Ayurvedic medicine remedy contains several ingredients theoretically used for different purposes. With only a small percentage of imported supplements being inspected by federal officials, the main issue for these products continues to be potential adulteration or heavy metal toxicity. Prescribers will remember the PC-SPES remedy for prostate cancer that contained warfarin (Coumadin®) and/or alprazolam (Xanax®) (9). More recently, an analysis of imported Ayurvedic formulations demonstrated potentially harmful level of heavy lead, mercury, and/or arsenic in 20% of the samples analyzed (10).

Nevertheless, dietary supplements do not always measure up to their label claims. The industry recognized this in 1995, after passage of the Dietary Supplement Health and Education Act in 1994, and submitted proposed Good Manufacturing Practice (GMP) Regulations to Food and Drug Administration which were approved only recently after a period of more than 10 years. The details of GMP regulation are detailed in chapter 16. In addition, several third-party organizations are currently providing supplemental avenues for content and GMP verification and these are further described in section X.

WHAT CAN THE CLINICIAN DO TO PROTECT HIMSELF WHEN RECOMMENDING DIETARY SUPPLEMENTS?

TABLE 14.1 Appropriate Recommendation of Dietary Supplements: Incorporating the HERBAL Mnemonic: A Legal Perspective

- **H**ear the patient out
  - regarding their goals for care including the rationale and motivation for the use of dietary supplements based on medical history, previous treatments, and symptoms
- **E**ducate the patient
  - on the benefits and potential risks of utilizing dietary supplements as well as how supplements compare to other treatment options in this setting
- **R**ecord/document
  - (A) the decision-making process
    - Describe both from the patient and clinician perspective regarding the decision to use dietary supplements based on the subjective and objective aspect of the evaluation
    - "Patient has failed other approaches for her postmenopausal symptoms and wishes to avoid hormonal replacement therapy."
    - "Patients with refractory knee arthritis requesting discussion of complementary and alternative approaches to treatment including dietary supplements."
    - If patient declines conventional care document that patient is aware of risks, benefits, and alternatives to use of dietary supplements for the stated condition
  - (B) specifics of the recommendation, examples:
    - Name and formulation of supplements with specific brand, if possible
    - Dosage and frequency of intake
    - Follow-up plans for reassessment
    - Special instruction or warnings
      - Timing of supplement(s) with food
      - Document discussion of typical side effects and potential interactions as appropriate
      - Document other prescription and nonprescription formulation patient is utilizing
- **B**e aware of potential reactions and interactions
  - by accessing trusted references and tell the patient what to watch for in specific scenarios and how to respond appropriately (See section 4 on Reactions and Interactions)
- **A**gree to discuss
  - Make yourself and staff available for questions or concerns regarding supplement use:
    - Handling possible or typical side effect
  - Further information regarding supplements:
    - Staff can provide handouts or links to reliable information (e.g., Natural Medicines Comprehensive Database patient handouts [www.naturaldatabase.com] or Office of Dietary Supplements fact sheets [http://dietary-supplements.info.nih.gov])
  - Request regarding how to obtain discussed supplement (chapter)

(continued)

TABLE 14.1 *(Continued)*

- Learn
  - about common dietary supplement that your patients are using or considering using including their safety and efficacy through trusted resources. Subscribe to some good resources about the clinical information. A full listing of resources is available in chapter 42. I recommend one such resource: *Natural Medicines Comprehensive Database* found at: http://www.naturaldatabase.com/
  - about your staff's understanding of what you mean by "dietary supplement," "herb," "botanic," and other terms. Train your staff to help you learn what your patients are taking
  - about your professional liability insurance to see what definitions are used regarding your prescribing coverage
  - about your state laws concerning dietary supplements. Know what is prohibited, limited, or considered investigational

In these pages, a lot of ground is covered to help you think of the essential legal areas when you prescribe *or recommend* dietary supplements. Professionals are people who keep up-to-date with the information in their fields. As long as you remain professional you will have no serious problems in prescribing dietary supplements.

References

1. Dietary Supplement Health and Education Act of 1994 (Public Law 103-417) 103rd Congress. http://ods.od.nih.gov/About/DSHEA_Wording.aspx. Accessed September 25, 2008.
2. American Society of Anesthesiologists. What you should know about herbs and dietary supplements and anesthesia. www.asahq.org/patientEducation/herbPatient.pdf/. Accessed June 22, 2007.
3. Reginster JY, Bruyere O, Neuprez A, et al. Current role of glucosamine in the treatment of osteoarthritis. *Rheumatology* 2007;46(5):731–735.
4. Bone health and osteoporosis: a report of surgeon general. www.surgeongeneral.gov/library/bonehealth/. Published October 2004. Accessed June 22, 2007.
5. Preventing Medication Errors: Quality Chasm Series (Free Executive Summary) at 117. Accessed June 6, 2007 at www.nap.edu/catalog/11623.html/ citing D'Arcy and McElnay, 1987. Accessed June 22, 2007.
6. California Case on Tea Tree Oil, *Melaleuca alternifolia*, injected to remove wart on a finger, *Katherine Meza v Southern California Physicians Insurance Exchange,* 73 Cal. Rep. 91 (Ct. App. 3rd March 26, 1998).
7. Texas Medical Board. Standards for physicians practicing complementary and alternative medicine. Chapter 200.1–200.3. www.tmb.state.tx.us/rules/rules/200.php/. Accessed May 30, 2007.
8. Pub L No. 109-462, Congressional research service summary. www.thomas.gov/. Accessed May 30, 2007.
9. Natural Medicine Law™ Newsletter, March 2002, Vol. 5, No.5. Free downloads and searches, except the most recent issue.www.natmedlaw.com/. Accessed June 22, 2007.
10. Saper RB, Kales SN, Paquin J, et al. Heavy metal content of ayurvedic herbal medicine products. *JAMA* 2004;292(23):2868–2873.

III

Regulation

CHAPTER 15

Evaluating Dietary Supplements: Regulation

Robert Alan Bonakdar

Even before passage of the Dietary Supplement Health and Education Act (DSHEA) of 1994, supplement regulation has been a strongly debated and evolving arena. Since passage, additional efforts have been recommended or enacted to expand the level of regulation. Unfortunately, consumers and physicians continue to be misinformed regarding the extent of supplement regulation and how it differs from that of prescription medications (1). In addition, the Food and Drug Administration continues to publish safety alerts regarding supplements with potential or documented regulatory abnormalities including adulteration (2).

The following section attempts to provide a foundational understanding of supplement regulation and the parties attempting to provide oversight in this expanding field. An understanding of these trends is crucial for the clinician both in familiarization of what is required of the supplements they may recommend and in educating patients who may be utilizing supplements. The section begins with an overview of the DSHEA as well as qualified health claims (chapters 16 and 17). This is followed by an international perspective on regulation which is helpful in placing US regulatory efforts in perspective (chapter 18). Next, the roles of the supplement industry and related organizations are reviewed (chapters 19 and 20). Last, a number of third-party verification programs have attempted to provide additional avenues of oversight. Several of the leading programs are featured (chapters 21–23) in an effort to familiarize clinicians with their efforts. In some cases they may provide clinicians the ability to more confidently identify and discuss specific evidence-based supplements and brands with patients.

References

1. Ashar BH, Rice TN, Sisson SD. Physicians' understanding of the regulation of dietary supplements. *Arch Intern Med* 2007;167(9):966–969.
2. The U.S. Food and Drug Administration. 2009 safety alerts for human medical products. http://www.fda.gov/medwAtch/safety/2009/safety09.htm#dietary. Accessed March 28, 2009.

CHAPTER 16

DSHEA and Beyond: An Overview of Dietary Supplement Regulation

Annette Dickinson

Dietary supplements are used by most American adults, according to national surveys (1). Health care providers are as likely as members of the lay public to be users of dietary supplements, and many of these professionals also recommend dietary supplements to their patients or clients (2). While users of dietary supplements may value and rely on these products as an integral component of their overall search for wellness, most users are not entirely clear about whether and how these products are regulated. Health care providers can help consumers understand important regulatory as well as scientific issues. Dietary supplements are not pharmaceuticals (drugs) and are not regulated as drugs. Nor are they "unregulated," as is sometimes charged. Dietary supplements are regulated as foods, and dietary supplement laws and regulations can best be understood in the context of overall food law and regulation.

Food law is not static but changes continually as Congress enacts new laws amending the basic Food, Drug, and Cosmetic Act of 1938 (FD&C Act). In 2002, for example, Congress enacted the Bioterrorism Act to help safeguard the US food supply by requiring the registration of all food manufacturing facilities and requiring companies to give prior notice before importing foods or food ingredients. These requirements apply to dietary supplement facilities and imports as well as to conventional foods. In 2004, Congress enacted the Food Allergen Labeling and Consumer Protection Act, which requires the labels of foods, including dietary supplements, to more clearly label food allergens that may be present, such as ingredients derived from milk, eggs, or nuts. Initiatives such as these update legal and regulatory requirements in response to health concerns or global challenges and affect the day-to-day operation of all food and dietary supplement marketers. The two major legislative initiatives that have shaped the dietary supplement market in the past two decades are the Nutrition Labeling and Education Act (NLEA) of 1990 and the Dietary Supplement Health and Education Act (DSHEA) of 1994.

FOODS FOR SPECIAL DIETARY USE

Dietary supplements are a subcategory of food and have been regulated as a category of food ever since the enactment of the basic FD&C Act in 1938. At that time, dietary supplements of vitamins and minerals were already wildly popular with the American public. Accordingly, there was specific discussion in Congress regarding how these products should be regulated under the new law. Since the main purpose of the supplements was to increase dietary intake of vitamins, minerals, and other food components, they were put squarely in the category of foods. Congress even created a special category of foods for "special dietary use" and specified that the labeling of such products must include "such information concerning its vitamin, mineral, and other dietary properties as the Secretary determines to be, and by regulations prescribes as, necessary in order fully to inform purchasers as to its value for such uses." Food and Drug Administration (FDA) regulations published in 1941, establishing the labeling requirements for vitamin and mineral supplements and other foods for special dietary use, represented the agency's first attempt at what we now know as nutrition labeling (3).

STANDARD OF IDENTITY

As the market for dietary supplements continued to expand, the medical and nutrition communities became concerned about the rationality of the formulations being offered to consumers. Throughout the 1960s and into the early 1970s, FDA worked on developing a "standard of identity" for vitamin and mineral supplements, which would have put a cap on maximum levels of these nutrients and would have also limited the combinations of nutrients that could be provided. The FD&C Act gave FDA authority to establish standards of identity for various product categories, in order to ensure product quality, and FDA had used this authority to establish standards for many product categories. The standards for enriched grain products including flours and breads, for example, specified the exact amounts of nutrients to be added. In 1973, FDA finalized regulations that would have established a standard of identity for vitamin and mineral supplements, limiting the amounts of vitamins and minerals to a range of roughly 50% to 150% of the recommended daily intake of each nutrient and also severely limiting the possible combinations of nutrients that could be marketed (4). The FDA rule created a storm of protest, and numerous legal challenges were filed, charging that the regulations were overly restrictive. The courts overturned the regulations in 1974, FDA revised them, and the courts overturned them yet again in 1978 (5, 6). In the meanwhile, in 1976 Congress passed legislation prohibiting FDA from restricting the quantity or combination of vitamins and minerals in dietary supplements, through means such as establishing a standard of identity (7). That legislation did not, however, alter FDA's authority over the safety of dietary supplement ingredients.

DIETARY SUPPLEMENT HEALTH AND EDUCATION ACT OF 1994

In the 1990s, FDA Commissioner David Kessler viewed the dietary supplement category as "unfinished business" and appointed an internal task force to make recommendations regarding an overall regulatory approach. Unfortunately, the task force came up with a plan that seemed to hark back to the agency's previous effort to impose its own view of nutritional rationality on the highly diverse dietary supplement category. An Advance Notice of Proposed Rulemaking published by FDA in 1993 favored putting caps on the permissible levels of vitamins and minerals, said amino acids should not be included at all, and suggested that herbal ingredients were inherently therapeutic (and therefore more druglike and perhaps inappropriate for marketing as dietary supplements) and possibly unsafe (8). This notice set off a new storm of protest which again led to the passage of new legislation—the Dietary Supplement Health and Education Act (DSHEA) enacted in October 1994 (9). DSHEA was meant to accomplish two main goals: preserving consumer access to a wide variety of dietary supplements and providing the public with more information about the intended uses of dietary supplements.

Dietary supplements under DSHEA continue to be defined as a category of foods, as they have been since 1938. DSHEA defined dietary supplements in terms of their intended use, permissible ingredients, and physical form. The law also "grandfathered" ingredients already in use in 1994, established a notification system for introducing new ingredients, added an additional safety standard for dietary supplements, and authorized FDA to develop new Good Manufacturing Practice (GMP) regulations for dietary supplements. DSHEA also permitted a broad range of label claims describing the effect of a dietary supplement on the structure or function of the body. (These label statements are discussed in chapter 17.)

DSHEA added a new Section 201(ff) to the FD&C Act, defining dietary supplements as products "intended to supplement the diet." Permissible ingredients are listed as part of the definition, and these include vitamins, minerals, herbs, or other botanics, amino acids, other dietary substances, or a concentrate, metabolite, constituent, extract, or combination of such ingredients. These ingredients are considered "dietary ingredients" and not food additives. Ingredients that were marketed before October 1994 are "grandfathered" and may continue to be used in dietary supplements. If a company wants to include "new dietary ingredients," then FDA must be notified at least 75 days in advance and the company must submit safety information, unless the ingredient is an ordinary food component that has not been chemically altered. FDA is actively reviewing the new dietary ingredient notifications it receives, and a large fraction of submissions have been rejected, often for failure to provide sufficient information on the identity or safety of the ingredient (10).

Dietary supplement ingredients must meet the same general safety standard as other foods. Section 402(a) of the FD&C Act provides that a food is deemed to be adulterated (unsafe) "if it bears or contains any poisonous or deleterious substance which may render it injurious to health." DSHEA added a new provision as Section 402(f), which deems a dietary supplement to be adulterated if it "presents a significant or unreasonable risk of illness or injury under (i) conditions of use recommended or suggested in labeling, or (ii) if no conditions of use are suggested or recommended in the labeling, under ordinary conditions of use." FDA used this new provision effectively in 2004 as the basis for banning dietary supplements containing ephedra, an herbal ingredient with naturally occurring ephedrine alkaloids, after such products were associated with numerous serious adverse events (11). FDA has and exercises broad authority to take action against any dietary supplements that are unsafe (adulterated) or misbranded, as illustrated by crackdowns on androstenedione and erectile dysfunction products (12, 13).

The definition of dietary supplements in DSHEA specifies that the products are intended for ingestion and that they may be marketed in the physical form of tablets, capsules, softgels, gelcaps, or powders. They may also be marketed as liquids intended for ingestion in small quantities such as drops, teaspoons, or other small units of measure (but not presumably as beverages to be consumed like soft drinks, although some dietary supplements in beverage form do seem to get into the marketplace). A dietary supplement may even take the physical form of conventional food (such as a wafer or a bar), provided it "is not represented for use as a conventional food or as a sole item of a meal or the diet." This means that the product label should say that the product is for use in supplementing the diet and should not suggest that the product is a substitute for conventional food. A label statement saying that a product is intended to be used as "part of a delicious meal," for example, could be considered to represent the product for use as a conventional food, rather than as a dietary supplement.

NUTRITION LABELING

In 1990, Congress passed the NLEA, which made nutrition labeling mandatory for virtually all foods, including dietary supplements, and also, for the first time, authorized FDA to permit "health claims" in the labeling of foods, including dietary supplements (14). (Health claims are discussed in chapter 17.)

NLEA required FDA to revise the format for nutrition labeling to move the primary focus away from vitamins and minerals and toward other components including fats, cholesterol, and fiber. FDA regulations ultimately established two separate formats for nutrition labeling for conventional foods and dietary supplements (15, 16). Both feature a simple and bold design with a "facts box" enclosing and highlighting the nutrition information. For conventional foods, the facts box is called **Nutrition Facts**. For dietary supplements, the facts box is called **Supplement Facts**. (There is also a "facts box" for drug product labeling, which is headed **Drug Facts**.)

The Nutrition Facts box for conventional foods must include a mandatory list of macronutrients (fat, carbohydrate, protein) and sodium, even if the product does not actually contain those substances. This results in nutrition labeling on bottled water and diet sodas, for example, prominently featuring numerous "zeroes." Moreover, while the Nutrition Facts box must include a listing of any vitamins and minerals *added* to a food, it cannot list other types of functional ingredients not specifically mentioned in the nutrition labeling regulation. For example, functional components or ingredients such as omega-3 fatty acids, nonvitamin antioxidants, herbs, and caffeine are not permitted to be listed in the Nutrition Facts box. For additional information on Labels, please see chapter12.

Why are these details about nutrition labeling important in this discussion of dietary supplement regulation? Initially, FDA regulations for nutrition labeling under NLEA were meant to apply to dietary supplements as well as conventional foods. However, the dietary supplement industry objected strenuously to the requirement to list macronutrients not actually present in the product and to the prohibition against listing of functional components other than vitamins and minerals. This would have been especially inappropriate for the labeling of botanic products or indeed for any dietary supplement that was not primarily composed of vitamins and minerals. The DSHEA of 1994 required FDA to develop a more appropriate approach to the labeling of such products, and today nutrition labeling for dietary supplements (21 CFR 101.36) features a list of all the components for which supplemental benefit is claimed. The macronutrients must be listed first but only if they are actually present in the product. The vitamins and minerals are listed next, and they must appear in the same order as required for conventional food labeling. Then a bold line is drawn below the vitamins and minerals, and all other components are listed below that line. There is no specified order of listing for these other components, which could range from botanics to antioxidants, from amino acids to caffeine, from glucosamine to bee pollen, and from soy isoflavones to zeaxanthin.

Nutrition labeling for dietary supplements requires the Supplement Facts box to include the name and quantity of every ingredient for which a supplemental benefit is claimed, with one exception. DSHEA specified that "proprietary blends" could be listed as such. The total quantity of the blend must be stated, and the components of the blend must be listed in decreasing order of predominance, but the actual quantity of each component does not have to be listed. This provision unfortunately detracts from the full information consumers have a right to expect in dietary supplement labeling.

REGULATION BY THE STATES AND BY AGENCIES OTHER THAN FOOD AND DRUG ADMINISTRATION

Every state in the United States has its own legislature, its own health department, and its own equivalent of the FDA. Thus, consumer products including dietary supplements are subject to regulation by the states as well as by the federal government. On some issues, federal law specifically preempts state law, and the states are not permitted to establish different requirements. This is the case with regard to nutrition labeling, because NLEA specifically prohibited the states from establishing different rules. In general, however, states can and sometimes do establish requirements that differ from federal laws and regulations, and companies marketing in those states must be in compliance. A classic example is California Safe Drinking Water and Toxic Enforcement Act of 1986 (Proposition 65), which establishes extremely stringent limits for environmental contaminants and requires products with higher levels to bear a label saying that the product contains a substance "known to the State of California" to cause cancer, birth defects, or reproductive harm (17). This requirement applies to water, air, and virtually all consumer products.

Dietary supplements are also subject to laws and regulations enforced by federal agencies other than FDA. For example, the Consumer Product Safety Commission regulates poison prevention packaging and requires child-resistant closures for all dietary supplements and pharmaceutical products containing iron to protect children from accidentally ingesting excessive and potentially dangerous amounts of iron (18). The United States Department of Agriculture has primary jurisdiction (shared with FDA) for keeping animal products that could carry bovine spongiform encephalopathy out of the US food supply (19). Regulations controlling the import of ingredients derived from animal products apply to all food manufacturers, including dietary supplement companies. They also apply to manufacturers of other products including pharmaceuticals, vaccines, and animal feeds.

The Federal Trade Commission (FTC) is an independent agency with a mandate to enforce the FTC Act, which prohibits advertising claims that are false or misleading. (FTC initiatives are discussed in chapter 17.)

GOOD MANUFACTURING PRACTICES

FDA has established Good Manufacturing Practices (GMPs) for many categories of products subject to its authority. GMP regulations describe the controls and procedures considered necessary to ensure that products have the appropriate identity and quality and that they are not adulterated by the presence of contaminants. Foods, including dietary supplements, have historically been subject to the general requirements of food

GMPs found in Title 21 of the Code of Federal Regulations, Part 110, although there are more comprehensive processing requirements for some food categories, including low-acid canned foods, infant formula, and bottled water. Moreover, there are separate and more stringent GMPs for drugs, in 21 CFR Part 211. As an example, drug GMPs include extensive requirements for validation of methods and processes as well as broader emphasis on quality control (QC) operations and written procedures.

GMP regulations provide companies as well as FDA inspectors with a template for judging the adequacy of manufacturing procedures and controls. Recognizing the importance of ensuring the quality of dietary supplements, DSHEA specifically authorized FDA to develop separate GMP regulations for dietary supplements. Industry trade organizations, including the Council for Responsible Nutrition, promptly offered to provide assistance in drafting GMP regulations, which FDA accepted. A comprehensive industry draft submitted to FDA in 1995 was published by the agency for public comment in 1997. This was followed in 2003 by a formal proposed rule which triggered numerous and extensive comments. These were evaluated by FDA, and a much improved final rule, consistent with recognized principles of QC, was published in 2007 (20). The final rule on dietary supplement GMPs became effective for large manufacturers in June 2008. Smaller companies (fewer than 500 employees) have until June 2009 to comply, and the very smallest companies (fewer than 20 employees) have until June 2010 to comply.

The core of FDA's final rule on dietary supplement GMPs is the requirement that every company have a system in place that ensures effective control over the quality of ingredients and over all stages of the production process. Personnel must be designated to fulfill the QC function, and their responsibilities include approving or rejecting all materials, processes, labels, and finished products, based on testing and established specifications. They must also review and approve all written procedures and specifications. Products must be manufactured in accordance with a master record. For every batch of product produced, there must be a batch record, and initials are required to document the date and time of performance of each step in the manufacturing process. Materials received at the plant must be quarantined until samples are collected and QC has approved materials for use, and the company must keep records that allow tracing of all materials to their suppliers and to the final product in which they are used. Manufacturing records must be kept for 2 years after the date of manufacture (or 1 year after the expiration date) and must permit tracing of the product throughout the distribution system. Product complaints must be investigated by qualified personnel. Any complaint that may be related to a failure of GMPs must be investigated, and the investigation must extend to related batches. Table 16.1 summarizes some of these key provisions.

To facilitate adequate control, the rule requires companies to have **written procedures** (Standard Operating Procedures) for most key operations, including calibration of instruments, cleaning and maintenance of equipment and utensils, QC operations, receiving of ingredients and packaging, laboratory operations and testing, manufacturing operations, packaging and labeling operations, holding and distribution, handling of returns, and handling of complaints. Final testing of finished products can be based on a statistically sound program of sampling and testing, provided the company documents the rationale for the sampling plan and the selection of tests to be done.

While many leading companies in the industry already have internal GMP procedures that meet or exceed the new requirements, the comprehensive new regulations

TABLE 16.1 Key Provisions of New Dietary Supplement Good Manufacturing Practices (GMPs)

Personnel	Adequate training, qualified supervision, health, cleanliness, hair covers, gloves
Plant and grounds	Water supply, trash disposal, pest control, plumbing, lighting, ventilation
Equipment	Designed to facilitate cleaning and maintenance and avoiding contamination of product
Process controls	Manufacturer must have a comprehensive system of production and process controls
Quality control unit	Approve or reject all materials, processes, labels, and finished products, based on testing and specifications; review and approve all written procedures
Receiving materials	Quarantine materials received until quality control collects samples and approves supplies for use; keep records that permit tracing of all materials to suppliers and finished products
Master manufacturing record	Specifies ingredients, quantities, controls, procedures, packaging, and labeling for each product
Batch record	Initials required to document date and time of performance of each step in process; control number for every batch
Laboratory operations	Must test or examine components, in-process materials and finished products against specifications; tests must be scientifically valid; may use statistical sampling plan
Manufacturing operations	Designed to ensure that specifications are consistently met and product is protected against contamination
Packaging and labeling	Must be kept in secure location; procedures must ensure that correct labels are used; records must permit labeled product to be followed throughout distribution chain
Product complaints	Must be reviewed by qualified personnel; complaint related to possible GMP failure must extend to related batches
Manufacturing records	Must be retained for 2 years, or 1 year beyond product expiration date, and be available for inspection
Written procedures	Required for all key operations, to ensure consistency, and to facilitate training of personnel

will raise the bar for product quality for the industry as a whole. One key to success will be effective enforcement by FDA and by regulatory authorities in the various states. Federal and state inspectors have been participating in educational and training programs in preparation for conducting inspections under the new GMPs.

ADVERSE EVENT REPORTING

Adverse events happen to people all the time, ranging from headaches to nausea, from dizziness to falls, from allergic reactions to strokes. If a person uses a food or drug and then suffers an adverse event, the two occurrences are related in time but may or may not be related in terms of causality. FDA encourages consumers and health professionals to report adverse events that are believed to be related to use of drug products or other FDA-regulated product categories, using the MedWatch reporting system. A series of adverse events may be a signal of a health or safety problem that requires FDA investigation.

If a consumer or a health professional contacts a company about a possible adverse event, the company may or may not be required to pass that report on to FDA. If the company is a food manufacturer, there is no reporting requirement. If the company is the manufacturer of a prescription drug and if the event is a "serious adverse event," then the pharmaceutical company must submit a report to FDA within 15 business days. Serious adverse events include those that result in death, a life-threatening experience, inpatient hospitalization, a persistent or significant disability or incapacity, or a congenital anomaly or birth defect. Serious adverse events also include those that require a medical or surgical intervention to prevent such outcomes.

In the 1990s, there was an explosion of interest in dietary supplements containing the herb ephedra, which contains naturally occurring ephedrine alkaloids with stimulant properties. The products were marketed for weight loss and for sports nutrition, and beginning in about 1992 some states and FDA began to receive reports of adverse events, including some serious events. The number of reported adverse events, including some deaths, mounted over a period of years. FDA called special meetings of its Food Advisory Committee in 1995 and 1996 in an effort to decide what should be done and published a proposed rule in 1997. Several Congressional committees held hearings on the issue, and it was discovered that one of the major marketers of ephedra had received thousands of consumer reports of adverse events. This led to calls for legislation, both at the federal level and in some states, to require mandatory reporting of adverse events by manufacturers of dietary supplements. FDA banned ephedra from dietary supplement products in 2004, but legislators continued to be concerned about the need for more information about any serious adverse events that might be occurring.

Ultimately, several trade associations representing not only manufacturers of dietary supplements but also manufacturers of over-the-counter (OTC) drugs cooperated with key Congressional offices to draft comprehensive legislation that would require the mandatory reporting by companies of serious adverse events relating to dietary supplements or to OTC drugs that were not already covered by a reporting requirement. The law requires mandatory reporting to FDA by manufacturing or marketing companies to whom a serious adverse event may be reported by a consumer or by anyone else, including health care providers.

The Dietary Supplement and Nonprescription Drug Consumer Protection Act was enacted by Congress in December 2006 and became effective as of December 2007 (21). Under the new law, manufacturers of dietary supplements or OTC drugs are required to report *serious adverse events* to FDA, using the MedWatch form, within 15 business days after the company learns of the event from a consumer or health provider or anyone else. In addition, companies are required to keep records of *all* adverse event reports they receive (not just serious adverse events) for 6 years, and those records must be made available to authorized FDA inspectors.

This new reporting requirement will help FDA monitor the safety of dietary supplements, since adverse events provide an important signal of potential safety issues that may require further evaluation by public health agencies.

PUTTING DIETARY SUPPLEMENTS IN PERSPECTIVE

Dietary supplements are frequently in the news, often for positive reasons but sometimes for negative reasons. Consumers may see stories on the Internet, on television, or in the newspaper claiming that dietary supplements are "unregulated." Critics who make this statement generally mean to point out that dietary supplements are not regulated like drugs, and this is a true statement, but it does not equate to being unregulated. Foods, including dietary supplements, are subject to extensive legal and regulatory requirements affecting every aspect of their production, labeling, and advertising. They are subject not only to FDA regulations but also to regulation by a variety of other federal agencies with responsibilities for safeguarding consumer health. In addition, the individual states have their own food and drug authorities and health departments, whose regulations must also be observed. Understanding how dietary supplements fit into the overall system of food regulation in the United States will help health professionals as well as consumers put these products in the proper perspective.

References

1. Radimer K, Bindewald B, Hughes J, Ervin B, Swanson C, Picciano MF. Dietary supplement use by U.S. adults: data from the National Health and Nutrition Examination Survey, 1999–2000. *Am J Epidemiol* 2004;160:339–349.
2. Council for Responsible Nutrition. Study finds physicians and nurses both take and recommend dietary supplements. http://www.lifesupplemented.org/articles/news/study_finds_physicians_and_nurses_both_take_and_recommend_dietary_supplements.htm. Published 2007. Accessed August 2008.
3. Food and Drug Administration. Definition of "special dietary uses" and label regulations for food represented for special dietary uses. *Fed Regist* 1941;6:5921.
4. Food and Drug Administration. Definition and standards of identity for food for special dietary use: dietary supplements of vitamins and minerals. *Fed Regist* 1973;38: 20730–20740.
5. *National Nutritional Foods Association v FDA*, 504 F2d 761 (2d Cir 1974), *cert denied,* 420 US 946 (1975).
6. *National Nutritional Foods Association v Kennedy*, 572 F2d 377 (2d Cir 1978).
7. Pub L No. 94-278, Title V, sections 501-502, 90 Stat 410-413; April 22, 1976. [The vitamin bill, adding a new Section 411 to the FD&C Act.]
8. Food and Drug Administration. Advance notice of proposed rulemaking regarding dietary supplements. *Fed Regist* 1993;58:33690.
9. Pub L No. 103–417, 108 Stat 4325-4335; October 25, 1994. [Dietary Supplement Health and Education Act of 1994.]
10. McGuffin M, Young AL. Premarket notifications of new dietary ingredients—a ten-year review. *Food Drug Law J* 2004;59:229–244.
11. Food and Drug Administration. Sales of supplements containing ephedrine alkaloids (ephedra) prohibited. http://www.fda.gov/oc/initiatives/ephedra/february2004/. Accessed August 2008.

12. Food and Drug Administration. FDA warns manufacturers to stop distributing products containing androstenedione. http://www.cfsan.fda.gov/~dms/dsandro.html. Accessed September 2008.
13. Food and Drug Administration. Buying fake ED products online. http://www.fda.gov/consumer/updates/erectiledysfunction010408.html. Accessed September 2008.
14. Pub L No. 101-535. [Nutrition Labeling and Education Act of 1990].
15. Code of Federal Regulations, Title 21, Section 101.9. Nutrition Labeling of Food.
16. Code of Federal Regulations, Title 21, Section 101.36. Nutrition Labeling of Dietary Supplements.
17. State of California Office of Environmental Health Hazard Assessment. Proposition 65 in plain language. http://www.oehha.org/prop65/background/p65plain.html. Accessed August 2008.
18. Code of Federal Regulations, Title 16. Poison Prevention Packaging. Section 1700.14, Substances requiring special packaging.
19. Food and Drug Administration. Commonly asked questions about BSE. http://www.cfsan.fda.gov/~comm/bsefaq.html. Accessed August 2008.
20. Food and Drug Administration. Current good manufacturing practice in manufacturing, packaging, labeling, or holding operations for dietary supplements: final rule. *Fed Regist* 2007;72:34752–34958.
21. Pub L No. 109-462, 120 Stat 3469. [Dietary supplement and nonprescription drug consumer protection act.]

CHAPTER 17

NLEA and DSHEA: Health Claims and Structure/Function Claims

Annette Dickinson

Foods are obviously essential to life and health, and food marketers are always eager to tell consumers about the benefits of their products. Dietary supplements by definition are intended to supplement the diet with specific nutrients and other functional components of food, and they exist solely to provide nutritional or health benefits. However, the ability of US marketers of foods and dietary supplements to convey information about health benefits to the public was historically hampered by the fact that health-related claims were generally deemed by the Food and Drug Administration (FDA) to be "drug claims." The advance of science and the emergence of a new appreciation of the intimate relationship between diet and health led policy makers to decide that it would be a good idea to harness the marketing power of the food industry to help educate the public about the critical importance of certain foods and food habits. The Food, Drug, and Cosmetic (FD&C) Act was amended in 1990 to permit FDA for the first time to authorize certain well-substantiated "health claims" for foods and dietary supplements to appear on product labels.

Once the door to health claims was opened, however, it became legally impossible to limit permissible health claims to a select few, and a new and broader category of "qualified health claims" came into being. And once the law had been amended to permit health claims, it became politically feasible to amend it further to permit additional types of claims describing the effects of dietary supplements on the structure and function of the body—commonly known today as "structure/function claims." Once these claims were permitted for dietary supplements, FDA also began permitting a broader range of structure/function claims for conventional foods. Thus, the current array of health-related claims permitted for foods, including dietary supplements, is the direct result of the interplay of advancing science and evolving public policy, leading to new laws and regulations as well as new FDA enforcement policies. The availability of health information in product labeling and advertising has exploded, bringing with it an expanded need for regulatory oversight.

FOOD VERSUS DRUG

Dietary supplements are defined and regulated as a category of foods. Foods are loosely defined in Section 201(f) of the FD&C Act, as "articles used for food or drink for man or other animals." Within this broad category of foods, the Act also recognized "foods for special dietary uses," a category that includes dietary supplements.

The Dietary Supplement Health and Education Act (DSHEA) of 1994 confirmed the food status of dietary supplements and added a more specific definition, as discussed in chapter 16.

Yet, it is possible for any food to be considered a drug, for purposes of enforcement, if drug claims are made for it. To understand this fact, it is necessary to consider the statutory definition of a "drug."

Drugs are defined on the basis of their use, and it is the *intended use* of a product that determines its legal classification. Section 201(g) of the FD&C Act defines drugs in part as "articles intended for use in the diagnosis, cure, mitigation, treatment, or prevention of disease in man or other animals." This aspect of the drug definition will be especially important in the discussion of health claims for foods, below. Drugs are also defined in part as "articles (other than food) intended to affect the structure or any function of the body of man or other animals." The parenthetical statement "other than food" recognizes that foods do in fact affect the structure and function of the body, and this recognition is the basis for permitting some label claims for dietary supplements, as further discussed below.

Foods, including dietary supplements, can legally be considered "drugs" for purposes of FDA enforcement, if they are labeled for disease prevention or treatment. For example, orange juice labeled for use as a "tasty and nutritious breakfast drink" is a food. However, that same orange juice could be seized by FDA as an unapproved drug if the labeling claimed that it would prevent or treat any disease—a minor disease such as the common cold or a major disease such as cancer. The label claim describes the "intended use" of a product, and its classification as a food or a drug flows from the intended use.

Interestingly, in today's marketplace it is possible for a product to be both a food and a drug, and to be labeled as both. Calcium carbonate tablets, for example, are commonly sold as dietary supplements, as a source of calcium. Exactly the same tablets are commonly sold as over-the-counter (OTC) drugs labeled for use as antacids. Some brands of calcium carbonate currently bear dual labeling as dietary supplements and antacids. Similarly, soluble fiber from psyllium is added to some breakfast cereals as a source of fiber and is marketed in tablet or wafer or powder form as a fiber supplement. Exactly the same ingredient is sold in some OTC drugs labeled for use as laxatives, and some brands currently bear dual labeling.

Some dietary supplement ingredients such as omega-3 fatty acids EPA and DHA (eicosapentaenoic acid and docosahexaenoic acid) are currently marketed also as prescription drugs, with FDA approval for specific drug uses. The active ingredients in this case are somewhat different structurally and in terms of concentration than the usual dietary supplement ingredients. Even if they were identical, however, the same physical product could not be labeled both as a prescription drug and as a dietary supplement, since the former can only be dispensed with a physician's prescription and the latter is by definition available to consumers for purchase and use at their own discretion.

DIET AND HEALTH

In the 1970s and 1980s there was increasing public and scientific interest in diet/health relationships, and this interest eventually resulted in major changes affecting the labeling of all foods, including dietary supplements. In 1976, the Senate Select Committee on Nutrition and Human Needs published a highly controversial report charging that 6 of the 10 "killer diseases" in the United States were related to poor dietary habits (1). Congress instructed the United States Department of Agriculture and the United States Department of Health, Education and Welfare (now the United States Department of Health and Human Services) to develop guidelines telling Americans how to eat for health and to review those guidelines every 5 years. This was the origin of the *Dietary Guidelines for Americans*, first published in 1980 and revised every 5 years since then (2). In 1982, the National Research Council published *Diet, Nutrition, and Cancer*, calling for major changes in the US diet (3). All of these reports emphasized similar concerns—people would be healthier and reduce their risk of many chronic diseases if they consumed less fat and if they got more fiber and an abundance of antioxidant nutrients from fruits, vegetables, and whole grains.

Companies that marketed foods consistent with these recommendations were naturally anxious to tell the public about the potential health benefits of their products. However, FDA was holding to the hard line that disease prevention claims were not permitted in food labeling. Something was bound to give.

Companies were not the only parties anxious to educate consumers about diet and health issues. In 1984, the National Cancer Institute was in the midst of a national educational campaign about the health benefits of fiber. In an unprecedented move, the Kellogg Company joined in this campaign, and the backs of cereal boxes carried the message that diets high in fiber were associated with reduced risk of many types of cancer. The cereal label provided an 800 number consumers could call to request a brochure from NCI about fiber and cancer. FDA considered the possibility of sweeping Kellogg high-fiber cereals off supermarket shelves on the grounds that they were "unapproved new drugs" intended for disease prevention. Instead, FDA began serious public discussion about the possibility of permitting some health claims for foods.

In 1988, the Surgeon General of the United States published *Nutrition and Health*, and this was followed in 1989 by the National Research Council's *Diet and Health*, reiterating and expanding the message that dietary habits were both the cause of debilitating disease and the potential source of salvation from it (4, 5). The stage was set for a major revolution in public policy regarding diet and health information.

HEALTH CLAIMS

The Nutrition Labeling and Education Act (NLEA) of 1990 brought about a fundamental change in food and drug regulation by authorizing FDA to approve "health claims" for foods and dietary supplements (6). FDA had previously enforced a bright line between the types of label claims permitted for foods and the types of claims permitted for drugs, and health-related claims for foods were very limited. In 1990, because of the growing recognition of the importance of some foods and dietary habits in promoting health and preventing disease, Congress decided that the time had come to permit health claims for food components scientifically demonstrated to reduce disease risk. This monumental change was accomplished by defining health claims in the food sections of the FD&C Act, specifying the conditions under which FDA was authorized to approve health claims for foods, and—very importantly—amending the drug definition. The drug definition in Section 201(g) of the FD&C Act was amended specifically to provide that a food or a dietary supplement making an FDA-approved health claim "is not a drug solely because the label or the labeling contains such a claim."

TABLE 17.1 FDA-Approved NLEA Health Claims

Food or Component	May Reduce the Risk of:
Foods low in total fat and saturated fat	Cancer
Foods low in saturated fat and cholesterol	Coronary heart disease
Foods low in sodium	Hypertension
Naturally good sources of dietary fiber	Cancer
Naturally good sources of soluble fiber	Coronary heart disease
Naturally good sources of vitamin C or beta-carotene	Cancer
Foods sweetened with sugar alcohols	Dental caries
Calcium (including supplements)	Osteoporosis
Folic acid (including supplements)	Neural tube birth defects
Specific soluble fiber components from oats, barley, or psyllium that reduce cholesterol (including supplements)	Heart disease
Soy protein (including supplements)	Heart disease
Stanol or sterol esters (including supplements)	Heart disease

A health claim is a statement that describes the relationship between a food substance and a disease or a health-related condition. The claim not only may but must include the name of the disease or condition affected by the food or food substance. Congress specified that FDA could approve health claims only after reviewing the scientific evidence and concluding that the claim was supported by "significant scientific agreement"—a very high standard. When FDA approves a health claim, the agency issues a regulation describing the evidence for the claim, specifying certain elements that must be included in the claim, and providing a model claim. Companies are not required to use the language of the model claim but can develop their own language, provided the required elements are included. Importantly, FDA requires health claims to use language referring to "reducing the risk" of disease and to avoid using terms that appear in the drug definition, such as "prevent" or "treat." The distinction is semantic but important.

FDA has approved 12 NLEA health claims, to date, as summarized in Table 17.1 (7). Three of the claims are for foods *low* in certain risk nutrients, including fat, cholesterol, and sodium. Three are permitted only for foods with certain naturally occurring nutrients, including dietary fiber, soluble fiber, and vitamin C or beta-carotene, on the assumption that these nutrients may be markers for healthy dietary habits and may not necessarily be responsible for the benefit. One is for foods sweetened with sugar alcohols. Dietary supplements are eligible for five of the approved NLEA claims, provided the products contain a threshold amount of the relevant substance. For example, the health claim regarding calcium and a reduced risk of osteoporosis can appear on the label of a food or supplement that provides at least 200 mg of calcium per serving (8). Another health claim advises women of childbearing age that an increased intake of the B vitamin folate (or folic acid) may reduce their risk of having a baby with a neural tube birth defect such as spina bifida (9). Dietary supplements are also eligible for several health claims for ingredients that have been shown to lower cholesterol levels and therefore are believed to reduce the risk of heart disease. These include claims for specific soluble fibers (from oat, barley, and psyllium), for soy protein, and for stanol or sterol esters.

QUALIFIED HEALTH CLAIMS

What happens if FDA evaluates a health claim, decides there is no "significant scientific agreement" supporting it, and therefore does not approve the claim? FDA's assumption and the apparent intent of the NLEA was that only FDA-approved health claims would be permitted in food labeling, and no other label information about diet/disease relationships would be permitted. The public might learn of exciting new "emerging evidence" from the media, but such new evidence was not to be mentioned in food labeling.

This approach was found by the courts to be in violation of First Amendment protections of freedom of speech, which apply to commercial speech as well as to individual speech (10). The FD&C Act clearly permits FDA to prohibit or ban false or misleading statements in food labeling, but the courts questioned whether a truthful statement about emerging scientific evidence would necessarily be misleading. Thus, in cases in which FDA concluded that a claim was not supported by "significant scientific agreement," the courts required FDA to go a step further and also consider whether it was possible to develop a modified claim that would truthfully describe the level of evidence supporting the claim, without misleading consumers about its significance. Such modified claims have come to be called "qualified health claims."

FDA's current approach to qualified health claims is to review the evidence submitted for a claim and then to select qualifying language that is tailored to the situation (11). If the scientific evidence is relatively strong, the qualifying language will be mild, but if the evidence is relatively weak, the qualifying language will be stronger. In some cases, the qualifying language may be so severe as to make the claim basically meaningless—a deliberate tactic to discourage the use of weakly supported claims. For example, FDA found the evidence regarding green tea and breast cancer or prostate cancer to be very weak but permitted a qualified claim referring to "weak and limited" studies and saying that "FDA concludes that it is highly unlikely" that green tea reduces risk of these cancers. Other parts of the green tea petition, relating to other types of cancer, were denied outright. Other petitions for qualified health claims that have been denied outright include those relating to lycopene and certain cancers, vitamin E and heart disease, lutein and macular degeneration, and glucosamine and osteoarthritis.

It should be noted that FDA does not actually "approve" qualified health claims. There is no formal rulemaking, as there is for a fully approved health claim. Instead, FDA evaluates the evidence and sends the petitioner for the claim a letter in which the agency agrees to "exercise its enforcement discretion" to permit a qualified claim, provided various criteria are met, and the letter is made publicly available on the FDA Web site. There are currently more than a dozen qualified health claims permitted under letters of enforcement discretion. A list of the qualified health claims permitted or denied is available on the Web site (12).

One of the stronger qualified claims currently being permitted relates to omega-3 fatty acids (EPA and DHA) and a reduced risk of heart disease. The claim is permitted for dietary supplements as well as conventional foods, and the language of the model claim is: "Supportive but not conclusive research shows that consumption of EPA and DHA omega-3 fatty acids may reduce the risk of coronary heart disease." FDA considers the phrase "supportive but not conclusive research" to be "qualifying language" that tells consumers that the evidence is still emerging on this issue. It is unclear, however, whether the public grasps the intended distinction between fully approved claims and qualified claims, let alone between stronger and weaker qualified claims (13).

FDAMA HEALTH CLAIMS

There is another category of health claims, permitted by the FDA Modernization Act (FDAMA) of 1997, called "FDAMA health claims" (14). Under this law, companies can petition FDA for health claims based on authoritative statements of scientific bodies such as the National Academy of Sciences, the Public Health Service, or the Centers for Disease Control and Prevention. FDA has 120 days to deny the claim, and if there is no agency action within that time frame, then the claim can be made. This provision was adopted because Congress was frustrated with FDA's delay in permitting the NLEA health claim about folic acid and neural tube defects, despite the existence of a Public Health Service recommendation based on the evidence for it. Congress therefore created a mechanism to provide a fast track to a health claim based on such a recommendation or conclusion by a recognized scientific body. FDA has permitted several FDAMA health claims in response to petitions submitted to the agency. Examples include a claim for whole grain foods to reduce the risk of heart disease and certain cancers and a claim for potassium-containing foods (such as orange juice) to reduce the risk of high blood pressure and stroke.

DIETARY SUPPLEMENT HEALTH AND EDUCATION ACT: STRUCTURE/FUNCTION CLAIMS

When the DSHEA was passed in 1994, FDA was still in the process of evaluating the first wave of health claims, and it appeared unlikely that many health claims would be approved for dietary supplements. However, it was considered important to provide consumers with more information about the intended uses of dietary supplements, and Congress decided to create a mechanism for accomplishing this goal. DSHEA defined a new class of label claims for dietary supplements called "statements of nutritional support" (15). There are four types of "statements of nutritional support," including statements describing the effect of a product on the structure or function of the body, statements describing the mechanism by which a product has such an effect, statements relating to nutritional deficiency, and statements about general well-being. By far the most important of these is the first type, today called "structure/function" claims.

As mentioned earlier, the drug definition implicitly recognizes that foods (as well as some drugs) affect the structure or function of the body. FDA has always permitted some structure/function statements in food labeling, especially statements that truthfully describe the recognized role of an essential nutrient.

DSHEA expanded the range of structure/function statements permitted to be used in the labeling of dietary supplements. Moreover, just as NLEA amended the drug definition in the FD&C Act to make it clear that a food would not be considered a drug solely because its labeling included an approved health claim, DSHEA amended the drug definition to provide that a food or a dietary supplement would not be considered a drug solely because its labeling included a truthful and not misleading structure/function claim.

While all label statements for foods are required under the FD&C Act to be truthful and not misleading, DSHEA specifically emphasizes the need for companies to have substantiation for structure/function claims for dietary supplements. There are also additional requirements that must be met under DSHEA. Companies must notify FDA within 30 days of any structure/function claim being made; the statements must not claim to "diagnose, mitigate, treat, cure, or prevent a specific disease or class of diseases;" and any structure/function statement on the label must be marked with an asterisk referring to a disclaimer. The disclaimer must be set off in a box and its text must read:

> **"This statement has not been evaluated by the Food and Drug Administration. This product is not intended to diagnose, treat, cure, or prevent any disease."**

Each sentence of this disclaimer has a specific purpose. The first sentence distinguishes structure/function claims from health claims, which by definition *have* been evaluated by FDA. The second sentence distinguishes structure/function claims from drug claims, which *do* relate to the prevention or treatment of disease.

Companies were quick to utilize structure/function claims under the conditions specified by DSHEA, and FDA has received many thousands of letters of notification. Many of these letters are duplicative, since each marketer must submit letters for its own brands and products, and the same product or ingredient may be marketed by many different companies. FDA does not approve structure/function claims but does sometimes object to claims. When FDA receives a notification for an inappropriate structure/function claim, the agency responds by sending the company a "courtesy letter," outlining the reason for the objection. In 1997, FDA established a public docket for the courtesy letters, which currently includes almost 1,000 entries (16). In general, companies have a good understanding of the limits for permissible structure/function claims, and it is estimated that FDA responds to only about 10% of the notifications.

One reason for the good industry understanding of the scope of structure/function claims is that FDA published a rule in January 2000, which included an extensive and instructive discussion of the scope of these claims and the nature of the dividing line between these claims and health claims or disease claims (17). For example, a health claim must specifically mention a disease condition such as heart disease or cancer or osteoporosis. A structure/function claim cannot mention a disease condition and instead should refer to supporting or maintaining normal function. The statement that "diets high in calcium may reduce the risk of osteoporosis" is a health claim; the statement that "calcium builds strong bones" is a structure/function claim. However, both statements effectively signal to the public that the product is related to bone health.

The rule on structure/function claims makes it clear that FDA continues to view certain structure/function statements as implied disease claims. This is particularly true with regard to claims about lowering cholesterol, blood pressure, or blood glucose levels. High cholesterol and high blood pressure are recognized surrogate risk factors for heart disease, and FDA considers any mention of reducing these levels to

TABLE 17.2 Examples of Acceptable Structure/Function Claims

Antioxidant effects	Provides powerful antioxidant protection, provides antioxidant protection for the eyes
Bones and teeth	Essential for building strong bones and teeth, strengthens and protects bones
Cognitive effects	Supports brain function, improves mental performance, reduces absentmindedness, enhances mental alertness
Gastrointestinal effects	Stimulates digestion, promotes regularity, adds bulk and supports colon health, soothing for the stomach or digestive tract, supports healthy intestinal function
Heart health	Helps maintain a healthy heart, contributes to cardiovascular health, maintains healthy cholesterol levels when already within the normal range
Immunity	Supports healthy immune function, helps boost the immune system, helps maintain natural resistance
Joints	Supports healthy joints, helps maintain healthy connective tissue and cartilage, maintains joint mobility
Prostate	Supports prostate health, maintains healthy prostate function
Sleep	Promotes restful sleep, aids in the regulation of circadian rhythms
Stress	Promotes relaxation, helps you feel calm and relaxed, eases normal anxiety, promotes serenity and a sense of well-being
Weight loss	Helps maintain normal body weight, part of a complete weight loss program

be equivalent to a direct claim to lower heart disease risk. While statements such as these are permitted in some approved health claims, they are not permitted in structure/function claims (17). Structure/function claims may, however, refer to maintaining healthy cholesterol or blood pressure or glucose levels when these are already in the normal range.

Table 17.2 lists some examples of apparently acceptable structure/function claims that are currently being used in dietary supplement labeling, without FDA objection.

Now that a broader range of structure/function claims is permitted for dietary supplements, FDA is also expanding its view of structure/function claims allowed for conventional foods. For example, the makers of a famous brand of frozen foods recently introduced different combinations of frozen vegetables prominently labeled with terms such as "Healthy Vision" and "Immunity Boost." Since conventional foods are not covered by DSHEA, they are not required to notify FDA when a structure/function statement is used and they are not required to use the DSHEA disclaimer on the label.

SUBSTANTIATION OF CLAIMS

The Federal Trade Commission (FTC) is an independent agency with a mandate to enforce the FTC Act, which prohibits advertising claims that are false or misleading. The advertising law applies not only to dietary supplements and conventional foods but also to all consumer products, ranging from pharmaceuticals or cosmetics to garden hoses or automobiles. Companies are expected to have substantiation for claims made in advertising *before* the advertisement is disseminated. The amount and kind of evidence required is related to the actual claim made in the advertisement. For example, if a company says two studies show a certain effect, FTC expects there to be two studies relevant to the claim and relevant to the product being advertised. When it comes to health-related advertising claims, FTC has high expectations and requires such claims to be supported by "competent and reliable scientific evidence" but does not specify exactly what kind of evidence or how much evidence is required to support a particular type of claim. This may vary from case to case, depending on the exact wording of the claim or the seriousness of the health implications of a false claim.

After the passage of DSHEA, trade associations representing the dietary supplement industry requested FTC clarification regarding the kinds of structure/function claims that would be considered acceptable in advertising and regarding the degree and type of substantiation required for such claims. In 1998, FTC responded by publishing a document called *Dietary Supplements: An Advertising Guide for Industry* (18). This guide, which is available on the FTC Web site, provides a thorough and very useful overview of the criteria for determining whether an advertisement is supported by "competent and reliable scientific evidence," as required for claims relating to health benefits. Numerous theoretical examples are provided of various scenarios illustrating adequately supported claims and explaining why some claims may be found to be false or misleading.

FTC requires advertisers to have substantiation for any implied claims as well as express claims made in advertising, and the substantiation must be appropriate to the claim. Studies cited should ideally relate to the same ingredient or product mentioned in the advertisement, and the quantity of the product used in the study to obtain the effect should be similar to the quantity recommended for consumer use. Studies should be of good quality, and the totality of the evidence should be considered. If there are positive and negative studies, the advertiser needs to be able to explain why a positive claim is justified.

FTC has been especially vigorous in pursuing misleading weight loss claims, whether made for dietary supplements, for conventional foods, or for various devices or programs promising easy weight loss (19). Penalties imposed by FTC can be very large and can include millions of dollars in fines or disgorgement of profits. In January 2007, for example, FTC announced penalties of $25 million against four companies making weight loss claims for products including Xenadrine, CortiSlim, Hoodia, and multivitamins (20). FTC and FDA and other US and international agencies also cooperate in massive Internet sweeps to identify and stop misleading marketing of a variety of products, including dietary supplements (21).

In 2004, FDA provided draft guidance for the industry regarding substantiation of structure/function claims (22). The document includes numerous examples of cases illustrating adequate or inadequate substantiation for theoretical claims. It emphasizes that a company should have scientific evidence that the product or ingredient has the effect being claimed. The evidence should relate to levels of intake comparable to those provided by the product in populations similar to those that will be using the product. The guidance also notes that, if there are positive as well as negative studies, the totality of the evidence needs to be evaluated to determine whether a positive claim can be supported. These provisions are similar to guidance provided by the FTC in 1998, discussed above.

LOOKING TO THE FUTURE

Dietary supplements are here to stay, and their use is increasing in the lay public and also among health care professionals. People make the decision to include dietary supplements in their personal wellness regimen because of scientific evidence suggesting possible benefits. The rate of appearance of new scientific research is ever-increasing, as more journals appear both in hard copy and online, and as the media seeks to provide the public with rapid access to the hottest news that might have an impact on health concerns. This is not a scenario that necessarily leads to balanced reporting or to sound decision-making. New research is often reported by the media as the last word on a particular topic and is not placed in the context of the overall evidence available on the subject. Consumers who have been taking a particular supplement for years may suddenly be confronted with a story saying that it failed to provide a benefit in a particular study. What are they to think? They may decide immediately to ignore the story or to abandon the supplement, or they may look for someone credible to ask for advice. Health care professionals can provide a valuable service by putting such stories in context. Was the study done in healthy people or in people who already had a disease? What have other studies shown? What is the overall evidence for benefit, and is there a potential for harm? Helping consumers understand the answers to these questions will help them evaluate and if necessary revise their own personal dietary supplement regimen.

References

1. Senate Select Committee on Nutrition and Human Needs. *Dietary Goals for the United States*. Washington, DC: Government Printing Office; 1977.
2. U.S. Department of Health, Education and Welfare (now U.S. Department of Health and Human Services) and U.S. Department of Agriculture. *Dietary Guidelines for Americans*. Washington, DC, 1980, 1985, 1990, 1995, 2000, 2005.
3. National Research Council. *Diet, Nutrition, and Cancer*. Washington, DC: National Academy Press; 1982.
4. U.S. Surgeon General. *Report on Nutrition and Health*. Washington, DC: U.S. Department of Health and Human Services; 1988.
5. National Research Council. *Diet and Health: Implications for Reducing Chronic Disease Risk*. Washington, DC: National Academy Press; 1989.
6. Pub L No. 101-535. [Nutrition Labeling and Education Act of 1990].
7. Food and Drug Administration. Health claims that meet significant scientific agreement. http://www.cfsan.fda.gov/~dms/lab-ssa.html. Accessed August 2008.
8. Food and Drug Administration. Food labeling: health claims; calcium and osteoporosis. *Fed Regist* 1993;58:2665–2681. (Codified in Section 101.72, Title 21, Code of Federal Regulations.)
9. Food and Drug Administration. Food labeling: health claims and label statements; folate and neural tube defects. *Fed Regis* 1996;61:8752–8781. (Codified in Section 101.79, Title 21, Code of Federal Regulations.)

10. U.S. Court of Appeals for the District of Columbia Circuit, *Pearson v Shalala*, 164 F3d 650 (DC Cir 1999).
11. Food and Drug Administration. Consumer health information for better nutrition initiative: task force final report. http://www.cfsan.fda.gov/~dms/nuttftoc.html. Published July 2003. Accessed August 2008.
12. Food and Drug Administration. Qualified health claims. http://www.cfsan.fda.gov/~dms/lab-qhc.html. Accessed August 2008.
13. International Food Information Council (IFIC). Qualified health claims consumer research project executive summary. http://www.ific.org/research/qualhealthclaimsres.cfm. Published March 2005. Accessed August 2008.
14. Food and Drug Administration. FDAMA claims. http://www.cfsan.fda.gov/~dms/labfdama.html. Accessed September 2008.
15. Pub L No. 103-417, 108 Stat 4325-4335; October 25, 1994. [Dietary Supplement Health and Education Act of 1994.]
16. Food and Drug Administration. Dietary supplements, courtesy letters. http://www.fda.gov/ohrms/dockets/dockets/97s0163/mostrecent.htm. Accessed August 2008.
17. Food and Drug Administration. Regulations on statements made for dietary supplements concerning the effect of the product on the structure of function of the body; final rule. *Fed Regist* 2000;65:999–1050.
18. Federal Trade Commission. Dietary supplements: an advertising guide for industry. http://www.ftc.gov/bcp/edu/pubs/business/adv/bus09.shtm. Published 1998. Accessed August 2008.
19. Federal Trade Commission. Weight loss advertising: an analysis of current trends. http://www.ftc.gov/bcp/reports/weightloss.pdf. Published 2002. Accessed August 2008.
20. Federal Trade Commission. FTC reaches "New Year's" resolutions with four major weight-control pill marketers. http://www.ftc.gov/opa/2007/01/weightloss.shtm. Accessed September 2008.
21. Federal Trade Commission. FTC and FDA act against Internet vendors of fraudulent diabetes cures and treatment. http://www.ftc.gov/opa/2006/10/diabetessweep.shtm. Accessed September 2008.
22. FDA guidance on substantiation of claims for dietary supplements. http://www.cfsan.fda.gov/~dms/dsclmgui.html. Accessed August 2008.

CHAPTER 18

International Perspectives on the Regulation of Herbs and Phytomedicines

Mark Blumenthal, Sue Akeroyd, Thomas Brendler, Simon Y. Mills, and Joel B. Taller

Herbs are regulated in numerous ways within various countries and regions of the world, along a continuum that can include both food and drug status. This spectrum can include spices and conventional foods, food additives, food supplements and dietary supplements (basically the same thing, depending on country), so-called functional foods and other categories on the food side of the equation, nonprescription medications (aka over-the-counter medicines or OTC drugs), and/or prescription drugs. In some of these countries, herbs and herbal preparations may be simultaneously regulated in more than one category, that is, depending on how the preparation is registered or licensed, the type of condition or indication for which it is intended and marketed, the type of preparation, etc. Table 18.1 shows many of these categories and how many countries use them.

This chapter provides a general overview of international regulations concerning herbs and herbal preparations sold for health-related purposes (conventional foods and cosmetics are not included). Furthermore, this chapter intentionally does not cover the regulatory status of herbal preparations in the United States, where

TABLE 18.1 Regulatory Categories for Herbs Worldwide[a]

Category	Countries
Nonprescription drug/OTC	97
Prescription drug	50
Dietary supplement	47
Self-medication only	40
Separate herbal-specific category	25
Health food	15
Functional food	9
No status	23

[a]From World Health Organization. *National Policy on Traditional Medicine and Regulation of Herbal Medicines: Report of a WHO Global Survey*. Geneva: World Health Organization; 2005.

most but not all of them are sold under the legal category known as "dietary supplements," a category of foods created by the Dietary Supplement Health and Education Act of 1994 (DSHEA). Some herbs are still approved as safe and effective ingredients in nonprescription/over-the-counter (OTC) drugs in the United States; however, during the past three decades OTC drugs have been reviewed for safety and efficacy and many herbs were removed due to a lack of adequate data submitted to the United States Food and Drug Administration to confirm their safety and/or efficacy. Hence, most herbal products in the Unites States are sold as dietary supplements as regulated under DSHEA. An extensive description of this law and related regulatory considerations related to herbs in the United States is discussed in chapter 16 of this book.

The scope of this chapter includes a global perspective as documented by the World Health Organization (WHO) as well as specific sections on the regulatory systems in other English-speaking countries, that is, Australia, Canada, and the United Kingdom. In addition, the regulatory system in Germany is explained since Germany was frequently touted by some proponents in the United States in the 1990s as a rational regulatory model, particularly for the documentation of the therapeutic (i.e., druglike) uses of herbs and medicinal plants. Finally, a brief explanation of the Traditional Herbal Medicinal Products (THMPs) regulatory initiative in the European Union (EU) is provided since this development is affecting the regulation and sale of many herbal preparations which do not meet the normal requirements for market authorization as approved medicines.

GLOBAL PERSPECTIVE—WORLD HEALTH ORGANIZATION SURVEY

In 2005, the WHO published a survey showing that many countries had made recent progress in the development and implementation of regulations on herbal medicinal products (HMPs) (1–3). WHO's *National Policy on Traditional Medicine and Regulation of Herbal Medicines: Report of a WHO Global Survey* provides information on the status of herbal regulations and laws worldwide as well as the state of national policies on the acceptance and regulation of traditional (i.e., indigenous, historical), complementary, and alternative medicine modalities (1, 2).

The WHO survey had been distributed to national health authorities of the 191 countries serving as WHO's member states in 2002. Survey responses were returned by 142 countries (74% response rate; the United States was not a responder). Before 1988 only 14 WHO member states had instituted regulations relating specifically to the manufacture and sale of HMPs; this number had grown to 53 member states (37%) by 2003. Forty-two countries (49%) without laws and regulations related to herbs claimed that such regulations were in the process of being developed. The majority of responding countries (92, or 65%) claimed to have laws or regulations dealing with herbal medicines, some of which are included in provisions related to conventional drug products.

According to the WHO survey, the most common regulatory status for herbal medicines is that of nonprescription/OTC drugs, a category used within 97 of the countries responding to the survey.[1] Other regulatory categories for the regulation of

[1]The term *OTC drug* is often synonymous with *nonprescription drug* in most countries. In Germany, for example, most herbal drugs are sold as nonprescription medicines in pharmacies only, but they are not allowed to be sold in many of the locations where OTC drugs may be sold in other countries, like in the United States, for example, grocery stores, convenience stores, hotel lobbies, vending machines.

herbal medicines include the following: prescription medications (50 countries), dietary supplements (47 countries), self-medication-only products (40 countries),[2] separate herbal-specific categories (25 countries), health foods (15 countries), and functional foods (9 countries). (Respondents were allowed to choose multiple categories if more than one status was in effect, so the total for each of the categories (283) exceeds the number of countries participating in the survey.) At the time of the survey, 23 countries had no regulatory status for herbs. These categories are summarized in Table 18.1.[1]

Different regulatory categories determine the types of health-related claims that are allowed for herbal products. In the WHO survey, the majority of respondents (73%; 103 countries) stated that they allow the use of health-oriented claims on the packaging and in the sale of herbal medicines. The strength of these claims is dependent on the regulatory category. OTC drugs generally deal with self-diagnosable, self-treatable, and self-limiting conditions and symptoms, whereas prescription drug status would allow claims for treatment of symptoms of more serious diseases (e.g., cardiac function and diabetes).

Quality control is a key factor in the development of any herbal product. Because botanics come from raw agricultural products, there are issues related to ensuring the proper identity of the plant material and determining whether there has been any (accidental or intentional) substitution or adulteration or contamination with foreign matter (including filth, pesticides, and/or heavy metals). The way that many countries routinely attempt to establish standards for the quality and identity for botanic materials (as well as conventional drugs) is through the development of a national pharmacopeia—a compendium containing officially recognized standards and methods of analysis for dietary supplement and/or drug materials.

According to the WHO survey, only 24% of countries (34 countries) indicated the existence and use of a national pharmacopeia. Of the 104 countries without such a document, 25% (26 countries) claimed that a (national or regional) pharmacopeia was in development (in 2002), and 56% (58 countries) responded that another (external) pharmacopeia is in use. A similarly small percentage of countries (33%, or 46 countries) claimed to have national monographs. Of the 84 countries lacking national monographs, 28% (25 countries) indicated that monographs were being prepared and 38% (34 countries) claimed to use other monographs from other sources. Of these, 27 countries without national monographs provided names of the other monographs utilized, some indicating the use of multiple compendia. The most commonly selected international monographs were those prepared by WHO[(1–3)] (12 countries), followed by the *European Pharmacopoeia* (8 countries), European Scientific Cooperative on Phytotherapy (ESCOP) monographs (4 countries), German Commission E Monographs (3 countries [Note: Commission E monographs are therapeutic monographs only; they do not provide standards for quality control]), and the *British Pharmacopoeia* (3 countries). Twelve countries indicated use of other sources for monographs. Of the 46 countries with national monographs, 52% (24 countries) identified them as being legally binding; of the 34 countries using other monographs, 44% (15 countries) reported those texts as legally binding (1).

Data regarding manufacturing regulations and safety assessment of herbal medicines were also collected through the global survey. Questions about manufacturing requirements were answered by 126 countries, and these countries were

[2]It is not clear how this differs from nonprescription/OTC drugs, which are usually self-selected.

allowed to select more than one response. The majority of respondents (73 countries) claimed that the same rules of good manufacturing practices (GMPs) required for conventional medicines are enforced for herbal medications. Fifty-nine countries indicated that they are required to adhere to the criteria, requirements, and other related information specified in pharmacopeias and official monographs, and 30 countries indicated that they use special GMP rules. Twenty-eight countries claimed to have no manufacturing requirements for herbal medicines.

Safety of herbal preparations is a key issue on which regulatory officials often express great concern. In the WHO survey, 130 countries responded to safety assessment questions. The majority of countries (82) claimed to use special requirements for safety assessments, wherein determining safety of an herbal material is different from determining that of a conventional pharmaceutical medication. For example, many herbs have been used for centuries and/or millennia in systems of traditional medicine, and such use may be documented in writing. (Most conventional pharmaceutical drugs, by contrast, are single chemical entities—some extracted and purified from plants, most of which are synthetic and have no prior history of use.) In many countries, to establish safety for an herbal material, particularly when a conventional drug-safety type of approach has not been conducted, regulators require documentation of traditional use without demonstrated harmful effects and/or references to scientific research (if such research is available). Fifty-seven countries claimed to use the same safety requirements as those related to establishing the safety of conventional pharmaceutical drugs, and 28 countries stated that they have no safety requirements for herbs. Furthermore, 59 of 114 responding countries indicated the existence of a postmarketing surveillance system for herbal medicines to collect and monitor adverse reaction reports, 53 (or 90%) of which also claimed to have a national system to monitor adverse effects. What is more, 44 of the 77 countries without postmarketing surveillance systems reported that such systems were under development.

REGULATION OF HERBAL MEDICINAL PRODUCTS IN SPECIFIC COUNTRIES

As noted above, the following section presents brief summaries of the regulation of HMPs in the following countries: Australia, Canada, Germany, and the United Kingdom. In addition, the THMPs regulatory system for the EU is included. Furthermore, the regulatory status in the United States is extensively covered in chapter 16.

AUSTRALIA

In Australia, herbal medicines are regulated as "therapeutic goods," a classification of drugs. Australia has maintained a national register of drugs/medicines since 1966. In 1991, the existing legislation was considerably amended to expand the range of products captured in the Australian Register of Therapeutic Goods (ARTG) (4). An amnesty period allowed for medicines on the market at the time to be submitted for inclusion; these came to be known as 'grandfathered medicines,' and many remain on the market today. For all new medicines (locally produced or imported), a preclearance gateway (premarket approval) has been in place ever since.

Australia regulates medicine on many levels from "registered" prescription and OTC conventional pharmaceutical drugs to "listed" "complementary" medicines (more at www.tga.gov.au). Complementary medicines are eligible for listing if their ingredients (active and/or inactive) are included on the Therapeutic Good Administration (TGA's) list of eligible ingredients and if the claims or "indications" are for nonserious medical conditions (5, 6). The "positive" list of eligible listable ingredients consists of ingredients enabled by Schedule 4 of the Therapeutic Goods Regulations 1990 (7) that were included in those medicines grandfathered in 1991 plus substances that have been applied for safety assessment since then (8).

Like most nations, Australia regulates medicines and foods. Products that are typically regulated as "dietary supplements" in other markets will mostly be regulated as (complementary) medicines (i.e., therapeutic goods) in Australia (5), unless they are foodlike in their presentation. Australian food regulations are complex; the Food Code (9) is developed jointly between Australia and New Zealand but administered by Australian states and territories. New Zealand has a provision under food law for dietary supplements (10); Australia does not.

Considering herbs and herbal preparations, there is a continuum between food and medicine ranging from beverage and culinary herbs to herbs used for medicinal applications. Medicinal products can be sold both as prepared medicines and for extemporaneous compounding. When determining whether an item will be regulated as a food or a medicine, the consumer-level presentation is considered, including form, claims, instructions for use, and novelty. Phrasing in the legislation takes into consideration the consumer's perception of the intention of the product, so omitting a health-related claim from the label is not generally an option to avoid stricter regulation as a medicine.

Extensive regulatory guidance is provided for all levels of Australian medicines. Australia draws its regulatory precedent for data requirements from the European Union's Committee for Proprietary Medicinal Products, the scientific committee of the European Medicines Evaluation Agency (EMEA), but edited for Australian purposes in consultation with industry. The Australian regulatory guidelines for complementary medicines (11) are comprehensive and cover both registered and listed complementary medicines as well as the data needs for new listable substance applications.

Australian medicines, including complementary medicines, are required by the Therapeutic Goods Order No. 69 (General requirements for labels for medicines Labeling Order) (12) to be labeled with a purpose statement and directions for use. This purpose statement (indication) could be a structure/function claim (as is allowed for dietary supplements in the United States under the terms of DSHEA) or symptom relief claim. For listed medicines, such purpose statements are required to be supported by "evidence," and the "level" of evidence is graded in accordance with the considered level of claim. More serious indications require a higher level of evidence of proof of efficacy. *The Guidelines for Levels and Kinds of Evidence to Support Indications and Claims* for Nonregisterable Medicines, including Complementary Medicines, and other Listable Medicines (13) also describes the circumstances in which traditional data are acceptable for claim support.

The preclearance process for listed complementary medicines requires that an electronic form be completed, which describes and mostly quantifies the formulation and indications. It is a "smart form" process which validates the eligibility of the medicine for listing. Only eligible ingredients can be selected from the drop-down menus. For herbal medicines, the electronic form will require the plant part, extract type, solvent details, and extract ratio, which, in turn, leads to consideration of when a change in extract triggers a determination of a medicine being "separate and distinct." A draft guidance on the topic of phytoequivalence was issued for consultation in November

2007, but at the time of this writing has not yet been finalized (14). This deals with whether a product is separate and distinct or perhaps not eligible for listing.

A specific requirement is that most Australian complementary medicines are required to be manufactured by licensed manufacturers (15). For products supplied from offshore, this may require inspection of the facility by the Australian authorities, unless there is a country-to-country agreement in place covering manufacture of that product type. For example, the Mutual Recognition Agreement between Australia and Canada does not cover the manufacture in Canada of natural health products (NHPs); a medicine/drug manufacturing license is required. Similarly, Australia does not recognize dietary supplement GMPs in the United States, including Food and Drug Administration inspection thereof. Australia would require at least a desktop audit, in addition to access to inspection reports from other (equivalent) regulators, but most likely an on-site inspection by Australian inspectors to Australian Good Manufacturing Practice requirements. Such inspections would be repeated at 2 to 3 yearly intervals.

The electronic process of listing a complementary medicine is a self-assessment by the applicant (sponsor) and carries with it commitments and obligations regarding regulatory compliance, including adverse reaction reporting, maintenance of distribution records, GMP agreements, and holding "evidence" compliant with the guidance described above. The legislated penalties are significant where harm has resulted. The electronic listing facility is supported by a random and targeted post-market review, at which time the product specification, certificate of analysis, table of evidence, and label copy will be assessed for compliance. Failure at that point can result in de-listing from the ARTG.

Promotion of herbal medicines in the mainstream media in Australia is required to be precleared (16). Officers of the respective trade associations have been delegated to perform that function upon application by the advertiser. Advertisements are checked for compliance with the Therapeutic Goods Advertising Code (17) and the corresponding ARTG record for the medicine. A preclearance reference is required to be shown when published.

The Australian regulation of herbal medicines is considered coregulatory. In addition to legislation, and a comparatively low barrier to market entry (cf. pharmaceuticals), sponsors are also held accountable by the multiple complaint mechanisms that exist. Trade associations each have a member Code of Practice. There is also the Complaints Resolution Panel, which is described as "an example of a partnership between government and non-government stakeholders to exercise controls" (18). The membership of the Panel consists of representatives from industry, consumers, advertising agencies, health care professionals, and government. It is chaired by a person elected by the Therapeutic Goods Advertising Code Council. The Complaints Resolution Panel maintains a publicly viewable Complaints log at www.tgacrp.com.au.

The Australian regulatory environment for complementary medicines, including herbal medicines, is constantly being fine-tuned by way of guidance development in concert with industry or by legislative amendment.

CANADA

The following summary is based on an article (19) published in 2003 by Joel B. Taller, a regulatory affairs attorney in Ottawa, Canada; it has been extensively revised to reflect changes since the new Canadian regulatory system became effective.

On January 1, 2004, Canada created a system for the regulation of NHPs, a new regulatory category that includes herbs and herbal preparations, which recognizes the therapeutic activity of this class of goods. However, rather than providing for a separate designation for NHPs in the *Food and Drugs Act* Canada, NHPs were defined to be a subset of drugs. To provide for a more appropriate regulatory model and rather than subsume the evaluation and regulation of NHPs under the existing drug regulations, the Canadian government established *Natural Health Product Regulations* (*NHP Regulations*) (20).

The *NHP Regulations* were published in the *Canada Gazette* (19) as the final regulatory step to control all aspects of the commercialization of NHPs, including their manufacture, importation, labeling, and packaging. NHPs include herbal and botanic supplements in dosage form (e.g., pills, tinctures) and even food formats, such as infused beverages (i.e., herbal teas), depending on the ingredients and claims. A more detailed definition is provided below.

Background

An interesting aspect of the Canadian regulatory situation was stated by the Standing Committee on Health (the "Committee") of the Federal Parliament in its 1998 review of the regulatory framework for NHPs. Noting the complexities of the regulation of NHPs, the Committee stated, "Although we feel the government has a responsibility to protect public health and safety, this should not be applied in a way that unreasonably denies consumers *access* [emphasis added] to products that they perceive to be necessary for their well being. Thus, a balance must be struck between safety and access (21)." Furthermore, the Committee noted, ". . . the framework must allow for more products to be marketed to provide people with that choice."

In the Canadian system, NHPs are regulated by a specially created and separate regulatory entity, the Natural Health Products Directorate (NHPD). The NHPD is at the same level within Health Canada as the Therapeutic Products Directorate, which regulates medical devices and drugs, and the Food Directorate, which regulates food. The intention of the Committee was that the NHPD was to be staffed with individuals with expertise and experience in the field of NHPs, agreeable to both government and NHP stakeholders (e.g., members of the NHPs industry).

NATURAL HEALTH PRODUCT DEFINITION

The definition of an NHP is based on (i) ingredients and (ii) claims (22). For a product to be an NHP, it must first contain the specific substances set out in Schedule 1 of the *NHP Regulations* (i.e., plant or plant material, bacteria, fungi [extracts and isolates of these materials provided there is no change in the molecular structure from that found in nature], certain vitamins, minerals, amino acids, essential fatty acids, and probiotics). Synthetic duplicate versions of these are also included.

In addition to the required ingredients, the NHP must be sold or represented for use in the following situations: (i) the diagnosis, treatment, mitigation, or prevention of a disease, disorder, or abnormal physical state or symptoms in humans; (ii) restoring or correcting organic functions in humans; or (iii) modifying organic functions in humans in a manner that maintains or promotes health. Excluded from the definition of an NHP or from the application of the *NHP Regulations* are prescription and injectable drugs, radiopharmaceuticals, tobacco products, and controlled substances. A health benefit claim is a mandatory requirement for all NHPs.

For example, a product previously marketed as containing 500 mg of St. John's Wort (*Hypericum perforatum*) but without any claim must now include language on its label about the product's health effect or therapeutic benefit.

NATURAL HEALTH PRODUCTS, INCLUDING CONVENTIONAL FOODS

While it is possible for an NHP to be sold in a (conventional) food format, Health Canada has struggled with how to regulate NHPs marketed in this way. A product is "in food format" if it is sold in a format and serving size consistent with food use. Examples include chewing gum, hard candies, candy bars, tea, juices, and other beverage. (The policy does not address the numerous drug products sold in food format, e.g., fruit juice [mineral supplement], chocolate-flavored chews [mineral supplement], frozen treats [cough, cold treatment], and night-time warm beverages [cough, cold treatment].)

For a brief period at the outset, NHPs in a food format were regulated as NHPs, and product license applications (PLAs) (see below) were reviewed as such. But shortly afterward, all reviews of PLAs for NHPs in food format were frozen for more than 2 years; Health Canada then announced that NHPs in food format would remain regulated as NHPs but be reviewed by the Food Directorate, not the NHPD. This resulted in a different set of review criteria being applied to NHPs in food format compared with the review criteria applied to all other NHPs. The difference was met with resistance from the industry.

On March 6, 2009, the NHPD released a new guidance document titled, "Classification of Products at the Food–Natural Health Product Interface: Products in Food Format (23)."

The Food–NHP Classification Committee will adjudicate and classify products in food format based on four criteria (20). The guidance document does not indicate which of these criteria have priority over the others and whether the ultimate classification as a food or NHP will be based on a majority of the four criteria, favoring one classification over the other. In addition, the criteria below appear to be best directed to clear situations, which for the most part is not the case. As such, it is suggested that the decision will continue to be resolved on a case-by-case basis, with little predictability in outcome.

These four criteria are as follows:

1. **Product Composition.** When a product or ingredient is present solely to provide nourishment, nutrition, or hydration or to satisfy hunger, thirst, or a desire for taste, texture, or flavor (typical food attributes), then such criteria are indicative that the product or ingredient is a food. Conversely, if a product is or has an added ingredient that has no known food purpose, and the ingredient has been added for its therapeutic use, then the ingredient or food is likely to be classified as an NHP.
2. **Product Representation.** A product that might, for composition or other reasons, be classified as a food may nonetheless be an NHP if it is represented or sold as a product having therapeutic uses. Claims that provide for a therapeutic use not based on the use of the product as a food suggest the product is an NHP.
3. **Product Format.** Product sold in a manner that lends itself to dosing, that is, sold in single dose units for measured amounts, is an indication that the product is an NHP.

4. **Public Perception and History of Use.** If a product has a historical pattern of use as a food or if public perception is that the product is a food, then these are indications that the product is to be classed as a food. This latter criterion appears to be a general catchall that, if desired, would allow the Food–NHP Classification Committee to classify a product in a food format as a food.

General Overview

The *NHP Regulations* provide for the following regulatory oversight:

1. A premarket review and approval process with respect to all aspects of the NHP, including safety, efficacy, claims, and product specifications;
2. A requirement to manufacture, package, and label NHPs in accordance with appropriate GMPs that apply to both domestically produced and imported NHPs;
3. The requirement for any domestic entity manufacturing, packaging, labeling, and importing NHPs in Canada to hold a site license, including requiring importers to provide evidence to support that the foreign manufacturing, packaging, and/or labeling sites from which it imports, and operate in accordance with equivalent GMPs (a foreign site is not licensed but must be included on the site license of an importer of those NHPs into Canada);
4. The regulatory oversight of the clinical trial process involving NHPs;
5. Requiring specific labeling, which includes a requirement to list each medicinal (active) ingredient in the product together with the amounts found in each dosage unit (one cannot list a proprietary blend without identifying on the label each ingredient in the proprietary blend and the amount of each contained in the product); and
6. A postmarket surveillance program to track and report certain potential adverse reactions.

PRODUCT LICENSE APPLICATION

The Canadian system relies on a premarket approval process in order for the seller of the NHP to obtain a product license. To obtain a product license, an applicant (i.e., a manufacturer, importer, or distributor) must submit a PLA to the NHPD. This application must include sufficient scientific and clinical information to support its safety and efficacy. The primary evidence must consist of human evidence. Animal and/or in vitro studies, while supportive, will not on their own support the approval of a PLA.

The type of evidence submitted will determine the types of claims that can be made in association with the NHP (i.e., a structure/function claim, along the lines of those claims being made for dietary supplements in the United States under DSHEA), risk-reduction (i.e., the reduction of risk of developing a disease, disorder, or abnormal physical state or its symptoms), or therapeutic claims (i.e., diagnosis, treatment, mitigation, or prevention of a disease, disorder, abnormal physical state, or its symptoms). There is theoretically a sliding scale in which the level of evidence required to support both safety and efficacy will vary depending on the nature of the claim (i.e., therapeutic compared with structure/function claims) or the inherent risk associated with the active ingredients. Theoretically, clinical trials are required for only therapeutic claims, while traditional references may suffice for traditional herbals. There have been situations in some NHPD reviews that question whether the NHPD adequately employs this sliding scale, that is, whether it may be more inclined to require at least two human studies to be submitted to support the safety of each medicinal ingredient and at least two human studies to be submitted for at least one medicinal ingredient to support the claims for the NHP.

ISSUANCE OF PRODUCT LICENSE

Following the review of a PLA and assuming the information submitted has been viewed as establishing the safety and efficacy of the NHP, the Minister of Health will issue a product licence and assign a natural product number (NPN) to the NHP.

The *NHP Regulations* provide for an abbreviated review process when the NHP is compliant with a compendium or monograph that has been published by the NHPD. To date (July 2009), NHPD has produced 107 monographs (24) and 15 product monographs (25). These monograph include, but are not limited to, data from previously published authoritative monographs, including the German Commission E Monographs, the monographs from ESCOP, the *British Herbal Pharmacopoeia*, and others. The minister must review and either approve or refuse compendial applications within 60 days. The NHPD will accept as support for the safety and efficacy of certain NHPs' compliance the established Labelling Standards and Category IV Monographs that previously applied to certain NHPs when classed as drugs (26). Only compliance with the NHPD monograph will provide a "fast track" 60-day review.

Predictably, the review process has been slow; for multiingredient products, it can take well more than 3 years. By the end of March 2009, the NHPD had received 36,127 PLAs, of which 22,227 have been dealt with, and of those, 11,007 NPNs were issued. The number of applications rejected by the NHPD appears to be increasing—likely a result of the current review of applications comprising multiple ingredient NHPs for which the applied claims are not limited to traditional use claims.

PHASING IN OF PRODUCT LICENSING

NHPs that had been provincially sold as drugs, with drug identification numbers, are permitted to be sold until December 31, 2009. Before that date, the holder of the drug identification numbers must complete and submit an abridged PLA and receive an NPN. All NHPs sold without a product license after January 1, 2004, while not legal, could continue to be sold without complying with the product licensing provisions in accordance with the NHPD's Compliance Guide and Policy on noncompliant NHPs (the "Compliance Policy"). The intention behind the Compliance Policy was to permit the continuation of the sale of the estimated 50,000 noncompliant NHPs while applicants sought the premarket authorization to sell. It was anticipated that all NHPs must be licensed and otherwise comply with the *NHP Regulations* by March 31, 2010. There has been concern within the industry regarding the actual date when Health Canada will begin enforcing the premarket authorization provisions of the *NHP Regulations*. There remain thousands of applications yet to review, and the concern is that these applications will not be reviewed prior to the March 31, 2010 deadline. In addition, as mentioned previously, it is believed that the standards of evidence an applicant is being asked to meet with respect to safety and efficacy exceed that which is reasonable and what was anticipated by the Committee at the time of the release of its report, which led to the establishment of the NHP category when the initial NHP legislation was passed.

SITE LICENSING (PART 2 OF THE REGULATIONS)

While product licensing deals with the efficacy and safety of the NHP, site licensing is intended to ensure that all levels of manufacturing, packaging, labelling, and importing of an NHP are performed in accordance with GMPs set out in the *NHP Regulations* or an equivalent GMP system. This is achieved by linking the issuance of a site licence to the provision of evidence to support that all regulated activities are conducted in accordance with GMPs. As of January 1, 2006, a site licence is required for all importers, manufacturers, packagers, and labelers of NHPs. The site licence is specific to any building in which any of the regulated activities are carried out. Importers must submit evidence to show that any regulated activities performed outside of Canada have been done in accordance with Canadian GMPs or equivalent GMPs. Evidence of this compliance is reflected on a foreign site annex on the importers' site licence, which refers to each foreign site from which NHPs are imported. To list the foreign site on the foreign site annex, the importer must submit evidence to the NHPD in the form of a quality summary report, with actual records (the same information domestic manufacturers have to supply) showing compliance by the foreign entity with GMPs as set out in the *NHP Regulations* or equivalent GMPs.

GOOD MANUFACTURING PRACTICES (PART 3 OF THE REGULATIONS)

GMPs deal with product specifications, the manufacturing/labelling sites, equipment used in the manufacturing/labelling/storage process, personnel, sanitation, operation procedures, quality assurance, stability, record keeping, sampling, and recall reporting. GMPs are drafted broadly without specificity. The NHPD has issued a GMP guidance document suggesting different ways in which compliance can be achieved (27) as well as a guidance document outlining the testing required to be done on finished products (28).

LABELING AND PACKAGING (PART 5 OF THE REGULATIONS)

Requirements

Section 86 of the *NHP Regulations* states that no person is permitted to "sell a natural health product unless it is labelled and packaged in accordance" with the Regulations. This requirement does not apply to NHPs sold to a manufacturer or distributor.

The information required on the label must be in either English or French with the exception of the following, which must be in French *and* English (29): recommended use or purpose; recommended route or administration; recommended dose; recommended duration of use; and risk information, including cautions, warnings, contraindications, or known adverse reactions.

Section 88 of the *NHP Regulations* states that the information required on an NHP label must be "clearly and prominently displayed; and readily discernible to the purchaser under customary conditions of purchase and use."

If there is only one label, then all the required information must be shown on that label.

Subject to the provisions for small container sizes, the inner and outer label must show the following information on the principal display panel (30): the brand name; the product number; the dosage form; if the product is sterile, the words "Sterile" and "Stérile"; the net amount of the immediate container in terms of weight, measure or number; and on any other panel (31): the name and address of the product licence holder; if the product is imported, the name and address of the importer; the proper name and the common name of each medicinal ingredient; the strength or potency of each medicinal ingredient as contained in each dosage unit; recommended use or purpose; recommended route of administration; recommended dose; recommended duration of use, if any; risk information including any cautions, warnings, contraindications, or known adverse reactions associated with the product's use; recommended storage conditions; lot number; expiry (expiration) date; and a description of the source material of each medicinal ingredient.

In addition to the prescribed content for the inner and outer labels, the outer label must show (32) a list of all nonmedicinal ingredients contained in the NHP and, if the product contains mercury or any of its salts or derivatives, a quantitative list by proper name that sets out all preservatives contained in the product.

As many NHPs are sold in small packages, the *NHP Regulations* provide that if the container is too small to accommodate an inner label with all the required information, the inner label may contain limited information (33).

GERMANY

Herbal products have a long tradition in Germany. Germany is probably the best example of how a modern industrialized nation can develop a system to evaluate the safety and efficacy of herbal preparations used for medicinal purposes. Depending on the category in which herbal products enter the health market, they need to comply with a variety of national rules and regulations.

- Herbal medicinal products (phytomedicines) are required to comply with the German Medicines Act (Arzneimittelgesetz [AMG]) (34) and need to be registered with and authorized by the Federal Institute for Drugs and Medical Devices (*Bundesamt für Arzneimittel und Medizinprodukte* [BfArM]) before being placed on the market. The same procedure applies to THMPs in accordance with the EU guidelines 2001/83/EG (35) and 2004/24/EG (36).
- Herbal food supplements are regulated by the German Food and Feed Code (*Lebensmittel-Bedarfsgegenstande-und Futtermittelgesetzbuch* [LFGB]) (37) and the Food Supplement Code (*Nahrungsergänzungsmittelverordnung* [NemV]) (38) and require notification from the Federal Office of Consumer Protection and Food Safety (*Bundesamt für Verbraucherschutz und Lebensmittelsicherheit* [BVL]).
- Herbal dietary products are regulated by the German Food and Feed Code and the German Regulations on Foods for Special Dietary Uses (*Verordnung über diätetische Lebensmittel* [DiätV]) (39) and require notification from the Federal Office of Consumer Protection and Food Safety.
- Marketing of herbal novel foods is regulated by the German Food and Feed Code (37) and the Novel Food Regulation (40, 41) and requires authorization or notification from the Federal Institute for Risk Assessment (*Bundesinstitut für Risikobewertung* [BfR]) and the European Commission.

A comprehensive German medicines act—superseding a variety of specific rules and regulations—was introduced in 1961 in accordance with the Treaties of Rome of 1957. These required national drug laws in a move toward harmonization of European legislation. This law made registration of industrially manufactured drugs obligatory and regulated manufacturing in industry and pharmacies. It did not, however, regulate the evaluation of efficacy and safety, which was left as the responsibility of the respective manufacturers. The revision of the German Medicines Act of 1976 (42) met stricter regulations and guidelines on a European level and henceforth included evaluation of drugs for quality, safety, and efficacy. At this point in time, the number of HMPs in the German market is estimated to have been around 20,000. Thus, phytotherapy, homeopathy, and anthroposophy[3] were explicitly incorporated into the medicines act. A transitory period of 12 years was introduced to give manufacturers the opportunity for "postregistering" their products in accordance with the new regulations.

To accommodate for the specifics of these "nonallopathic" forms of therapy, scientific and empirical evidence was to be evaluated by ad hoc established expert bodies: Commission C for anthroposophic, Commission D for homeopathic, Commission E for HMPs, and a commission for traditional medicinal products according to §109a AMG (43). During the registration and "postregistration" process, more than 2,400 HMPs were positively evaluated in accordance with the 1976 drug law, comprising about 1,900 mono preparations and more than 500 combinations.

"Post-registration" of HMPs was introduced in 1978. For products based on known substances, it required full documentation of quality for ingredients and final products. With regard to safety and efficacy, however, the manufacturer was permitted to refer to the findings of the relevant commission of experts, the Commission E Monographs. Some 380 monographs for herbal substances, mono preparations, and fixed combinations were published in the *Federal Gazette* (*Bundesanzeiger*) from 1980 to 1994. In 1998, these monographs were translated, cross-referenced, and published by the nonprofit American Botanic Council as a book (44) and as a database available on the American Botanic Council Web site (www.herbalgram.org). The Commission E produced monographs until 1994, at which time its role was changed to one of an advisory capacity to the BfArM. This was mainly because the development of national monographs by individual countries in the EU gave way to a more pan-European model where herbal drugs (as well as conventional drugs) are now reviewed and assessed by the EMEA.

While the Commission E monographs represented all available scientific evidence at the time of publication, they did not set quality standards, nor did they get updated post 1994 or include reference bibliographies. This work has been continued by Kooperation Phytopharmaka, but has since been superseded by the publication of ESCOP monographs, and recently, by EMEA's community monographs. Herbal monographs including quality standards, however, can also be found in the *German Pharmacopoeia* and its supplements (*Deutsches Arzneibuch* [DAB] and Ergänzungsbücher [EB]), the *German Drug Codex* (*Deutscher Arzneimittel Codex* [DAC]), as well as the *European Pharmacopoeia*.

A simplified "postregistration" procedure was established for herbal medicines with a long tradition of use in 1994. Manufacturers were required to document the traditional use of these products with bibliographical evidence. Documentations were evaluated by the §109a commission (see above), which compiled a list of substances and substance combinations approved for specific indications. Claims and labeling had to explicitly reflect the fact that efficacy of these products was based on experience and tradition only.

Recently, with the ratification of the European guideline on traditional herbal medicines and its inclusion into the German Medicines Act (§§39a–d) (45–48) in 2005, herbal medicines can be registered in a simplified procedure as THMPs,

---

[3]Anthroposophy or anthroposophic medicine (AM) is a "complementary system of medicine founded by Rudolf Steiner and Ita Wegman, which includes active (AM art and eurhythmy therapy) as well as passive therapy modalities (massage, medications, and herbal and dietary supplements)." (Hamre H, Witt C, Kien G. Anthroposophic therapy for children with chronic disease: a two-year prospective cohort study in routine outpatient settings. *BMC Pediatrics* 2009;9:39. doi:10.1186/1471-2431-9-39.)

including those containing vitamins and/or mineral, if they have been used traditionally for at least 30 years, 15 of which must have been in the EU. Manufacturers have to present a quality dossier and bibliographic summaries for safety and plausibility of pharmacological actions or efficacy. Previous registrations as traditional herbal medicines in accordance with §109 AMG expire in 2011, unless licensing or registration documentations have been submitted to BfArM before January 2009.

The total number of HMPs in the German market that are either registered or obtained postmarketing approval is around 2,400—1,900 mono preparations and 500 fixed combinations. In addition, there are some 2,500 homeopathic and anthroposophic products available (49).

Herbal medicinal products can be marketed in Germany as either nonprescription OTC or as prescription medicines. Before the reform of the German health care system in 2004, the majority of herbal medicines were available by prescription (as well as nonprescription) and thus eligible for reimbursement by the public health insurance system. Reimbursement was abolished for all herbal medicines except standardized preparations of ginkgo (*Ginkgo biloba*), Hypericum (aka St. John's Wort, *H. perforatum*), and mistletoe (*Viscum album*), which led to a significant drop in prescriptions being issued. The total value of herbal medicines sold in Germany in 2008 was about one billion euros, which amounts to 36% of all nonprescription sales. Seventy-three percent of the German population use herbal medicines either regularly or occasionally, the majority for cough and cold-related indications (50).

Under the German Medicines Act, medicinal products can principally be sold only in a pharmacy (*Apotheke*). Prescription-only status is determined in consideration of drug safety, that is, potential health hazards or abuse. However, under certain conditions nonprescription (e.g., sometimes available over-the-counter) sales are permitted in retail drugstores (*Drogerie*), supermarkets, and health-food stores but only for those medicines that are prophylactic or intended for treatment of minor health disorders. OTC sales outside pharmacies are permitted only if the sales outlet employs personnel with the required and obligatory expert training and knowledge.

TRADITIONAL HERBAL MEDICINAL PRODUCTS IN THE EUROPEAN UNION

Until 2004, most HMPs sold in the EU required authorization to be sold as drugs or, depending on national laws and requirements, were marketed unlicensed altogether. Because of the premarket approval requirements of such, this process excluded many herbal preparations that have been used traditionally in Europe as well as those traditional herbal products that have found increased popularity in Europe in the past 20 to 30 years, for example, herbal formulations based on Traditional Chinese Medicine.

EU Directive 2001/83/EC (51) determines that no medicinal product may be placed on the market without having obtained a marketing authorization. The application for such a marketing authorization must contain the results of laboratory tests on quality and pharmacology as well as clinical trials on safety and efficacy of the product. However, data relating to safety and efficacy need not be presented where it can be demonstrated by detailed references to published scientific literature that the product has a well-established medicinal use (in Article 10(1)(a)(ii) of Directive 2001/83/EC, as defined in Part 3 of Annex I to Directive 2003/63/EC) (52).

For many HMPs, however, sufficient published scientific data are not available to demonstrate a well-established medicinal use, despite the fact that they have been used for a long period of time.

EU regulators found themselves faced with the rising popularity and regular usage of unlicensed herbal medicines, and, correspondingly, an increasing number of reports of adverse drug reactions. While many unlicensed herbal medicines were already made to reasonable and even full GMP standards, without some form of approval by a regulatory body, consumers could not identify which products are manufactured to acceptable standards. These concerns led to the EU Directive on Traditional Herbal Medicinal Products (THMPD).

The following are the key regulatory steps that evolved to create the procedure for the registration as THMPs; this procedure is incorporated into the process of harmonization within the EU, thus applying to all EU nations (53–55):

- Directive 1999/83/EC of 8 September 1999 with regard to "well-established use" (56)
- Directive 2003/63/EC of 25 June 2003, an updated Annex I to Directive 2001/83/EC with specific provisions for HMPs for "well-established" use (52)
- Directive 2004/24/EC of 31 March 2004 introducing the simplified registration of THMPs (37)
- Regulation 726/2004/EC of 31 March 2004 establishing the Committee on Herbal Medicinal Products (HMPC) (57)

The main purpose of the HMPC is to ensure the safe use of HMPs by patients and to facilitate access to safe HMPs. It establishes community herbal monographs (58) and entries to the "list of herbal substances, preparations and combinations thereof for use in traditional medicinal products" (59). Furthermore, the Committee has issued a number of procedural and regulatory documents as well as scientific guidelines for various aspects of HMP development, documentation, and registration, such as quality, safety, etc.

In 2004, Directive 2004/24/EC (THMPD) introduced a new pathway for marketing THMPs—the "simplified registration"—whereby manufacturers of good quality herbal medicines can register their products as actual medicines, rather than classifying them as food supplements, thus allowing them to make restricted medicinal claims. The registration scheme will help protect public health by requiring specific standards of safety and quality for traditional herbal medicines in contrast to unlicensed products.

The normal requirement for conventional medicines to be proven as efficacious, as required under Directive 2001/83/EC, is now replaced for THMPs by a requirement to produce bibliographic or expert evidence on the "safety" of the herbal medicine or "corresponding" (i.e., comparable) product(s) by providing bibliographic evidence of a minimum of 30 years of traditional use for the product, of which at least 15 of the 30 years must have been within the EU. Thus, adequate evidence of traditional use replaces the requirement to demonstrate efficacy.

The requirement of medicinal use to be shown for 30 years can also be satisfied where the number or quantity of ingredients has been reduced over that period of time. Where the product complies with a community monograph or the ingredient(s) listed in the community list as established by the HMPC (58, 59), the requirement to demonstrate traditional use is removed.

According to Directive 2004/24/EC, corresponding products are those that have the same active ingredients, the same or similar intended purpose, the same or similar route of administration, and equivalent strength. Directive 2004/24/EC also states that a corresponding product "is characterized by having the same active ingredients, irrespective of the excipients used, the same or similar intended purpose, equivalent strength and posology [dosage regimen] and the same or similar route of administration as the medicinal product applied for." Moreover, article 16c (3) outlined that the requirements to show medicinal use throughout the period of 30 years are satisfied "if the number or quantity of ingredients of the medicinal product has been reduced during that period." Thus, traditional use of an herbal combination can be documented with corresponding products that contain more active ingredients than the product applied for.

THMPs may exist as mono preparations but also as combinations of several herbal substances/preparations and/or vitamins and minerals. These are products with one single herbal substance or herbal preparation that will be found in community herbal monographs and on the list of herbal substances, preparations, and combinations thereof for use in traditional medicinal products.

Under THMPD, the herbal product must comply with the normal rigorous quality standards required for all other medicines with a marketing authorization. It must therefore be manufactured under GMP, and pharmacovigilance (i.e., adverse event reporting) requirements apply. As for any other nonprescription medicine, patient information must be provided along with a statement on the label and in advertisements that the medicinal claim and indications are based on traditional use only (60, 61).

UNITED KINGDOM

There has been little formal regulation of the practice of herbal medicine in the United Kingdom. In British legislature (applying to England, Wales, Scotland, and Northern Ireland and also in part to former colonies like Australia, New Zealand, and Canada), rights of common law have prevailed in individual's choice of health care. Under these ancient rights, health care is a personal choice and, unlike most other modern countries, there has been no licensing or other proscription of activities for those providing herbal medicine. Until 1968, the only statutory regulation of this practice dates back to an Act of Parliament signed by King Henry VIII in 1542 (sometimes referred to as *The Herbalists' Charter* or even *The Quacks' Charter* in some histories of medicine). This Act has, however, little relevance to modern times.

The Medicines Act of 1968 was the first legislation in modern times to regulate the supply of herbal remedies, though even here there was almost no reference to practice itself. In the subsequent conversion of UK with European law, this Act has become progressively superseded by European Union directive 65/65/EC (62) and in turn by its successor 2001/83/EC (51). This has led to progressive reduction of earlier opportunities to supply herbal remedies in the United Kingdom.

Under the 1968 regulations, there were two regulatory avenues for herbal medicines to be marketed: (i) "licensed herbal medicines" and (ii) "herbal remedies exempt from licensing." Around 600 herbal products in retail trade in 1971 successfully achieved licensed status ("marketing authorization") by 1990. Medicinal claims are allowed for such licensed herbal medicines. The Medicines and Healthcare products Regulatory Agency enforces the same GMPs rules for licensed herbal medicines as those required for conventional pharmaceutical medicines. Enforcement is conducted via the licensing and inspection of manufacturing facilities. Safety requirements for licensed herbal medicines are the same as those for conventional pharmaceutical drugs. Under the Medicines Act, manufacturers were able to establish efficacy based on bibliographic evidence of established use.

Herbal preparations can claim exemption from licensing requirements if they adhere to criteria established in Section 12 of the 1968 Act. This permits either the sale without labeled medicinal claims or even branding (section 12.2) or supply on a one-to-one basis by one individual to another (section 12.1). Herbal practitioners have been able to maintain their common law protection under section 12.1, although this did not define herbal practice itself.

Previously, unlicensed herbal remedies were not required to comply with any specific requirements of quality or safety. However, in 2004 the EU passed the Traditional Herbal Medicinal Products Directive (THMPD; 2004/24/EC) (37), which raised the regulatory requirements for such unlicensed herbal products. This includes the introduction of a simplified *registration* process (not licensure) in which THMPs will be required to comply with the same specific standards of quality and safety as those for licensed HMPs. However, instead of requiring a conventional drug standard for efficacy, THMPs will merely have to demonstrate history of traditional use (30 years worldwide; 15 years use in the United Kingdom).

Licensed HMPs must comply with compendial quality standards, ideally those published in the *European Pharmacopoeia*, which currently has almost 200 monographs for HMPs published or in preparation. The *British Herbal Pharmacopoeia*, revised from the original 1983 version in 1996 by the British Herbal Medicine Association, an industry trade group, also contains quality monographs for 169 herbal materials, serving as quality guidelines on a voluntary basis (63).

In 1996, unlicensed herbal medicines were included in the United Kingdom's national postmarketing surveillance system (the pharmacovigilance and adverse event reporting system for medicines, established in 1964), which already also included licensed herbal medicines as a part of the licensure process.

In the United Kingdom, herbal medicines are sold in pharmacies as prescription and nonprescription medicines and in other retail outlets without restriction. They are also supplied by practitioners.

The final enactment of the THMPD in 2011 will see the effective end of the herbal practitioner exemption (section 12.1) under the 1968 Act. In anticipation of this, there is a concerted process to statutorily regulate (or license) herbal practitioners and allow them to supply herbal products as "authorized health professionals" in European terms. Herbalists can already receive extensive professional training at one of five universities offering degrees in herbal medicine and may then join one of the professional bodies currently seeking registration through the European Herbal & Traditional Medicine Practitioners Association (EHTPA: www.ehtpa.eu).

ACKNOWLEDGMENTS

The first author gratefully acknowledges Ms. Courtney Cavaliere, managing editor of *HerbalGram*, the journal of the American Botanic Council, whose article on the WHO international regulations survey provides the basis for the WHO section of this chapter. Also, Simon Y. Mills for his review and edits of the section on the United Kingdom.

References

1. World Health Organization. *National Policy on Traditional Medicine and Regulation of Herbal Medicines: Report of a WHO Global Survey*. Geneva: World Health Organization; 2005. http://whqlibdoc.who.int/publications/2005/9241593237.pdf. Accessed April 27, 2006.
2. World Health Organization. Executive Summary: *National Policy on Traditional Medicine and Regulation of Herbal Medicines: Report of a WHO Global Survey*. Geneva: World Health Organization; 2005:iii–vii.
3. Cavaliere C. WHO surveys worldwide patterns of herbal regulations. *HerbalGram* 2006;71:58–59.
4. Therapeutic Goods Administration. Australian register of therapeutic goods medicines. http://www.ebs.tga.gov.au/ebs/ANZTPAR/PublicWeb.nsf/cuMedicines?OpenView.
5. Therapeutic Goods Administration. The regulation of complementary medicines in Australia—an overview. http://www.tga.gov.au/cm/cmreg-aust.htm. Published April 2006.
6. Therapeutic Goods Advertising Code Council. Appendix 6. www.tgacc.com.au.
7. Therapeutic Goods Administration. Therapeutic Goods Regulations 1990. http://www.comlaw.gov.au/comlaw/management.nsf/lookupindexpagesbyid/IP200400127?OpenDocument.
8. Therapeutic Goods Administration. Substances that may be used in listed medicines in Australia. http://www.tga.gov.au/cm/listsubs.htm. Published December 12, 2007.
9. Food Standards Australia New Zealand. Australia New Zealand Food Standards Code. http://www.foodstandards.gov.au/thecode/foodstandardscode/. Published 2009.
10. New Zealand Dietary Supplements Regulations 1985 (SR 1985/208) (September 3, 2007). http://www.legislation.govt.nz/regulation/public/1985/0208/latest/link.aspx?search=ts_regulation_dietary_resel&p=1.
11. Therapeutic Goods Administration. Australian regulatory guidelines for complementary medicines (ARGCM). http://www.tga.gov.au/docs/html/argcm.htm.
12. Therapeutic Goods Administration. Therapeutic goods order No. 69 (general requirements for labels for medicines labelling order). http://www.tga.gov.au/docs/html/tgo/tgo69.htm. Published September 12, 2001.
13. Therapeutic Goods Administration. Guidelines for levels and kinds of evidence to support indications and claims. http://www.tga.gov.au/docs/html/tgaccevi.htm. Published October 2001.
14. Therapeutic Goods Administration. Guidance on equivalence of herbal extracts. http://www.tga.gov.au/cm/drequiv.pdf. Published November 2007.
15. Therapeutic Goods Administration. eBS Australian register of therapeutic goods; Australian approved manufacturers. http://www.ebs.tga.gov.au/ebs/MIS/bluebook.nsf/AustralianManufacturers?OpenView.
16. Therapeutic Goods Administration. Advertising medicines to consumers. http://www.tga.gov.au/docs/html/advmed.htm.
17. Therapeutic Goods Administration. Therapeutic Goods Advertising Code 2007. http://www.comlaw.gov.au/ComLaw/Legislation/LegislativeInstrument1.nsf/all/search/F767C1377721F31CCA257291001B8CDA?OpenDocument.
18. Complaints Resolution Panel. About US. http://www.tgacrp.com.au/index.cfm?pageID=2.
19. Taller JB. Canada issues final natural health product regulations. *HerbalGram*. 2003;60:62–65. http://cms.herbalgram.org/herbalgram/issue60/article2599.html.
20. Natural Health Products Regulations, S.O.R. [Statutory Orders and Regulations]/2003-196.
21. Health Canada, Standing Committee on Health. *Natural Health Products: A New Vision*. 1998:69. available at Health Canada Guidance Documents at http://www.hc-sc.gc.ca/dhp-mps/prodnatur/legislation/docs/index-eng.php
22. Natural Health Products Regulations, S.O.R. [Statutory Orders and Regulations]/2003-196, S.1.

23. Health Canada. Classification of products at the food-natural health product interface: products in food formats. http://www.hc-sc.gc.ca/dhp-mps/prodnatur/legislation/docs/food-nhp-aliments-psn-guide-eng.php. Published March 2009.
24. Health Canada. Drugs and health products. Single ingredient monographs. http://www.hc-sc.gc.ca/dhp-mps/prodnatur/applications/licen-prod/monograph/mono_list-eng.php.
25. Health Canada. Product monographs. http://www.hc-sc.gc.ca/dhp-mps/prodnatur/applications/licen-prod/monograph/product_mono_produit-eng.php.
26. Health Canada. A summary of NHP/DRUG classification of TPD category IV labelling standards ingredients. http://www.hc-sc.gc.ca/dhp-mps/prodnatur/applications/licen-prod/monograph/list_mono4-eng.php.
27. Health Canada. Good manufacturing practices guidance document. Version 2.0. http://www.hc-sc.gc.ca/dhp-mps/prodnatur/legislation/docs/gmp-bpf-eng.php. Published August 2006.
28. Natural Health Products Directorate. Evidence for quality of finished natural health products. Version 2. http://www.hc-sc.gc.ca/dhp-mps/prodnatur/legislation/docs/eq-paq-eng.php. Published June 2007.
29. Natural Health Products Regulations, S.O.R. [Statutory Orders and Regulations]/2003-196, s. 93(1)b.
30. Natural Health Products Regulations, S.O.R. [Statutory Orders and Regulations]/2003-196, s. 93(1)(a).
31. Natural Health Products Regulations, S.O.R. [Statutory Orders and Regulations]/2003-196, s. 93(1)(b).
32. Natural Health Products Regulations, S.O.R. [Statutory Orders and Regulations]/2003-196, s. 93(2).
33. Natural Health Products Regulations, S.O.R. [Statutory Orders and Regulations]/2003-196, s. 94(1)(1).
34. German Medicines Act [*Gesetz Über Den Verkehr Mit Arzneimitteln*]. http://bundesrecht.juris.de/amg_1976/index.html.
35. Directive 2001/83/EC of the European Parliament and of the Council of 6 November 2001 on the Community code relating to medicinal products for human use. http://eur-lex.europa.eu/LexUriServ/LexUriServ.do?uri = CONSLEG:2001L0083:20070126:EN:PDF.
36. Directive 2004/24/EC of the European Parliament and of the Council of 31 March 2004 amending, as regards traditional herbal medicinal products, Directive 2001/83/EC on the Community code relating to medicinal products for human use. http://eur-lex.europa.eu/LexUriServ/LexUriServ.do?uri=OJ:L:2004:136:0085:0090:EN:PDF.
37. German Food and Feed Code. [*Lebensmittel-Bedarfsgegenstande-und Futtermittelgesetzbuch*]. http://bundesrecht.juris.de/bundesrecht/lfgb/gesamt.pdf.
38. German Food Supplement Code. [*Nahrungsergänzungsmittelverordnung*] http://bundesrecht.juris.de/bundesrecht/nemv/gesamt.pdf.
39. German Regulations on Foods for Special Dietary Uses [*Verordnung Über Diätetische Lebensmittel*]. http://bundesrecht.juris.de/bundesrecht/di_tv/gesamt.pdf.
40. Regulation (EC) No 258/97 of the European Parliament and of the Council of 27 January 1997 concerning novel foods and novel food ingredients. http://eur-lex.europa.eu/smartapi/cgi/sga_doc?smartapi!celexapi!prod!CELEXnumdoc&lg=EN&numdoc=31997R0258&model=guichett.
41. Commission Recommendation of 29 July 1997 concerning the scientific aspects and the presentation of information necessary to support applications for the placing on the market of novel foods and novel food ingredients and the preparation of initial assessment reports under Regulation (EC) No 258/97 of the European Parliament and of the Council (Text with EEA relevance) (97/618/EC). http://eur-lex.europa.eu/smartapi/cgi/

sga_doc?smartapi!celexapi!prod!CELEXnumdoc&lg=EN&numdoc=31997H0618&model=guichett.

42. German Medicines Act of 1976. [Arzneimittelgesetz – AMG]. http://bundesrecht.juris.de/bundesrecht/amg_1976/gesamt.pdf.
43. §109a AMG [German Medicines Act]. http://www.jusline.de/index.php?cpid=f92f99b766343e040d46fcd6b03d3ee8&lawid=207&paid=109a.
44. Blumenthal M, Busse WR, Hall T, et al., eds. Klein S, Rister R (trans). *The Complete German Commission E Monographs—Therapeutic Guide to Herbal Medicines*. Boston: Integrative Medicine Communications; 1998. www.herbalgram.org.
45. §39a AMG. [German Medicines Act]. http://www.jusline.de/index.php?cpid=f92f99b766343e040d46fcd6b03d3ee8&lawid=207&paid=39a.
46. §39b AMG. [German Medicines Act]. http://www.jusline.de/index.php?cpid=f92f99b766343e040d46fcd6b03d3ee8&lawid=207&paid=39b&mvpa=53.
47. §39c AMG. [German Medicines Act]. http://www.jusline.de/index.php?cpid=f92f99b766343e040d46fcd6b03d3ee8&lawid=207&paid=39c&mvpa=54.
48. §39d AMG. [German Medicines Act]. http://www.jusline.de/index.php?cpid=f92f99b766343e040d46fcd6b03d3ee8&lawid=207&paid=39d&mvpa=55.
49. Bundesinstitut für Arzneimittel und Medizinprodukte [German Federal Institute for Drugs and Medical Devices]. Statistics of Division "Licensing 5." http://www.bfarm.de/cln_028/nn_1049954/EN/drugs/2__Authorisation/types/pts/statistics__licenses.html.
50. Gesundheitsberichterstattung des Bundes. Pflanzliche Arzneimittel. [German Federal Government Health Report. Plant Drugs] http://www.gbe-bund.de/oowa921-install/servlet/oowa/aw92/dboowasys921.xwdevkit/xwd_init?gbe.isgbetol/xs_start_neu/365244046/66180411.
51. Directive 2001/83/EC of the European Parliament and of the Council of 6 November 2001 on the Community code relating to medicinal products for human use (consolidated text). http://www.emea.europa.eu/pdfs/human/pmf/2001-83-EC.pdf.
52. Commission Directive 2003/63/EC of 25 June 2003 amending Directive 2001/83/EC of the European Parliament and of the Council on the Community code relating to medicinal products for human use. http://www.emea.europa.eu/pdfs/human/pmf/2003-63-EC.pdf.
53. Keller K. Die europäische Direktive zu traditionellen pflanzlichen Arzneimitteln. [The European directive on traditional herbal drugs]. *Bundesgesundheitsbl-Gesundheitsforsch-Gesundheitsschutz* 2003;46:1046–1049.
54. Vlietinck AJ. New European legislation for herbal medicinal products (HMPs)—new opportunities for African pharmaceutical industries? Presentation at Africa Herbal Anti-malarial Meeting organized by World Agroforestry Centre (ICRAF) and Association for the Promotion of traditional medicine (PROMETRA), Nairobi, Kenya. March 20–22, 2006.
55. Knöss W, Stolte F, Reh K. Europäische Gesetzgebung zu besonderen Therapierichtungen. [The regulatory framework for complementary and alternative medicines in Europe.] *Bundesgesundheitsbl-Gesundheitsforsch-Gesundheitsschutz* 2008;51:771–778.
56. Directive 1999/83/EC of 8 September 1999 amending the Annex to Council Directive 75/318/EEC on the approximation of the laws of the Member States relating to analytical, pharmacotoxicological and clinical standards and protocols in respect of the testing of medicinal products. http://eur-lex.europa.eu/LexUriServ/LexUriServ.do?uri=OJ:L:1999:243:0009:0011:EN:PDF.
57. Regulation 726/2004/EC of the European Parliament and of the Council of 31 March 2004 laying down Community procedures for the authorisation and supervision of medicinal products for human and veterinary use and establishing a European Medicines Agency. http://ec.europa.eu/enterprise/pharmaceuticals/eudralex/vol-1/reg_2004_726/reg_2004_726_en.pdf.

58. European Medicines Evaluation Agency. HMPC community herbal monographs. http://www.emea.europa.eu/htms/human/hmpc/hmpcmonographs.htm.
59. European Medicines Evaluation Agency. HMPC community list. http://www.emea.europa.eu/htms/human/hmpc/hmpclist.htm.
60. Vlietinck AJ, Pieters L, Apers S. Legal requirements for the quality of herbal substances and herbal preparations for the manufacturing of herbal medicinal products in the European Union. *Planta Medica* 2009. DOI 10.1055/s-0029-1185307.
61. Brendler T, Phillips LD, Spiess S. *A Practical Guide to Licensing Herbal Medicinal Products*. London: Pharmaceutical Press; 2009.
62. The Council of the European Economic Community. Directive 65/65 EC. Council Directive 65/65/EEC of 26 January 1965 on the approximation of provisions laid down by Law, Regulation or Administrative Action relating to proprietary medicinal products. http://www.ikev.org/docs/eu/365L0065.htm.
63. British Herbal Medicine Association. *British Herbal Pharmacopoeia*. Bournemouth, England: BHMA; 1996.

CHAPTER 19

The Role of Industry

Carolyn Sabatini

THE CHALLENGE

For many health care practitioners and their patients, navigating the world of dietary supplements can be an enormous challenge. Common hurdles include

- Understanding dietary supplement regulations and marketing guidelines
- The vast array of product offerings
- The growing body of science exploring nutrient benefits and limits
- Limited patient disclosure of dietary supplement use
- Lack of trusted resources for professionals and patients
- Lack of familiarity with reputable products, brands, and companies

Your patients enter the office armed with the latest news reports or recommendations from family and friends, making your role in determining which products are individually appropriate even more crucial. Added to these challenges is the variety of choices among different dietary supplement brands that are sold at numerous types of outlets such as

- Retail stores (food, drug, mass and club stores)
- Health food stores
- Internet
- Direct to consumer/multilevel
- Health practitioners' offices

THE GOOD NEWS

Industry self-regulation efforts have increased in recent years addressing product certification efforts and product advertising. More recently, increased enforcement by the Food and Drug Administration (FDA) and the Federal Trade Commission (FTC) of existing laws has helped differentiate responsible companies from those unwilling to abide by the law.

More Good News

In June 2007, the FDA released the dietary supplement Good Manufacturing Practices (GMPs). By 2010 all companies, regardless of size, will be required to follow the GMP guidelines, which cover manufacturing safeguards and extensive quality, equipment, and record-keeping requirements for dietary supplement manufacturers. Large companies such as Pharmavite are required to be in compliance by June 2008. Many companies such as Pharmavite have been following similar voluntary guidelines for many years.

In this chapter, you will read how one dietary supplement company, Pharmavite LLC, approaches the business of dietary supplements. You will learn how this company views its responsibility to the industry, to its consumers, and to health care practitioners. Pharmavite sells its Nature Made® brand products through retail stores—food, drug, mass and club stores, and select online retail outlets.

HOW CAN WE HELP

The purpose of this chapter is to provide you with information to help you answer these questions:

- What should my patients know before choosing a dietary supplement?
- How should my patients select reputable brands?
- What resources are available to me as a health care professional and to my patients?

Pharmavite is a leader in best practices and joins many other reputable manufacturers in the industry who sell products through various distribution channels. The industry has a long record of safety and a strong future in the preventive health care field. To be considered a responsible manufacturer, a company should

- offer scientifically supported products with substantiated product claims.
- develop and manufacture products to the highest quality and safety standards (e.g., FDA GMPs or beyond).
- provide quality process control from the beginning of the manufacturing process to the end—not "tested-in" afterward.
- market and promote products that abide by legal and ethical guidelines.
- educate health care professionals and consumers about the benefits of dietary supplements, the role of supplements in the diet, the state of the science, and important appropriate cautions.
- be proactive in advocacy and self-regulation.
- provide easy access for consumers and health care professionals via 800# and a Web site.

A PHARMAVITE SNAPSHOT

For more than 35 years, Pharmavite has been considered a leader in the wellness industry, manufacturing high-quality vitamins, minerals, herbs, and other dietary supplements, under its Nature Made brand name. As a result, the Nature Made brand is trusted by retailers and consumers and has become the nation's number one best-selling brand of vitamins, minerals, herbs, and supplements in food, drug, mass, and club stores.

For more than 25 years, Pharmavite has worked closely with the premier industry trade association, the Council for Responsible Nutrition, to foster the highest industry standards and encourage an industry climate of the highest integrity. Since

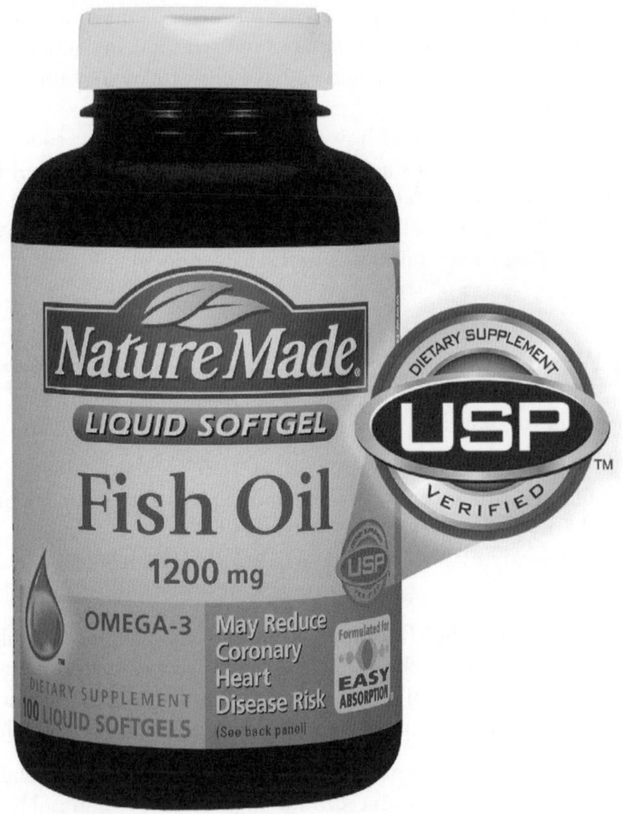

Figure 19.1 • Fish Oil Supplement with USP label.

1994, Pharmavite has advocated for the release of GMPs by the FDA. While waiting for its publication (June 2007), Pharmavite was the first to participate and be certified in the United States Pharmacopeia's (USP) Dietary Supplement Verification Program—a standard-setting program developed by the nearly 200-year-old, nonprofit organization. The Nature Made brand currently has more than 90 products certified which carry the USP seal (Fig. 19.1).

Beyond its primary focus developing and marketing consumer products, Pharmavite also invests in programs which support

- Retailers—with award-winning category management and education programs
- Consumers—with online education resources and detailed product information available at NatureMade.com and access to attentive and knowledgeable Consumer Affairs representatives at 800-276-2878.
- Health care professionals—with online, live, and print educational resources Pharmavite's parent company, Otsuka Pharmaceutical Co. Ltd., is a global health care company dedicated to the research and development of innovative medical, pharmaceutical, and nutritional consumer products. One of the largest privately held firms in the world, Otsuka has a presence in 15 countries, employs more than 22,000 individuals, and operates 17 research facilities worldwide.

Through this international network, Otsuka and Pharmavite share a vision to enhance the quality of human life.

The following is an overview of the key components of Pharmavite's commitment to produce and provide safe, high-quality dietary supplements.

PRODUCTS: FROM CONCEPT THROUGH RESEARCH AND DEVELOPMENT

From start to finish, Pharmavite is committed to offering safe, science-based supplements that work. The product development process begins by looking at today's scientific findings and how they can be transformed into tomorrow's innovative products. The entire product development process involves a cross-functional team, which includes representatives from scientific affairs, marketing, regulatory affairs, production, purchasing, and an independent Scientific Advisory Board. A new product can originate from a variety of sources. Pharmavite may tap into the knowledge banks of its parent company. It also seeks input from its Scientific Advisory Board, whose members represent a variety of health and nutrition-based disciplines at leading universities. Key insights from nutrition thought leaders at distinguished institutions provide new product ideas from emerging science and supply chain partners continuously present new ingredients and technologies.

The scientific data supporting ingredients and potential products are then analyzed. This data can include randomized controlled clinical trials as well as large observational studies. Pharmavite is also involved with advancing science by providing product for various government and educational institutions' clinical trials.

Once a potential product has gained approval from this cross-functional team, Pharmavite begins to develop product formulations and testing methods at its advanced research and development laboratory. This laboratory houses some of the industry's most sophisticated analytical equipment. Here, small-scale tablet and capsule machines enable researchers to mirror full-scale production runs.

Products that do not meet adequate safety or scientific criteria are not approved for development. Concepts supported by solid science are earmarked for development and undergo a series of stability and consumer and quality assurance (QA)/quality control (QC) testing before commercialization.

ENSURING QUALITY AND SAFETY

Once a product receives approval for commercialization, quality and safety continue to be the top priority. Pharmavite's production facilities include more than 600,000 square feet of manufacturing, packaging, distribution, and research and development space in four state-of-the-art facilities in San Fernando and Valencia, California. Through these facilities, more than 11.5 billion tablets, capsules, and softgels are produced annually.

The quality department works with manufacturing, packaging, technical operations, research and development, procurement, regulatory affairs, and marketing to ensure consumer satisfaction with all products.

Pharmavite adheres to manufacturing guidelines recommended by the USP and FDA's recently released GMP guidelines and has a core quality and technical unit responsible for QA, QC and technical operations (TO) functions.

The QA unit supports the manufacturing process by conducting audits, sampling, and inspections, and providing final product approval and release. The QA unit manages a vendor certification program that ensures that only the highest-quality raw material suppliers are used. The program sets strict guidelines that define the physical, chemical, microbiological, and functional characteristics of each raw material. Audits are also conducted to make sure suppliers follow appropriate manufacturing practices to ensure that all raw materials are safe and produced to Pharmavite's high standards.

After arriving at the manufacturing facility, raw materials are immediately quarantined, sampled, and tagged for computer-assisted tracking throughout the manufacturing process. Materials are released for production only after passing a comprehensive set of purity and potency tests. Sophisticated software is used to track every test result generated in the QC laboratory and ensure that only high-quality product is released.

The QC laboratory is one of the most advanced in the country and runs more than 300 tests daily using state-of-the-art equipment. QC laboratory testing also ensures that products are stable so that consumers receive 100% of the active ingredients through the product's expiration date.

Finally, the TO unit continually evaluates its systems and processes to assess how it can make good products even better. To this point, the QE unit develops guidelines for maintaining a high standard of manufacturing quality and efficiency and ensures that the company is prepared for random internal inspections, as well as inspections by outside parties, such as FDA and third-party auditors.

RESPONSIBLE MARKETING: A TEAM APPROACH

Comprehensive marketing, sales, and category management teams work together to make sure that product information is communicated to the retailer and consumer appropriately and ethically.

Product Claims

The marketing team works closely with regulatory affairs and scientific affairs to make sure the product claims used in packaging, labeling, and advertising are accurate and follow FDA and FTC guidelines and regulations. A common misperception is that there are few or no regulations guiding the dietary supplement industry. Quite the contrary is true. Nearly all aspects of dietary supplement manufacturing, labeling, marketing, and advertising are covered by extensive regulations issued and enforced by FDA and FTC. Dietary supplements have always been regulated as a special category of foods. The Federal Food, Drug, and Cosmetic Act of 1938 referred to this category as "foods for special dietary use." In addition, in 1994 dietary supplements received specific regulatory guidance under the Dietary Supplement Health and Education Act(DSHEA). Responsible marketing includes following all guidance for so-called structure/function claims, avoidance of disease claims, and use of appropriate warnings and other labeling guidelines. If products contain dietary ingredients not in use before 1994, the FDA must be notified 75 days in advance of marketing such "new dietary ingredients." If FDA deems the scientific evidence to be inadequate to support the safety of a new dietary ingredient, it may object to the use of such an ingredient before it is used in product formulations.

Sales

A national sales force works closely with retailers to understand their business and strategically develop plans to grow their business and respond to consumer demands. The sales force helps retailers stay up-to-date on industry trends, consumer research, scientific trends new product developments, current legislative changes and government regulations.

Product Marketing

Once a product is ready for the store shelves, advertising, marketing, and public relations support begins—all designed to help educate consumers about the benefits of dietary supplements. Pharmavite uses a variety of methods to reach consumers—from multimedia advertising, use of expert spokespeople, product sampling, and event sponsorships to direct mail sampling, event sponsorships, direct mail marketing, in-pack offers, sweepstakes, in-store point of purchase, and innovative trade marketing programs. All programs are carefully reviewed with regulatory and/or legal departments.

Category Management

The category management team analyzes a retailer's specific nutritional supplement business, evaluating the sales performance of current branded and private label products. Periodic audit reports provide retailers with comprehensive detailed assessments of all aspects of merchandising to help optimize retail sales and profits. To achieve that, Pharmavite uses both point-of-sale data and household purchasing data. The team also helps tailor products, promotions and marketing support to the very specific requirements of a retailer's operations.

EDUCATIONAL RESOURCES

At Pharmavite, educational resources and information are developed to meet the specific needs of each audience.

Health Professionals: The award-winning resource, Vitamin & Herb University (VHU) found at www.VitaminHerbUniversity.com, provides data on more than 70 dietary ingredients, including the latest scientific studies, suggested dosage, benefits, classic deficiency symptoms, dietary sources, warnings, a drug-nutrient interaction database, and information about populations with special needs for each nutrient (Fig. 19.2). VHU, a strictly nonbranded site, also features an accredited continuing education program with the University of Georgia for pharmacists. To date, over 18,000 pharmacists have received credits from VHU's continuing education program. Educational programs for other health care professionals (physicians, nurse practitioners, and registered dietitians) have also been supported by Pharmavite through educational grants.

Consumers: NatureMade.com was developed to help the more than 100 million Americans in the United States who use the Internet as a health education resource. With more than 2 million registered users and 5.6 million first time unique visitors since the site launched in 2002, NatureMade.com provides free access to the latest health information, details on Pharmavite products, personal wellness profiles, advice from experts, and a Wellness Rewards program, which allows members to accumulate points that can be redeemed for coupons for free products. Through a toll-free number found on every product,

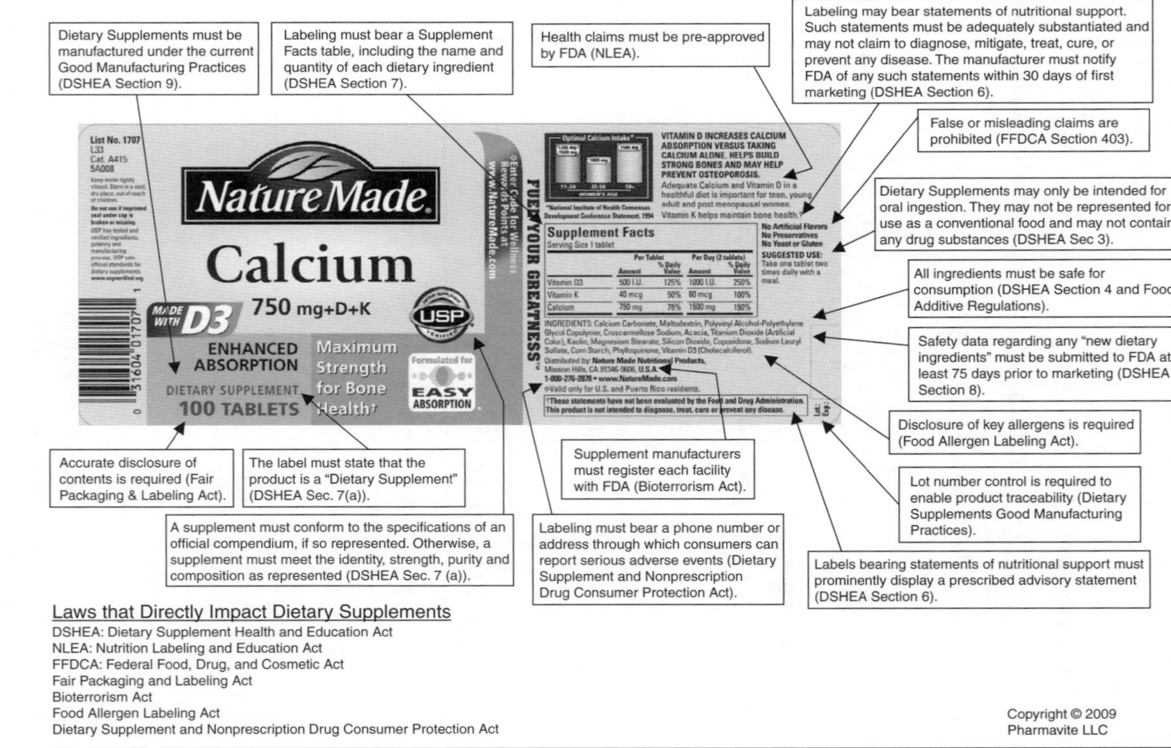

How Dietary Supplements Are Regulated
Dietary Supplements must be manufactured under the current Good Manufacturing Practices (DSHEA Section 9).
Labeling must bear a Supplement Facts table, including the name and quantity of each dietary ingredient (DSHEA Section 7).
Health claims must be pre-approved by FDA (NLEA).
Labeling may bear statements of nutritional support. Such statements must be adequately substantiated and may not claim to diagnose, mitigate, treat, cure, or prevent any disease. The manufacturer must notify FDA of any such statements within 30 days of first marketing (DSHEA Section 6).
False or misleading claims are prohibited (FFDCA Section 403).
Dietary Supplements may only be intended for oral ingestion. They may not be represented for use as a conventional food and may not contain any drug substances (DSHEA Sec 3).
All ingredients must be safe for consumption (DSHEA Section 4 and Food Additive Regulations).
Safety data regarding any "new dietary ingredients" must be submitted to FDA at least 75 days prior to marketing (DSHEA Section 8).
Disclosure of key allergens is required (Food Allergen Labeling Act).
Lot number control is required to enable product traceability (Dietary Supplements Good Manufacturing Practices).
Labels bearing statements of nutritional support must prominently display a prescribed advisory statement (DSHEA Section 6).
Labeling must bear a phone number or address through which consumers can report serious adverse events (Dietary Supplement and Nonprescription Drug Consumer Protection Act).
Supplement manufacturers must register each facility with FDA (Bioterrorism Act).
A supplement must conform to the specifications of an official compendium, if so represented. Otherwise, a supplement must meet the identity, strength, purity and composition as represented (DSHEA Sec. 7 (a)).
The label must state that the product is a "Dietary Supplement" (DSHEA Sec. 7(a)).
Accurate disclosure of contents is required (Fair Packaging & Labeling Act).
List No. 1707
L33
Cat. A415
5A008
Nature Made
Calcium
750 mg+D+K
MADE WITH D3
ENHANCED ABSORPTION
DIETARY SUPPLEMENT
100 TABLETS
Maximum Strength for Bone Health†
USP
Formulated for EASY ABSORPTION
◊Enter Code for Wellness Rewards Points at www.NatureMade.com
FUEL YOUR GREATNESS™
VITAMIN D INCREASES CALCIUM ABSORPTION VERSUS TAKING CALCIUM ALONE. HELPS BUILD STRONG BONES AND MAY HELP PREVENT OSTEOPOROSIS.
Adequate Calcium and Vitamin D in a healthful diet is important for teen, young adult and post menopausal women.
Vitamin K helps maintain bone health.†
Supplement Facts
Serving Size 1 tablet
No Artificial Flavors
No Preservatives
No Yeast or Gluten
SUGGESTED USE: Take one tablet two times daily with a meal.
Distributed by: Nature Made Nutritional Products, Mission Hills, CA 91346-9606, U.S.A.
1-800-276-2878 • www.NatureMade.com
◊Valid only for U.S. and Puerto Rico residents.
†These statements have not been evaluated by the Food and Drug Administration. This product is not intended to diagnose, treat, cure or prevent any disease.
Copyright © 2009
Pharmavite LLC

	Per Tablet Amount	% Daily Value	Per Day (2 tablets) Amount	% Daily Value
Vitamin D3	500 I.U.	125%	1000 I.U.	250%
Vitamin K	40 mcg	50%	80 mcg	100%
Calcium	750 mg	75%	1500 mg	150%

Laws that Directly Impact Dietary Supplements

DSHEA: Dietary Supplement Health and Education Act
NLEA: Nutrition Labeling and Education Act
FFDCA: Federal Food, Drug, and Cosmetic Act
Fair Packaging and Labeling Act
Bioterrorism Act
Food Allergen Labeling Act
Dietary Supplement and Nonprescription Drug Consumer Protection Act

Figure 19.2 • Drug–nutrient interaction database. Available at VitaminHerbUniversity.com.

consumers can also access a live consumer affairs representative to answer any product questions. These tools allow Pharmavite to obtain immediate consumer feedback on its product development efforts, current health trends, and retailer activities.

Media: With health news constantly being reported, health care professionals and their patients are understandably confused. The Pharmavite New Bureau (PNB) was developed to be on call 24 hours a day to assist the media. Through the PNB, media can request expert sources, clinical studies, and product information immediately. The PNB monitors the latest science and helps the media put the most recent clinical study into perspective. Company information and announcements are also accessible through the corporate Web site, Pharmavite.com.

Government and Regulatory Officials: Recognizing the importance of ongoing Congressional education in Washington, DC, Pharmavite's government affairs team regularly meets with members of Congress and their staff about the value and health benefits of dietary supplements. Pharmavite has sponsored Congressional briefings, participated in industry-led lobby days, and provided tours of its facilities to educate members about the high-quality manufacturing practices within the industry. Representing responsible industry is a role Pharmavite takes seriously.

Pharmavite also works to support legislation that positively impacts and builds trust in the industry. From the long-term support of the release of FDA's GMPs to the recently passed OTC and Dietary Supplement Consumer Protection Act (2006), Pharmavite is committed to educating lawmakers at the federal and state levels on the value, benefits, and important role of dietary supplements in preventive health care.

A BRIGHT FUTURE

Health care practitioners understand firsthand the daunting challenges facing the health of our nation. Responsible dietary supplement manufacturers recognize the role their products play in supporting health, in addition to a balanced diet, regular exercise, and preventive health checkups. They are an important tool to help individuals maintain overall health and well-being over the course of many years and help address nutritional needs of patients who take prescription medications that may reduce levels of certain nutrients. Responsible manufacturers also recognize the exciting ways that expanding scientific research is shedding new light on the value and benefit of dietary supplements and are committed to responsibly bringing them to market.

The 2007 release of dietary supplement GMPs is an important milestone for the industry. Companies like Pharmavite see this as a positive transition to further raise the bar for all companies and their products. Through a single-minded focus on science, innovation, quality, and education, the industry can thrive and offer people significant tools to enhance their health.

ACKNOWLEDGMENTS

This chapter was written with assistance from Paul Bolar, Vice President, Regulatory Affairs; Doug Jones, Manager, Corporate Communication; and Carroll Reider, M.S., R.D., Director, Scientific Affairs and with editing assistance from the Pharmavite News Bureau.

CHAPTER 20

The Role of Trade Associations

Andrew Shao

INTRODUCTION

Trade associations (also referred to as trade groups or industry advocacy groups) play a vital role in every regulated industry, and many exist and operate all over the world. In general, the main function of trade associations is to monitor and influence the environment within which their respective industries operate and serve as the collective voice of the industries which they represent. Established in 1973, the Council for Responsible Nutrition (CRN) is the leading trade association representing the mainstream dietary supplement industry (1). CRN is predominantly supported through member dues, with membership consisting primarily of dietary supplement manufacturers and ingredient suppliers. CRN member companies produce a large portion of the dietary supplements marketed in the United States and globally, including popular national brands as well as the store brands marketed by major supermarkets, drug stores, and discount chains. These products also include those marketed through natural health food stores and mainstream direct selling companies. CRN members agree to adhere to CRN's Code of Ethics and other voluntary guidelines for manufacturing, labeling, and marketing of their products. The work that CRN and other associations (Table 20.1) do is important to maintain a proper balance between policy and regulation and an open marketplace, while ensuring that the best interests of the consumer are met.

TRADE ASSOCIATION ACTIVITIES

CRN's heritage and identity are grounded in science, and the tagline *The Science Behind the Supplements®* is taken extremely seriously by both the organization's staff and member companies. CRN's mission is "To enhance and sustain a climate for our member companies to responsibly market dietary supplements and their ingredients by maintaining and improving confidence among consumers, media, government leaders, regulators, healthcare professionals and other decision makers with respect to our members' products." That mission is influenced by CRN's five guiding principles that articulate the values of the organization (Table 20.2). All the association's initiatives and activities contribute to this mission and the five principles. These activities involve regularly interfacing with regulators, policymakers, academic researchers, practitioners, the media (both trade and consumer-based),

TABLE 20.1 Dietary Supplement Industry Trade Associations

Trade Association	Web Site
Council for Responsible Nutrition	www.crnusa.org
Natural Products Association	www.naturalproductsassoc.org
American Herbal Products Association	www.ahpa.org
Consumer Healthcare Products Association	www.chpa-info.org

and consumers. The ultimate objective of CRN, and indeed the other trade associations in the dietary supplement sector, is to allow the industry to flourish responsibly and ensure that consumers have open access to safe, regulated, and high-quality dietary supplements.

Supporting Reasonable Legislation and Regulation, Championing Industry Self-Regulation

CRN is a strong supporter of reasonable legislation and regulation aimed at dietary supplements—policies that protect the public health but are not inappropriately restrictive (Table 20.3). CRN, in collaboration with other trade associations, was instrumental in the passage of the 1994 Dietary Supplement Health and Education Act (DSHEA), the law that governs the dietary supplement industry, as we know it today. The act included a mandate from Congress that the Food and Drug Administration (FDA) promulgate regulations for dietary supplement-specific Good Manufacturing Practices (GMPs). GMP regulations are a set of federally mandated standards for the manufacturing of specific categories of FDA-regulated products, including food, drugs, biologics, medical devices, and dietary supplements (Table 20.4). CRN and its member companies were among those that lobbied both FDA and Congress from 1995 urging the government to issue these critical regulations for dietary supplements up until the release of the Final Rule in June 2007 (2). The industry, through the leadership of CRN and other trade associations, submitted multiple comments and proposals and participated in various meetings and workshops, all of which provided substantial contributions to the final regulation released by FDA. The regulation is being phased in over time, and all dietary supplement manufacturers will need to be in compliance by June 2010.

TABLE 20.2 CRN's Strategic Principles

1	*Shaping the industry's operating environment is always CRN's first priority.*
2	*CRN's unquestioned commitment to science is the source of its influence and credibility with key audiences and stakeholders.*
3	*CRN plays a critical role in building and sustaining consumer confidence to create a more favorable climate for the industry's products.*
4	*CRN's growth through innovative means is an integral element of building strategic capacity and for making the organization sustainable over time.*
5	*CRN can strengthen the standing of its industry by encouraging responsible behavior among its members.*

TABLE 20.3 Dietary Supplement-Relevant Laws and Regulations Supported by CRN

Law/Regulation	Year Passed/ Implemented
Nutrition Labeling and Education Act	1990
Dietary Supplement Health and Education Act	1994
FDA Modernization Act	1997
Bioterrorism Act	2002
Anabolic Steroid Control Act	2004
Food Allergen Labeling Consumer Protection Act	2004
Nonprescription Drug and Dietary Supplement Consumer Protection Act	2006
Good Manufacturing Practices, Final Rule	2007
Mandatory Folic Acid Fortification	1996
Prohibition of the Sale of Dietary Supplements Containing Ephedrine Alkaloids	2004

CRN was also instrumental in the passage of the 2006 Nonprescription Drug and Dietary Supplement Consumer Protection Act (known as "the AER law"), a law requiring manufacturers of over the counter drugs and dietary supplements to notify FDA of any reports they receive involving serious adverse events associated with the use of their products. Previously, these two classes of products were exempted from mandatory reporting and thus FDA received such reports from companies only voluntarily. Because of the efforts of CRN and other trade associations over several years, this landmark legislation received strong bipartisan support. Now implemented by FDA, this law, which was opposed by many activists, is seen by the mainstream dietary supplement industry as important for fostering consumer confidence as well as demonstrating the relative safety of dietary supplements.

CRN has also actively opposed onerous or overly restrictive policies. Legislation proposed at both the federal and state levels intended to restrict access to safe and beneficial dietary supplements has been met with staunch opposition by the trade associations. CRN has successfully tamed concerns over the supplement dehydroepiandrosterone (DHEA) on the part of Congress, which erroneously characterized this important supplement for seniors as an anabolic steroid allegedly abused by teenagers and athletes. CRN has been successful in educating members of Congress and many state legislatures that DHEA and another supplement, creatine, are both effective and safe when used as directed, and that banning or restricting access to these products is unnecessary and would fail to address the potential issue of product misuse or abuse while unfairly punishing those who use the products appropriately. CRN member companies have even voluntarily pledged to refrain from marketing DHEA as providing a general anabolic steroidlike response and not to target those younger than 18 years of age in marketing or advertising of their DHEA-containing products (3).

TABLE 20.4 Categories of Regulation for FDA-Regulated Products

FDA-Regulated Products	Premarket Approval	Premarket Notification	Labeling	Mandatory Adverse Event Reporting*	GMPs	Facility Registration	Advertising[a] (FTC or FDA)
Foods		✓	✓		✓	✓	✓
Dietary supplements		✓	✓	✓	✓	✓	✓
Drugs	✓		✓	✓	✓	✓	✓[a]
Biologics	✓		✓	✓	✓	✓	✓[a]
Medical devices	✓		✓	✓	✓	✓	✓[a]

[a] FDA regulates prescription drug advertising; FTC regulates all other consumer-focused advertising. For more information visit www.fda.gov and www.ftc.gov.
*Food and Drug Administration Amendments Act of 2007 created the requirement that conventional food manufacturer must report incidents of contaminated food to a Reportable Food Registry established by FDA.

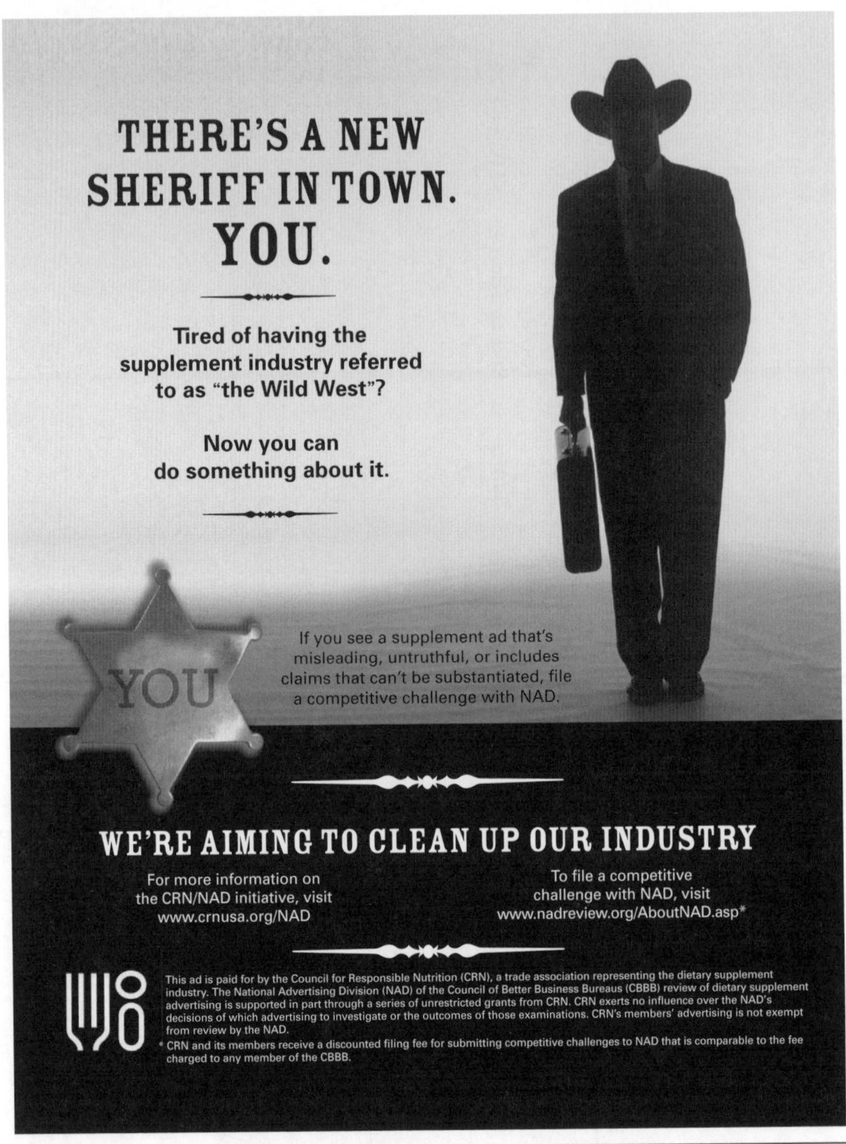

Figure 20.1 • A. An ad campaign appearing in the dietary supplement trade press describing the CRN and NAD initiative to increase scrutiny of dietary supplement advertising. In the three years since its inception, the initiative has increased NAD's dietary supplement advertising case load nearly five-fold (from six cases per year to nearly 30). Visit www.crnusa.org for more information.

Perhaps one of CRN's greatest contributions has been its fostering of industry self-regulation. There are countless examples from various regulated industries in which all members prosper when the companies police themselves and each other rather than having burdensome legislation and regulation imposed upon them. For the dietary supplement industry, CRN has been the leader of self-regulatory initiatives, starting with product advertising. In 2006, CRN pledged a 3-year unrestricted grant of nearly $500,000 to the National Advertising Division (NAD) of the Council of Better Business Bureaus to assist the organization in increasing its scrutiny of dietary supplement advertising (Fig. 20.1) (4). That agreement has recently been extended through 2014. Thus far, the CRN–NAD program has increased the NAD's normal caseload nearly five-fold. Cases can be generated from the NAD's own monitoring of national advertising or by companies filing competitive challenges of advertising claims. The NAD review process involves identification of the claims made to consumers and a complete review of companies' substantiation for those advertising claims in question. If the NAD determines that the substantiation is inadequate to support the claims, the company may be asked to modify or eliminate the claims. Although the entire process is voluntary, if companies refuse to participate in any aspect of the review process, their cases can be referred to the Federal Trade Commission (FTC). While the NAD process provides companies the opportunity to resolve issues related to advertising (either by modifying the advertisement or by bolstering the substantiation), the FTC process allows no second chance; extensive investigation, fines, disgorgement of profits, injunctions, and consent decrees are common outcomes. Hence, it is in the industry members' best interest to participate in this self-regulatory program.

Product quality is an important topic to all. The evolving global supply chain has brought with it complexities that require vigilance on the part of manufacturers, regulators, and consumers. When it comes to enforcing the laws governing foods and dietary supplements, FDA is woefully understaffed and underfunded. Through its affiliation with the Alliance for a Stronger FDA, CRN has lobbied Congress to dramatically increase appropriations for the agency (5). Recognizing this important limitation, CRN has led a multiassociation effort in the development of a tool to assist manufacturers of dietary supplements in their quest to source quality ingredients from raw material suppliers. The Standardized Information on Dietary Ingredients (SIDI) protocol (Fig. 20.2), launched in 2006, is a tool that can be used by ingredient suppliers as a guideline for the type and scope of information they provide to their customers (or potential customers) concerning their ingredient(s) (6). The protocol prompts ingredient suppliers to provide information such as how the ingredient is manufactured, from where it is sourced, what potential contaminants or allergens it may contain, and so on. This information assists in the qualification of the ingredient supplier and is critical to help manufacturers decide whether and to what extent they may want to source the ingredient from the supplier. The same information is pertinent to auditors and regulators who are inspecting a manufacturing facility and desire information on the ingredients that have entered the facility. While its use is voluntary, more and more companies are implementing the SIDI protocol, which has received critical acclaim by both the industry and regulators.

Resource for Dietary Supplement Research

One of CRN's five strategic principles states "CRN's unquestioned commitment to science is the source of its influence and credibility . . . " and the organization serves as an important resource for dietary supplement-related research for stakeholders. In 2008, CRN launched *Research Watch*, a monthly e-newsletter for member companies that highlights the very latest published human clinical trials involving dietary supplements or ingredients. Often, these are studies in the online publication phase, and have yet to appear in print. Also in 2008, CRN established a series of research awards through the American Society for Nutrition (ASN), the largest nutrition research society in the world, to recognize important research contributions

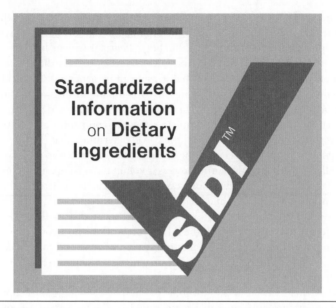

Figure 20.2 • B. The trademarked logo for the Standardized Information on Dietary Ingredients (SIDI) protocol, a voluntary initiative intended to assist dietary supplement manufacturers in the sourcing of high-quality ingredients. Use of the logo is encouraged so as to promote awareness and recognition of the self-regulatory program. Visit www.crnusa.org for more information.

in the field of nutrition. Presented annually at the Experimental Biology conference, the Mary Swartz Rose Awards are named after the late founder and president of the past American Institute of Nutrition (now known as ASN). The awards are given to a senior and young investigator for outstanding preclinical and/or clinical research on the safety and efficacy of dietary supplements as well as essential nutrients and other biologically active food components that might be distributed as supplements or components in functional foods.

When it comes to interpreting dietary supplement or nutrition research and providing the industry perspective, CRN and other trade associations serve as an important resource for the media, both the trade and consumer press. Results of controversial studies, whether positive, negative, or neutral, are often not reported in the proper context and are erroneously conveyed as "the final word." This results in confusion or even frustration as the public perceives the diet and nutrition pendulum swinging from benefit to harm and back again. Whether it is through by-lined articles in trade publications or quotes in mainstream magazines and newspapers, CRN always attempts to provide a balance by placing studies in their proper context and emphasizing that dietary supplements are supplements to—not substitutes for—a healthy lifestyle.

Educating Stakeholders

Educating stakeholders is another critical aspect of CRN's activities. Each year CRN hosts a series of symposia and online Webinars to educate members and the industry aimed primarily at how science drives nutrition and dietary supplement policy, the issuance of new or pending regulations, and emerging research. Many of

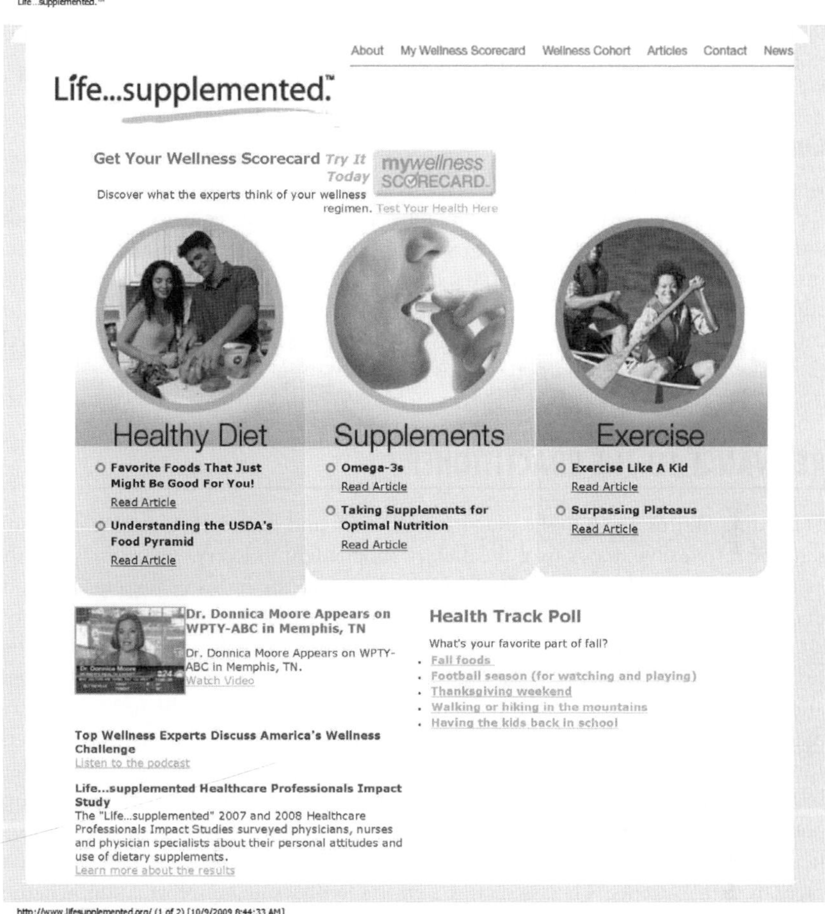

Life...supplemented.™
About My Wellness Scorecard Wellness Cohort Articles Contact News
Life...supplemented.™
Get Your Wellness Scorecard Try It Today
mywellness SCORECARD
Discover what the experts think of your wellness regimen. Test Your Health Here
Healthy Diet
Favorite Foods That Just Might Be Good For You!
Read Article
Understanding the USDA's Food Pyramid
Read Article
Supplements
Omega-3s
Read Article
Taking Supplements for Optimal Nutrition
Read Article
Exercise
Exercise Like A Kid
Read Article
Surpassing Plateaus
Read Article
Dr. Donnica Moore Appears on WPTY-ABC in Memphis, TN
Dr. Donnica Moore Appears on WPTY-ABC in Memphis, TN.
Watch Video
Health Track Poll
What's your favorite part of fall?
Fall foods
Football season (for watching and playing)
Thanksgiving weekend
Walking or hiking in the mountains
Having the kids back in school
Top Wellness Experts Discuss America's Wellness Challenge
Listen to the podcast
Life...supplemented Healthcare Professionals Impact Study
The "Life...supplemented" 2007 and 2008 Healthcare Professionals Impact Studies surveyed physicians, nurses and physician specialists about their personal attitudes and use of dietary supplements.
Learn more about the results
http://www.lifesupplemented.org/ (1 of 2) [10/9/2009 6:44:33 AM]

Figure 20.3 • C. A screen shot from the homepage of the Web site for the Life . . . supplemented consumer wellness campaign. The campaign is focused on helping individuals create a healthier lifestyle by offering actionable suggestions and educational information about the three pillars of a smart wellness regimen: healthy diet, supplements, and exercise. Visit www.lifesupplemented.org for more information.

the workshops are intended to assist members and the industry in general with the interpretation and implementation of new legislation or regulations, such as the GMPs or mandatory adverse event reporting. An annual conference is also hosted each year which brings together industry executives, regulators, policy makers, and business leaders to discuss topics of interest, some of them controversial. CRN's *The Workshop*: A Day of Science is an annual event focused solely on highly relevant scientific topics. The day-long workshop features presentations from expert academics, clinicians, and government officials. Past topics include nutrigenomics, the role of dietary supplements in integrative medicine, optimal design and interpretation of randomized trials for nutrients and chronic disease and validation of analytical methods.

CRN staff are also frequently featured speakers at various industry events, trade shows, and scientific conferences, and often contribute to by-lined articles in the various trade publications. CRN scientists have authored or coauthored nearly 70 peer-reviewed scientific publications.

Consumer Outreach

Recognizing that the consumer is a critical stakeholder, CRN in 2007 launched *Life . . . supplemented* (Fig. 20.3), a wellness campaign that focuses on helping individuals create a healthier lifestyle by offering practical suggestions and educational information about the three pillars of a smart wellness regimen: healthy diet, supplements, and exercise. The Web site (www.lifesupplemented.org) contains educational information, interactive tools, and survey results of consumers and practitioners and their usage and perceptions of dietary supplements.

RELEVANCE TO THE PRACTITIONER

What does all this mean to the practitioner? CRN and its member companies represent the responsible majority of the dietary supplement industry. The efforts that the association undertakes on behalf of its members and the industry help instill confidence in practitioners and their patients that dietary supplements *are* regulated (Table 20.3), and that consumers' best interests are the number one priority. By encouraging reasonable legislation and regulation, by actively lobbying for adequate enforcement and tirelessly promoting self-regulation, CRN helps maintain the integrity of the dietary supplement industry in the eyes of all stakeholders, including practitioners. Initiatives focused on product quality, responsible advertising, and the science underlying dietary supplements are just a few of the many projects the organization supports and/or leads. CRN's message that dietary supplements are not substitutes for a healthy lifestyle resonates with practitioners and is consistent with their own messages to their patients. The association's efforts to disseminate information, whether for regulatory compliance, to ensure that member companies keep abreast of the latest research involving dietary supplements, or to help place complex and controversial information in the proper context for the media not only instill confidence but also ultimately assist practitioners. CRN is actively engaged in efforts to encourage consumers and patients to discuss their dietary supplement use with their practitioners and periodically sponsors continuing education for health care professionals who rank highly among consumers as a trusted source for information on dietary supplements (7).

When it comes to dietary supplements, CRN, both directly and indirectly, serves as a reliable and credible resource for practitioners and their patients.

SUMMARY

Trade associations serve a vital role for the industries they represent, for practitioners, and consumers. For the dietary supplement industry, these organizations help balance the operating environment such that consumers are protected but are allowed open access to the marketplace. Ultimately, the most important goal is to build and sustain a high level of consumer (and practitioner) confidence in the industry and the products it provides.

References

1. *Fact Sheet*: Who is CRN? Washington, DC: Council for Responsible Nutrition; Accessed http://www.crnusa.org.
2. 21 CFR Part 111. *Current Good Manufacturing Practice in Manufacturing, Packaging, Labeling, or Holding Operations for Dietary Supplements; Final Rule*. Federal Register / Vol. 72, No. 121 / Monday, June 25, 2007, pg 34752, Docket No. 1996N–0417. Department of Health and Human Services, Food and Drug Administration.
3. Council for Responsible Nutrition's Voluntary Program for the Marketing Dehydroepiandrosterone (DHEA). Council for Responsible Nutrition, Washington, DC.
4. Council for Responsible Nutrition. Council for Responsible Nutrition/National Advertising Division initiative. Washington, DC. Accessed http://www.crnusa.org or http://www.nadreview.org/AboutNAD.asp.
5. Alliance for a Stronger FDA, an education and advocacy group dedicated to increasing the appropriated resources available to FDA. Silver Spring, MD. http://www.strengthenfda.org/.
6. Standardized Information on Dietary Ingredients (SIDI™) protocol. Silver Spring, MD: American Herbal Products Association; Washington, DC: Consumer Healthcare Products Association; Washington, DC: Council for Responsible Nutrition; Washington, DC: Natural Products Association.
7. The 2007 Consumer Confidence Survey. Online survey of 2,153 people consisting of a random sample of U.S. adults aged 18+ and the results were weighted to represent the U.S. adult population. Conducted by Ipsos-Public Affairs August 2007. Washington, DC: Council for Responsible Nutrition.

CHAPTER 21

USP Verified Dietary Supplements

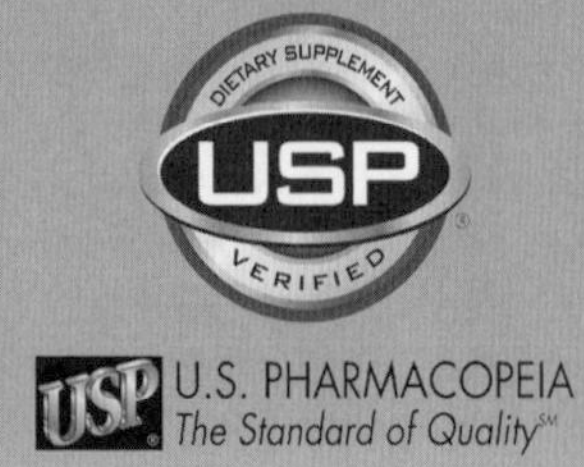

V. Srini Srinivasan and Laura N. Provan

UNITED STATES PHARMACOPEIA: THE STANDARD OF QUALITY FOR DIETARY SUPPLEMENTS

The United States Pharmacopeial (USP) Convention is an official standard-setting authority for all prescription and over-the-counter medicines and other health care products manufactured or sold in the United States. USP standards for the identity, quality, purity, strength, and consistency of these products are recognized and used in more than 130 countries. Our mission is to improve the health of people around the world through public standards and related programs that help ensure the quality, safety, and benefit of medicines and foods.

USP is a private, nonprofit organization whose independent, volunteer experts work under strict conflict of interest rules to set its scientific standards. Our contributions to public health are enriched by the participation and oversight of volunteers representing pharmacy, medicine, and other health care professions as well as academia, government, the pharmaceutical, dietary supplements, and food industries, health plans, and consumer organizations.

USP was founded in 1820 by a group of physicians concerned about the lack of consistency and quality in American medications, which at that time were compounded by individual physicians and pharmacists. They created the first *United States Pharmacopeia*, a book of standard recipes for medicines. Since that time, the pharmaceutical industry has grown and evolved dramatically, but the need for science-based, consistent standards for the quality of medications has remained constant.

Following a public health crisis in 1937 when a popular medication sulfanilamide vaginal (Elixir Sulfanilamide) was contaminated with the industrial chemical diethylene glycol—resulting in more than 100 deaths in the United States—USP's role as an official source of pharmaceutical standards was written into the Food, Drug, and Cosmetic Act of 1938. This means that all drugs sold in the United States must comply with the standards published in the *United States Pharmacopeia–National Formulary* (*USP–NF*). USP also sets widely recognized standards for food ingredients and dietary supplements. Food ingredient standards are published in the *Food Chemicals Codex*; a growing number of standards for dietary supplements have been published in the *USP–NF*. In the spring of 2009 USP published the new *Dietary Supplements Compendium*, containing quality specifications drawn from both the *USP–NF* and the *Food Chemicals Codex*. Supplements that claim adherence to USP standards on their labels, but which do not in fact conform, are liable to charges of misbranding under the Dietary Supplement Health and Education Act (DSHEA) of 1994. It is important to note that USP has no role in enforcement of any regulations, which (for drugs, supplements, and food ingredients) is the sole responsibility of the Food and Drug Administration (FDA).

Many of USP's written or documentary standards include physical reference standards for drugs (these are official standards), food ingredients, and dietary supplements. To help manufacturers with compliance, USP provides Pharmacopeial Education courses. Because the supply chains for drugs, supplements, and food ingredients are global, USP has built facilities in Switzerland, China, India, and Brazil as well as its headquarters near Washington, DC.

USP started the USP Verified program for dietary supplements in 2001 to help assure consumers of product quality, and as a way for manufacturers and distributors to publicaly demonstrate their commitment to quality. Under this voluntary, for-fee program, manufacturers submit products and ingredients to USP's rigorous independent testing. Those that pass earn the right to display the distinctive USP Verified mark. At a time when there is far too much news about accidental contamination or deliberate adulteration of food and drugs, USP Verified can be an important component of the safety nets that help protect public health.

WHY USP VERIFIED?

USP Verified helps assure consumers of the integrity, strength, purity, potency, and quality of the supplements they take. We do this through an independent process that includes a Good Manufacturing Practices audit, product and ingredient testing, and manufacturing documentation review. The dietary supplement and herbal product industries are not as closely regulated in the United States as are drugs, leaving ethical manufacturers and distributors with limited ways to distinguish themselves from those that may cut corners.

Recent data show that more than 77% of American adults use dietary supplements and herbals. Of these, more than 10 million buy an average of four supplement products each month, resulting in an industry that exceeded $23 billion in 2007 (1). Because of the proliferation of brands and outlets for supplements and herbals, many patients and consumers turn to their health care providers—physicians, pharmacists, nurses, dieticians—for advice about which supplements to take and which brands are best. But medical education in the United States often does not include thorough information about supplements. How can you help your patients make good choices?

FDA requires supplements to carry an ingredients label but does not verify the information or oversee manufacturing. DSHEA provisions essentially treat supplements as if they were foods. They are defined as products taken by mouth that contain an ingredient intended to supplement the diet—even though many supplements have well-known pharmacologic effects. FDA approved a set of Good Manufacturing Practices for supplements in 2007, but leaves it up to manufacturers to police their own products. Patients and consumers (and sometimes clinicians) often assume that supplements and herbals are held to the same standards for quality as drugs. But this is not the case. In fact, some supplements do not contain the amounts of ingredients stated on the label; others do not release properly in the body;

and some contain harmful levels of contaminants such as lead, mercury, pesticides, mold, or even prescription drugs.

Given that so many Americans turn to supplements and herbals seeking health benefits, it is important for them to be able to trust the quality of these products—and for clinicians to feel confidence as well, in the interest of providing the best possible care. Counseling patients to seek "USP Verified" brands offers both clinician and patient added confidence that the product contains the ingredients stated on the label; has the declared amount and strength of ingredients; dissolves properly in the body; has been screened for certain harmful contaminants; and has been manufactured using safe, sanitary, and well-controlled procedures. It is important to note that the USP Verified program includes postmarket surveillance, in which we randomly select product samples off store shelves to see whether they adhere to program testing requirements once they have left the factory.

WHAT IS "QUALITY?"

While a number of organizations and for-profit companies have tried to help consumers make better choices when buying supplements and herbals, USP is the only organization in the United States that has a full verification program and is also recognized in US federal law as an official standard-setting body for dietary supplements. Some manufacturers cite inclusion of "USP" ingredients, but that does not mean the product has been through independent third-party verification. Only the green and gold USP Verified mark provides that assurance.

It is an additional challenge for clinicians and patients to sort among the certifiers as well as among the supplements. USP has been protecting public health through quality standards for nearly 200 years. Our dedication to the best, most current, unbiased science in our standards-setting mission is the foundation of our other programs as well, including USP Verified. We provide a basis of trust for physicians, pharmacists, healthcare professionals, governments, manufacturers, and consumers throughout the world. USP Verified is cited by Consumer Reports Health, the Natural Medicines Comprehensive Database, and Pogo Health, among others, as the most reliable quality mark.

WHO PARTICIPATES IN DSVP?

The manufacturers and distributors who choose to participate in the USP Verified program do so as a way of demonstrating their commitment to product quality—and to the consumers who buy their products. To date, USP Verified appears on more than 200 million products,[1] which can be found on the shelves of US national and local pharmacies, wholesale clubs, and retail outlets. This includes 10 companies and numerous supplement categories, including vitamins, minerals, amino acids, botanics, and others (e.g., co-enzyme Q10, chondroitin sulfate sodium, glucosomine, fish oil, etc.). A complete list can be found on the USP Web site at http://www.usp.org/USPVerified/dietarySupplements/supplements.html.

[1]Nearly all the USP Verified products are dietary supplements (such as multivitamins, magnesium, fish oil, calcium); at this time, just two are herbal products.

HOW CAN CLINICIANS INCORPORATE UNITED STATES PHARMACOPEIA RESOURCES IN THEIR PRACTICE?

Physicians, pharmacists, and other health care professionals to whom patients turn for advice owe it to their patients to be informed about dietary supplements as well as about drugs. To this end, USP provides resources on our Web site (noted above) to help clinicians and patients make better dietary supplement choices. Among these is the interactive "Choosing a Dietary Supplement" module, which provides detailed information about examining dietary supplement choices, including talking with clinicians, reviewing the evidence, understanding labels, and utilizing other resources.

A good example of utilizing USP resources in practice would be the importance of insuring use of well-regulated folic acid supplementation for pregnant women in protecting against spina bifida and anencephaly. Prenatal vitamins are often given by prescription, but when they are bought off the shelf, it is vital that they be of good quality. Counseling patients to use the available USP resources when examining their prenatal vitamin choices, including looking for the USP Verified mark, can be a tangible and responsible part of providing the quality of care that patients deserve.

Reference

1. 2008 Nutrition Industry Overview. *Nutr Bus J* 2008;13(6/7).

CHAPTER 22

Third Party Dietary Supplement Testing: ConsumerLab.com

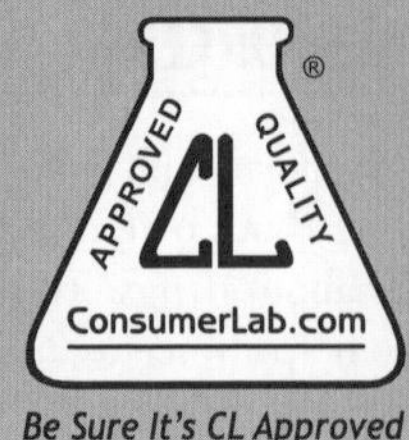

Tod Cooperman, MD

HOW CONSUMERLAB.COM BEGAN

In the late 1990s reports appeared in the press indicating that certain dietary supplements were found to provide little of their claimed ingredients. Consumers had no way of knowing what their dietary supplements contained.

To address this apparent problem, I started ConsumerLab.com in 1999 and immediately recruited from the US Food and Drug Administration (FDA) Center for Food Science and Nutrition, Dr. William Obermeyer, a natural products chemist. We began purchasing and testing hundreds of supplements to determine whether products met their ingredient claims and other quality standards. The results were shocking: About one quarter of the products did not pass the evaluations. This was particularly disturbing because many of these supplements are taken for months or years.

Ten years later, having tested more than 2,400 products, it is disappointing to report that the average failure rate remains the same. On the other hand, consumers and health professional now have an independent resource for finding products that are of high quality and for avoiding those that are not. We hear of many physicians and nutritionists who recommend a type of supplement, but advise patients to check with ConsumerLab.com before choosing a brand.

HOW CONSUMERLAB.COM TESTS DIETARY SUPPLEMENTS

For its Product Reviews, which are published online, ConsumerLab.com selects supplements commonly sold in the United States (and, most often, Canada) sampling from a wide variety brands (more than 350 brands to date). It currently reports on more than 60 popular product categories, including most vitamins, minerals, herbals, as well as specialty supplements such as chondroitin, CoQ10, fish oil, glucosamine, methylsulfonylmethane (MSM), red yeast rice, and resveratrol. It purchases products on the market, as a consumer would, through retail stores, online retailers, catalogs, health care professionals, and multilevel marketing companies. It purchases multiple samples of each product, all representing a single lot rather than averaging results across multiple lots, which can yield misleading results.

The products are evaluated using what ConsumerLab.com considers to be the most accurate and reliable testing methods and applies what it considers to be the best standards from a consumer perspective. Consequently, many of the tests surpass requirements of the FDA. For example, ConsumerLab.com applies the California Prop 65 limit on lead contamination (0.5 μg per daily serving with a 1.0 additional allowance for calcium supplements). Although this is an achievable level, other third party testing organizations that work more closely with industry tend to use more lenient standards, such as 10 μg or even 20 μg per daily serving, despite the fact that children should not be exposed to more than 6 μg of lead per daily serving from all dietary sources combined. Moreover, unlike other testing organizations, the specific testing methods and standards are made freely available on the Web (at www.ConsumerLab.com/methods_index.asp).

All products are tested to determine whether they contain the main ingredient(s) specified on the label. In addition, all herbs and minerals are checked for lead contamination and herbs are also tested for pesticide contamination. Tablets and caplets (unless chewable or timed-release) undergo disintegration testing to be sure that they break apart properly in a simulated gastric environment. For supplements containing ingredients known to have specific problems, additional tests are performed. Supplements made from fish oils or seed oils, such as flaxseed and borage oils, are tested for spoilage. Fish oils are tested for mercury and polychlorinated biphenyls (PCBs). All testing is conducted by outside laboratories and, whenever possible, product identities are not disclosed to those laboratories. Whenever possible, products that fail testing are also retested in a second laboratory for confirmation.

In addition to the products that ConsumerLab.com selects to test for its published Product Reviews, manufacturers and distributors may request testing of their products through ConsumerLab.com's Voluntary Certification Program, which predates similar programs offered by United States Pharmacopeia and NSF international. Companies pay a fee for this testing but are not allowed to send samples nor specify the lot to be purchased and tested. Products undergo the same evaluation as those in the Product Reviews. Those that pass testing in the Voluntary Certification Program are included in the Product Reviews with a footnote for having come through this program.

Companies whose products meet ConsumerLab.com's standards can license the flask-shaped CL Seal of Approved Quality for use on labels and in promotional materials for the approved products. To ensure continuing compliance with ConsumerLab.com's standards, these products must be periodically reevaluated.

Companies whose products fail our tests can contact us and obtain the test results at no charge. We also provide reserve sample at no cost for retesting at a third-party laboratory if the manufacturer is willing to publish the findings, which we will also do. While companies have attempted to discredit our results, it is rare that any has taken us up on this offer of retesting or has produced results that contradict our findings.

If a company believes that it has fixed a problem, it is welcome to have the improved product tested in our Voluntary program. If it passes, it will be added to our report along with the original failure and information to help consumers differentiate between the old and new products.

Every 2 to 3 years, reports on categories that are still popular are replaced with a new set of test results representing then-current products.

WHY PRODUCTS FAIL

There are a variety of potential quality problems with supplements. The most common problem we encounter is that a product delivers less ingredient than promised, or substandard ingredient. Other problems include too much active ingredient, the wrong ingredient, harmful or illegal ingredients, contamination (with heavy metals, dangerous pesticides, or pathogens), unexpected ingredients ("spiked" products), spoilage, poor disintegration (which affects absorption), misleading or insufficient product information, and misleading or unsupported health claims.

Recent examples of problems found with supplements include the following:

- Chondroitin supplements containing little (<20%) or no chondroitin. (We have also found this in supplements for pets).
- 44% of probiotics containing fewer viable organisms than claimed or generally known to be effective.
- Ginkgo supplements apparently adulterated with the compound "quercetin" to disguise the lack of proper ginkgo extract.
- Double the claimed amount of vitamin A (as retinol) in a cod liver oil supplement, putting it above the safe limit (UL) for children up to 13 and pregnant woman. A similar problem was found in a children's multivitamin.
- A soy isoflavone supplement containing as little as 30% of claimed isoflavones.
- Lead contamination in a women's multivitamin as well as in turmeric, black cohosh, iron, and other herbal and mineral supplements.
- An iron supplement with only 37% of its iron and a potassium supplement with only 18% of its potassium.

Many of these problems persist year after year. Some improve. For example, in 2000, ConsumerLab.com found that nearly half of 13 SAMe products selected for testing contained less ingredient than claimed. In 2003, the situation had improved to where one product had only 30% of its SAMe but seven others met their claims. All products passed the testing in 2007.

SOME SUPPLEMENTS FARE BETTER THAN OTHERS

Products that have failed our evaluations come from every type and size of company. Where the products were purchased—pharmacy, health food store, catalog, or other outlet—has had no bearing on whether they passed the tests. No channel of distribution seems immune to failure. Some brands tend to do better than others; but all products from a manufacturer or distributor are not necessarily of equal quality.

Some categories of supplements fair worse than others: 10% of nutritionals, 21% vitamins and minerals, 21% of the specialty supplements, and 51% of herbals have *failed* our most recent testing. Some specific categories, such as multivitamins, perform even worse: 56% of the products tested had problems in our tests; whereas others perform better: less than 10% of fish oil, vitamin C, and magnesium, and CoQ10 supplements failed recent testing. The particularly high failure rates for herbals and multivitamins relate to their complexity compared to single-ingredient vitamins or minerals, for example. Herbals are complex mixtures of phytochemicals and may be contaminated by their growing environment. Multivitamins must contain precise amounts of multiple ingredients, all remaining at more than 100% of their claimed levels until their expiration dates.

Sometimes (but certainly not always) after ConsumerLab.com identifies a problem, a manufacturer will upgrade manufacturing practices, secure a more reliable ingredient supplier, and correct labeling deficiencies. We have seen this, for example, with chondroitin supplements made with ingredient that actually contained little if no chondroitin but came with certificates of analysis showing 100%. These certificates, however, were based on nonspecific tests easily tricked by sulfer-containing compounds other than chondroitin.

Although not an ingredient quality issue, ConsumerLab.com's reports also identify products with suggested daily servings that exceed the Upper Tolerable Intake Levels (ULs) established by the Institute of Medicine. Among third-party verifiers, only ConsumerLab.com provides this information. Too much of certain nutrients, such as vitamin A in the retinol form, can be toxic. While it is sometimes appropriate to exceed these levels (e.g., in treating deficiency), many products deliver "mega" doses that may not be desirable.

THE ROLE OF REGULATORS

In 1994, the government passed the Dietary Supplement Health and Education Act (commonly referred to as DSHEA or "de-shay"). This law did not classify dietary supplements as drugs and, therefore, allowed them to fall outside the realm of FDA's regulation of prescription drugs. In some other countries, most notably Germany, supplements are classified as drugs and are regulated as such.

US law also distinguishes supplements from foods. Consequently, the United States Department of Agriculture, which regulates agricultural products, including most foods and beverages, does not regulate or oversee supplements. For example, though the United States Department of Agriculture routinely inspects most imported meats, no one routinely inspects imported supplements or their raw ingredients.

Before a drug can be sold in the United States, it must be proven safe and effective. Drug packaging must indicate exactly what the product contains and include extensive literature explaining the drug's approved uses, potential adverse effects, and risks including known interactions with foods or other drugs.

Dietary supplements, on the other hand, do not require proof that they work or that they are safe. Although supplement labels are supposed to state exactly what is in the package, governmental agencies do not routinely check for compliance—not even after a problem has been identified by ConsumerLab.com or others.

It is rare that a supplement is recalled—voluntarily or by the FDA. Adverse event reporting only began in earnest after being required in 2008—resulting in a tripling of the number of events over the year before. Second, the FDA has little authority to force a recall, relying instead on voluntary recalls by manufacturers. Even when a recall occurs, it is often done "quietly" through a letter to distributors and retailers but without public announcement. (Recalls about which ConsumerLab.com learns are reported on its Web site under Warnings at www.consumerlab.com/recalls.asp.)

THE GOOD MANUFACTURING PRACTICES—WILL THEY HELP?

Unlike prescription drugs, only recently have supplements been required to be manufactured under specific standardized conditions—Good Manufacturing Practices (GMPs)—and this requirement is being phased in over a 3-year period that does not require compliance from all companies until mid-2010.

Even at their best, the GMPs cannot fix all problems. Bad products can still be manufactured because the GMPs allow for a manufacturer's discretion as to product content (including the amount of key ingredient and use of untested combinations of ingredients), contamination limits, and how ingredient quality is determined, that is, the tests and standards. It is also unclear how often manufacturers will be inspected and how tightly the rules will be enforced. A 2009 Government Accounting Office report on Dietary Supplements showed that out of a total of 14,328 FDA inspections of domestic manufacturing facilities in 2008, only 65 were of supplement manufacturers—not even one-half of 1% of the total.

CHAPTER 23

NPA: Industry Self-Regulation

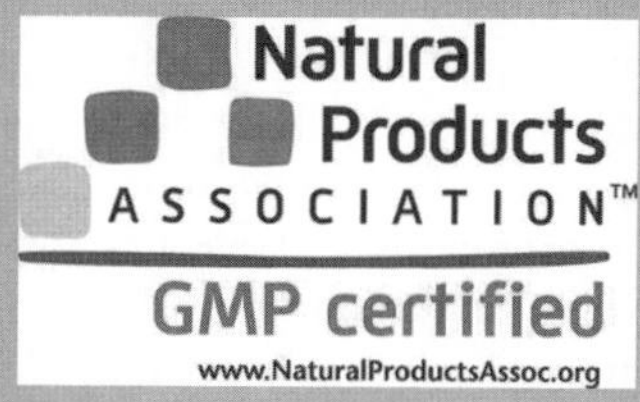

Daniel Fabricant

The Natural Products Association (NPA), formerly the National Nutritional Foods Association (NNFA), is the oldest and largest trade association representing the natural products industry. The association was founded in 1936, and its mission has long since been to advocate for the industry (1). When many envision a trade association they generally think of men in suits and Capitol Hill, but that does not accurately tell the whole story. While the NPA is committed to advocating for the rights of manufacturers, suppliers, and retailers to have a marketplace in which to sell products, we are also committed to consumers having access to products that will maintain their health and well-being. To assist in balancing the two, often times associations develop self-regulatory initiatives that demonstrate industry transparency and provide the consumer valuable information that can be used to evaluate products. The public and private benefits of industry self-regulation are numerous. First, self-regulatory initiatives may establish product standards that often assure safety. In turn, these standards may facilitate the emergence of markets by establishing baseline levels of product quality and safety and result in improved consumers' understanding and trust of new products (2).

Standard setting also can lower the cost of production. For example, a standard can be established to assist manufacturers in producing interconnecting or interchangeable parts. Especially in high-tech industries, standards assure a manufacturer that if its product conforms, the product will interconnect with complementary or rival products of similar specifications. But most important in the days of the global marketplace is that industry self-regulation helps consumers evaluate products and services by providing information about the qualities and characteristics of the seller's products.

Legitimate and fair self-regulation is becoming much more important considering that the global economy generally grows faster than government regulation. An industry group or trade association may engage in self-regulation to enhance its reputation for fair and honest service by establishing ethical standards and disciplining those who do not abide by the standards. Trade associations, for example, often exclude unqualified applicants to assure the public that practitioners possess a minimum level of competence and to protect the associations' reputation as well.

In addition, self-regulation often may deter conduct that would be universally considered undesirable but that the civil or criminal law does not prohibit or for which enforcement, for a variety of reasons, has been lacking. This is one reason that from a public policy perspective, self-regulation can offer several advantages over government regulation or legislation. It often is more prompt, flexible, and effective than government regulation. Self-regulation can bring the accumulated judgment and experience of an industry to bear on issues that are sometimes difficult for the government to define with bright line rules. Finally, government resources are limited, thus many government agencies have sought to leverage their limited resources by promoting and encouraging self-regulation. In considering all of these points, it is not surprising that a histories association, as the NPA is, has a long and diverse array of self-regulatory initiatives.

TRULABEL

The first self-regulatory program in the dietary supplement industry which continued currently is TruLabel. TruLabel was adopted by the then NNFA in 1990 as a registration and random-testing program for suppliers of dietary supplements. It was made an Association membership requirement for suppliers in 1995. The TruLabel program is required of all supplier members who manufacture under their own label. Currently, industry-wide there are more than 25,000 products registered with TruLabel, the Association maintains copies of all of the current registered product labels (3).

In order for a firm to maintain its membership in good standing with the Association, it must register new finished products within 90 days of introducing them into the market for resale and consumption. Moreover, products that have gone through formula revisions or ingredient changes must also be resubmitted for registration. Only products that fall under the category and are clearly labeled as dietary supplements must be registered. In addition, products must be registered to be displayed at the annual Natural Marketplace trade show. As an adherence tool unregistered products are removed from display shelves on the show floor. TruLabel is overseen internally by the Scientific and Regulatory Affairs department of the Association and at present does not authorize use of the TruLabel name or logo in product advertising. At one point the Association considered allowing the use of a TruLabel symbol on bottles to encourage members to join the TruLabel program; however, considering the problems of monitoring products, possible misuse of the symbol, and potential liability ramifications, the symbol use was discarded. The TruLabel program continues to be viable without a seal.

TruLabel policies are governed by the NPA's Committee for Product and Label Integrity (ComPLI) and the Association's board of directors. The purpose of the TruLabel program is to provide confidence among retailers and consumers that the supplements that they purchase are accurately labeled; in order to do so, TruLabel registered products are also subject to random testing conducted by independent laboratories for consistency between contents and labels. Categories and priorities for TL random supplement testing are determined by need according to the industry, the membership, specifically the BOD, and appropriate committees of the Association. Typically, the category chosen is one of current significance and impact within the supplement community. For example, they might select a product to test if there has been a considerable increase in sales or if the product has shown some inconsistencies in its quality; therefore, the testing of products will benefit the industry and be of value to both the supplier and the consumer. Should a test reveal a product or ingredient deficiency, the member company is contacted and given a brief period to correct the product or label. A company that fails to comply is expelled from membership and is thus unable to exhibit at the NPA's annual convention and trade show, Natural Marketplace. In addition, per the Association bylaws if a matter discovered through TruLabel testing is not appropriately remedied in a reasonable amount of time, Association membership can be suspended or revoked altogether.

The purpose of the TruLabel program is to provide confidence among retailers and consumers that the supplements that they purchase are accurately labeled. More importantly, it promotes self-regulation, which demonstrates maturity, responsibility, and reputability within the supplement industry and to other government organizations. A good example of how TruLabel is valuable to governmental organizations is the development of the Dietary Supplement Label Database (DSLD). On August 1, 2008, the National Institutes of Health's Office of Dietary Supplements (ODS) and the National Library of Medicine (NLM), the world's largest medical library, announced a pilot study to determine the feasibility of developing a Web-based database to catalog the labels of all dietary supplements sold in the United States (4). If the pilot project is successful, DSLD will continue to meet consumer-related informational and educational needs that NLM is addressing, while accomplishing the ODS's enhanced research goals. The DSLD will provide comprehensive label information in a format that is user-friendly for both consumers and researchers. The information included in the database will be determined by federal and stakeholder user groups. If findings from the pilot study demonstrate that such a project is feasible, then ODS and NLM will consider the development of a full-scale application that includes label information on virtually all dietary supplements sold in the United States. Because TruLabel provides the most comprehensive product database and hard copies of labels for dietary supplement products, NPA was selected as a subcontractor for the pilot study.

NATURAL PRODUCTS ASSOCIATION GOOD MANUFACTURING PRACTICES CERTIFICATION

While TruLabel has been and continues to be very influential for self-regulation, it is not the only Association program. In 2009, the NPA's Good Manufacturing Practices (GMPs) Certification Program entered its 10th year of verifying to consumers that dietary supplements are manufactured according to the highest standards. In 1994, the Food and Drug Administration (FDA) gained the power to develop manufacturing standards for dietary supplements as a result of the passage of the Dietary Supplement Health and Education Act, but did not offer the final GMP rules for dietary supplements (21 CFR Part 111) until June 2007 (5). In the meanwhile, dietary supplement manufacturers were only required to adhere to Good Manufacturing Practices for foods (21 CFR Part 110), which were largely enforced by local and state health departments. The Association recognized that while food GMPs are certainly significant in regard to controlling general sanitation practices they do not drill down on product quality with regard to specifications including identity, purity, strength, composition, as well as incorporate quality control features to prevent mix-up and contamination which could potentially render a product adulterated. Along with the American Herbal Products Association, the Council for Responsible Nutrition, and the Utah Natural Products Alliance, the then NNFA developed a model for the GMP regulations and passed it to FDA in late 1995 (6). This model served as the basis of the 1997 FDA proposed GMPs in the form of an advanced notice of proposed rulemaking (ANPR). Following the publishing of the ANPR, it became apparent to the leadership at NNFA that it would take the FDA a significant amount of time to finalize the GMPs for dietary supplements. Rather than waiting for FDA, the Association began developing its own GMPs incorporating the ANPR and hiring appropriate consultants and experts in inspection of FDA-regulated products to ensure that the necessary quality assurance aspects were present. The program, which was the first large-scale effort of its kind in the supplement industry, was launched in January of 1999 with the first certifications issued in July of that year. The program can mark its progress to date by having awarded certification to more than 70 member companies, ranging from some of the largest manufacturers to the smallest in the industry, including both domestic and foreign firms, representing more than 30,000 finished products and thousands of raw materials.

When the Association rolled out a GMP program in January 1999, it was initially intended to be a membership requirement similar to TruLabel but that policy was not enforced. In addition, when the program was first launched, it allowed for the use of the GMP seal on product labels; in 2002 the association no longer authorized the use of the seal on the product label but rather just on their advertising and marketing materials. A member supplier must receive an "A" rating in order to be certified. Those who receive either a "B" or "C" rating must correct deficiencies and submit for a reaudit. Certified companies are currently audited every 2 years to verify continued compliance with NPA GMPs (7).

When the program was first launched, the goal of the GMP Certification program was to ensure that all elements of the manufacturing process are reviewed so that products meet their intended quality. Third-party on-site inspections of manufacturing facilities cover such areas as disease control and cleanliness, establishment of a quality control unit, test methods, expiration dating, and procedures for storage and distribution. The third-party certification program includes inspections of dietary supplement manufacturing facilities to determine whether specified performance standards on a number of measures—including quality control, cleanliness, receiving and testing of raw materials—are being met.

Now, while the program still stays true to the initial goals of the program as specified above, the program was adapted in 2008 to incorporate the requirements put forth in the long awaited final FDA cGMPs for dietary supplements (21 CFR Part 111). We believe that the program still holds great value for the industry for a number of reasons but none more significantly than reducing exposure to regulatory vulnerability. It is important to note that a product that fails to be manufactured according to cGMP is considered adulterated (8). FDA is not going to help a manufacturer get prepared for the GMP inspection, nor is it offering certification. The objectives of the GMPs from FDA's perspective are to provide the general public with unadulterated products, which are not misbranded and meet their respective label claims. Thus, those manufacturing firms that seek to evaluate their state of compliance, have an expert third-party review their facility in preparation for an FDA inspection, or need very skilled and detailed assistance with their quality system to bring it to a state of compliance, can use a third-party certifier to do just that.

Some certifiers will go beyond GMP demands as part of their standard service, whereas others seek to more closely match the regulation to the letter. Knowing exactly what is required and what each certifier offers can save companies both time and money. For example, with our program, we know from our membership that retailers favor products with expiration dating, so it has been maintained in our program even though it is not a part of the FDA GMPs for dietary supplements. In addition, one of the key pieces for compliance is the ability to comprehend what has been put forth in the rule, considering the FDA GMPs have arrived in the United States in the form of an 815-page document that spells out the FDA's view on how to go about the manufacture of an estimated $22 billion worth of dietary supplements each year; there is a significant amount of information to digest. To assist firms with that digestion the Association has offered GMP education and training alongside the certification program since 1999. While the education sessions usually take place at industry events and trade shows in the United States, they have also been conducted individually for firms, and in Asia, Europe, and South America.

Previously, NPA and NSF had an alliance regarding GMP certification. The terms of the alliance were that NSF licensed and paid a royalty on NPA's GMP audit materials which NSF used as the basis of its plant inspection process. In addition, NSF recognized NNFA's GMP audits as meeting the requirements for NSF's Dietary Supplements Certification Program. One of the major factors the association considered in entering the alliance is that it provided a way for nonmember companies to be GMP certified to the NPA standard through NSF. Whether manufacturers use NPA's GMP certification or NSF's, the alliance indicated that the Association believed that GMPs are good for the entire industry.

This sentiment was shared by legislators at the time the alliance was put into effect in 2001 (9). Senator Tom Harkin (D-Iowa) commended the two organizations for "their commitment to ensure dietary supplements are produced to high standards and are accurately labeled." According to Harkin, "These organizations have picked up the ball that the FDA dropped in not issuing GMP regulations. Both these programs represent another important step toward the dietary supplement industry's goal of ensuring product quality and consumer safety." It is notable that the alliance was carried out as a private sector initiative at no direct cost to the public and on a substantially faster track than is usually the case in government-sponsored programs; however, following the promulgation of the final FDA GMPs (21 CFR Part 111) from FDA, NSF terminated the alliance with the NPA and no provisions were offered by NSF at the time they terminated the alliance to continue mutual recognition of the two programs.

NATURAL PRODUCTS ASSOCIATION CHINA RAW INGREDIENT TESTING INITIATIVE

In 2006 the association opened a branch office in Beijing, the Peoples Republic of China. The goals of that office are twofold. The first, which ties in to our overall mission is to grow the marketplace for natural products in China, the second is that with so much of the industry dominated by commodity ingredients originating from China, we wanted to play a role in strengthening the supply chain. While some Chinese suppliers are currently undergoing NPA GMP certification, with much of the recent press on the heels of melamine in pet foods, diethylene glycol in toothpaste, and tainted milk protein materials all originating from China, the association wanted to have the ability to display transparency not only for manufacturing practices but also for ingredients. The program is in response to industry efforts to maintain product quality and reliability as competition to supply ingredients and raw materials to the industry grows. In 2007, the association launched another industry first by offering a program for testing Chinese raw materials for purity and composition. While testing materials in China is nothing new, instead of having to rely either on tests provided by China or on postshipment tests, US manufacturers can

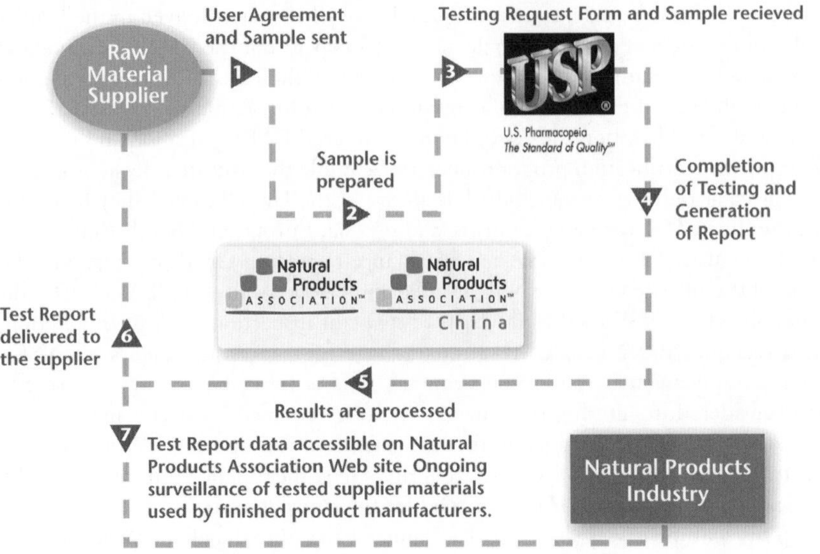

Figure 23.1 • NPA Raw Ingredient Testing Program Lifecycle.

test the quality of Chinese raw materials prior to shipment, and members have access to a database of suppliers' test results for consideration when making contractual decisions (10). The association's program also offers suppliers a competitive edge as well as a chance to demonstrate the quality of their products. How the program works is detailed in Figure 23.1. The NPA has a contract with United States Pharmacopoeia (USP) to test dietary supplement raw ingredients. The tests may be used to confirm the identity, strength, and purity of the ingredient, or they may be limited to searching for the presence of contaminants. USP scientists in Shanghai, China, perform the tests for the NPA in most cases. In some instances in which USP does not have highly specialized equipment to run some tests, such as microbiological evaluations, USP will subcontract these test to laboratories that USP has inspected and audited.

While the program does not have the storied past of TruLabel or the GMP certification program it has enjoyed much of the same success in its brief history. Recently, the program along with the GMP certification program was featured in the July 2008 Action Update Plan of the Presidential Working Group on Import Safety (11). Both programs were cited as private sector engagement highlights that help strengthen and secure the supply chain. Another example of the success of the program is that in October 2007, the Association was awarded a grant from the United States Department of Commerce (USDOC), receiving both financial and collaborative support from USDOC through the department's Market Development Cooperator Program in large part due to this initiative (12).

SUMMARY

While the dietary supplement industry is not the largest industry and while the NPA is certainly not the largest trade association in Washington DC, we have been able to grow membership and maintain a leadership position in the dietary supplement industry in large part due to our self-regulatory programs. They have afforded the manufacturers, suppliers, and retailers with the tools to gain and maintain consumer confidence. While we represent other sectors of the natural products industry, for example, personal care, we now have self-regulatory programs for them, specifically the first and only natural standard/natural seal for personal care products (13). The knowledge, respect, and recognition gained not only from the consumer but also from the federal government as indicated above is part of the reason the association and natural products industry are as viable and credible as they are today.

References

1. www.naturalproductsassoc.org.
2. http://www.ftc.gov/speeches/pitofsky/self4.shtm.
3. http://www.naturalproductsassoc.org/site/PageServer?pagename = ic_bg_trulabel.
4. http://ods.od.nih.gov/News/DSLDPilotAnnouncement.aspx.
5. http://www.fda.gov/bbs/topics/NEWS/2007/NEW01657.html.
6. American Botanical Council. *HerbalGram* 1996;38:27. http://content.herbalgram.org/iherb/herbalgram/articleview.asp?a = 1216.
7. http://www.naturalproductsassoc.org/site/PageServer?pagename = ic_gmp.
8. FFD&CA§ 402(g)(1).
9. http://www.supplementquality.com/news/NSF_NNFA_GMPs.html.
10. http://www.naturalproductsassoc.org/site/PageNavigator/abt_China_purity.
11. http://www.importsafety.gov/report/actionupdate/actionplanupdate.pdf.
12. http://www.naturalproductsassoc.org/site/News2?abbr = pc_&page = NewsArticle&id = 9095.
13. http://www.naturalproductsassoc.org/site/PageServer?pagename = naturalseal_index.

IV

Reactions and Interactions

CHAPTER 24

Herbal and Dietary Supplements: Important Reactions and Interactions

Robert Alan Bonakdar

No book on herbal and dietary supplements is complete without a section on adverse effects, reaction, and interactions. Unfortunately, this is one of the most difficult to handle and often-mishandled concepts in dietary supplementation. In discussing dietary supplements with clinicians, there are several scenarios, especially for clinicians who are new to discussing or managing dietary supplements, which can made them hesitant to bring up the topic with patients. One scenario is the case report of a potentially bad outcome reported in a medical journal attributed to a particular supplement. This is especially true if all the clinician hears about the supplement is that it can cause a serious adverse effect without readily available and realiable information with which to balance this negative potential.

The next two chapters hopefully provide the tools to proceed into this discussion with the needed reinforcement. The pharmacists asked to contribute have important perspectives to provide. First, they are involved with response to poison control issues that sometimes involve dietary supplements. In this scenario, multiple tools are needed to understand the likelihood of the reaction/interaction to determine the best response. Second, their work with the Natural Medicines Comprehensive Database provides examples of point-of-care resources available to discuss the benefit of a supplement with what is known about reactions/interactions.

In developing a balanced perspective it is important to know a potential is just that. Thus, a patient on ginkgo is not immediately at high risk for bleeding. In fact, if the clinician is aware of concomitant medications/supplements and goes on to making sure the supplement is well dosed and characterized as one which has been studied in a numerous clinical trials that did not demonstrate a significant risk of bleeding, then the potential can be seen very differently with a higher confidence to consider this treatment.

Similarly, a clinician not familiar with the popular European antidepressant St John's Wort (SJW) can view its use very cautiously. In the right setting, studies have demonstrated that standardized extracts can perform as well as selective serotonin reuptake inhibitor in the setting of mild to even severe depression and can have a lower side effect profile as compared to synthetic antidepressants (1, 2). However, in the wrong setting, it has also been shown in well-controlled trials to interact negatively with important medications (3).

SO, IS SJW GOOD OR BAD FOR THE DEPRESSED PATIENT?

The answer is in the discussion and understanding of the patient scenario as well as education regarding the benefit of specific formulations. The clinician must first understand the medical history, previous treatments, and goals for medical therapy. The clinician must begin to realize that not all supplements (SJWs in this case) are good or bad but, based on the evidence, certain formulations may be as well-tolerated and effective as other therapies (depression in this case) previously prescribed.

Putting these two factors together can change the picture dramatically and allow a frank and mutually beneficial discussion regarding the use or nonuse of particular supplements. In the end, previous studies, including the recent Mayo Clinic trial, have shown that the actual rate of adverse interactions is quite low and the most likely scenarios are easy to categorize:

> A small number of prescription medications and dietary supplements accounted for most of the interactions. The actual potential for harm was low. (4)

The clinician, in triaging cases, still needs to be very cautious in the scenario of well-documented reaction or interaction, such as the patient on HIV medication considering an antidepressant. In other cases, such as those noted in the chapters to follow, the clinician can quickly access the likelihood and significance of potential reactions/interactions that are less well-known. Lastly, there are still many cases exemplifying the art of medicine in which there is simply not enough information to place the supplement squarely on the risk/benefit radar. In this case, the clinician and the patient must truly engage in the art of medicine to figure out whether the supplement in question is the best choice for the issue at hand. Monitoring and reporting the benefit or not of such therapy is also essential in advancing medicine and our collective knowledge base.

References

1. Anghelescu IG, Kohnen R, Szegedi A, Klement S, Kieser M. Comparison of Hypericum extract WS 5570 and paroxetine in ongoing treatment after recovery from an episode of moderate to severe depression: results from a randomized multicenter study. *Pharmacopsychiatry* 2006;39(6):213–219.
2. Schulz V. Safety of St. John's Wort extract compared to synthetic antidepressants. *Phytomedicine* 2006;13(3):199–204.
3. Piscitelli SC, Burstein AH, Chaitt D, et al. Indinavir concentrations and St John's wort. *Lancet* 2000;355(9203):547–548.
4. Sood A, Sood R, Brinker FJ, Mann R, Loehrer LL, Wahner-Roedler DL. Potential for interactions between dietary supplements and prescription medications. *Am J Med* 2008;121(3):207–211.

CHAPTER 25

Herbal Adverse Reactions

Philip J. Gregory and Rajul Patel

INTRODUCTION

An important concept in pharmacology is that any substance that can produce a beneficial effect can also produce a harmful effect, also known as a side effect or an adverse reaction. This concept holds true whether the pharmacological effect is produced by a conventional drug or an herbal product. Whether a drug or herbal product produces a beneficial or harmful effect is often a matter of dosing and administration. At one dose a product may cause maximal benefit and minimal side effects. However, as the dose changes, usually as it goes higher, the potential benefit levels off or declines, while the risk of side effects increase.

Conventional drugs are highly concentrated- purified substances with relatively potent pharmacological effects. When such drugs are used, the balance between beneficial and harmful effects can be very delicate. Although herbal products have pharmacological effects, these products tend to be significantly less potent than conventional drugs. As a result, the tolerable dosing range tends to be wider, resulting in fewer significant side effects for such products when compared to conventional drugs.

Many herbal products are available as extracts in pill form. These extracts often concentrate active constituents of herbal products. Herbal products that are concentrated may increase the potency of the product but can also have adverse consequences such as decreasing the range of tolerable doses, and potentially increasing the chance of harmful side effects.

Adverse reactions or side effects from drugs and herbal products often occur because of improper dosing; however, there are a variety of types of adverse reactions (1):

Pharmacological reactions: Adverse reactions that occur because of dosing.

Drug interaction: Adverse reactions that occur when two or more substances are combined, resulting in an outcome that would not be expected if one of the substances were used alone.

Intolerance: A significant overreaction in response to an unusually small dose of a substance.

Hypersensitivity: An allergic reaction that cannot be explained by the pharmacology of the substance.

Idiosyncratic: An uncharacteristic response to a substance that is not allergic in nature and usually does not occur upon administration.

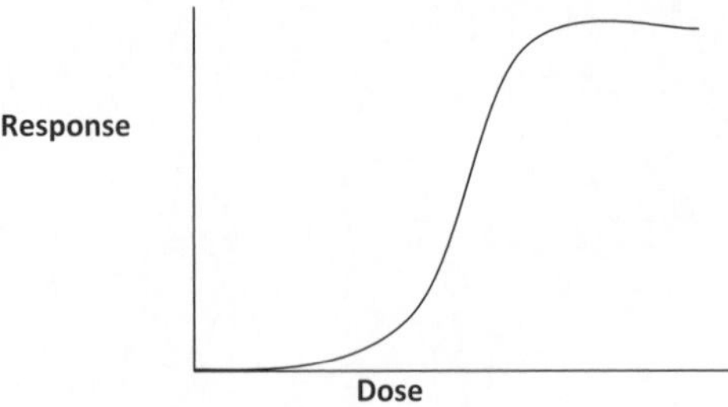

Figure 25.1 • Dose-response curve.

ASSESSING CAUSALITY OF HERBAL ADVERSE REACTIONS

Key Clinical Pearls

Suspected adverse reactions to herbal products need to be assessed to determine causality. When an adverse event occurs, it may be due to the herbal supplement, but it could also be due to a drug, a life event, or a concomitant disease state. Several key questions should be asked about an adverse reaction to get a better understanding of how likely it is that a specific substance caused the event. Examples of such questions may include the following:

Timing: Is the timing of the event consistent with the administration of the substance? For example, if the reaction consistently occurs shortly after the substance is administered, it is more likely that the substance caused the event.

De-challenge: Does the adverse reaction subside or improve when the substance is discontinued? If yes, then it is more likely that the substance is causative. A similar concept, re-challenge, addresses whether the reaction reappears when the substance is readministered. If so, again, it is more likely that the substance caused the reaction.

Dose response: Did the reaction occur when the dose of the substance was increased? If yes, it is more likely that the reaction was caused by the substance (see Fig. 25.1).

Alternate causes: Are there other feasible explanations for the reaction? If other plausible explanations exist, it is less likely that the substance caused the event.

Previous reports/studies: Has the reaction been previously reported and if so, in what number and strength (an isolated case study or controlled clinical trial). Searches for previous reports can be performed in database sources such as those noted in Table 25.1. If previously reported, is the phenomenon consistently noted with a specific formulation or extract or population (see the "Kava ⇔ Hepatotoxicity" section), and does the scenario encountered parallel that seen in the literature?

These questions, along with others, have been implemented in various tools in an attempt to more objectively assess whether a drug or another substance is the cause of an event. The most commonly used of these tools is called the "Naranjo Algorithm" (see Fig. 25.2) (47). By completing a series of questions and scoring each response, an estimate of the likelihood that an adverse reaction is caused by a substance can be determined. Causality is classified as "definite or highly probable," "probable," "possible," or "doubtful."

If examination of the scenario, research literature, and resource tools implicate an adverse effect, the clinician should take appropriate steps including:

TABLE 25.1 Selected Resources That Collect and Evaluate Information About Adverse Reactions and Interactions Related to Natural Products

- Alternative and Allied Medicine Database (www.ovid.com/site/catalog/DataBase/12.jsp)
- Embase (www.embase.com/)
- International Bibliographic Information on Dietary Supplements (grande.nal.usda.gov/ibids/index.php)
- Natural Medicines Comprehensive Database (www.naturaldatabase.com)
- PubMed (www.ncbi.nlm.nih.gov/pubmed)
- Reactions Database (http://www.ovid.com/site/products/fieldguide/adre/About_Reactions_Database.jsp)

discontinuation of the agent(s), laboratory/clinical evaluation, and specialty referral. In addition, the clinician should use available tools, including the MedWatch and Natural Medicines Watch™ programs, for systematic reporting. Lastly, submission to scientific publications is suggested so that experts in the field can peer review the findings and examine the case in the context of other available evidence.

Naranjo Algorithm

	Yes	No	Don't Know	Score
1. Are there previous conclusive reports of this reaction?	+1	0	0	
2. Did the adverse event appear after the suspect drug was administered?	+2	–1	0	
3. Did the adverse reaction improve when the drug was discontinued?	+1	0	0	
4. Did the adverse reaction reappear when the drug was readministered?	+2	–1	0	
5. Are there alternate causes (other than the drug) that could on their own have caused the reaction?	–1	+2	0	
6. Did the reaction appear when a placebo was given?	–1	+1	0	
7. Was the drug detected in the blood (or other fluids) in concentrations known to be toxic?	+1	0	0	
8. Was the reaction more severe when the dose was increased or less severe when the dose was decreased?	+1	0	0	
9. Did the patient have a similar reaction to the same or similar drugs in any previous exposure?	+1	0	0	
10. Was the adverse effect confirmed by any objective evidence?	+1	0	0	
			Total Score:	

Score Interpretation:
Definite or highly probable ⇔ ≥ 9
Probable ⇔ 5–8
Possible ⇔ 1–4
Doubtful ⇔ ≤ 0

Figure 25.2 • The Naranjo Algorithm (47).

OVERVIEW OF IMPORTANT HERBAL ADVERSE REACTIONS

The exact rate of adverse reactions due to herbal products is not known with any certainty. This is primarily because of a lack of rigorous scientific study, poor surveillance, and the underreporting of such events by health professionals.

Information about potential adverse reactions to herbal products is primarily derived from two sources: clinical trials and case reports. A secondary outcome of most clinical trials is an assessment of side effects experienced by patients receiving treatment. Clinical trials serve as the best source of data to determine fairly commonly experienced adverse reactions. However, adverse reactions that are fairly uncommon are rarely detected in clinical trials because the trials simply are not large enough to identify events that are rare in occurrence. For example, an event that occurs in only 1 out of 500 treated patients is very likely to go undetected in a trial with 100 patients. Case reports that are published in the literature or reported to adverse reaction surveillance systems (e.g., FDA's MedWatch) represent much of what we know about potentially severe adverse reactions to herbal products. Unfortunately, these reports can have serious limitations. Many of the reports lack enough detail to adequately assess causality. In many case reports, other potential causes of the event or reaction cannot be ruled out, making it difficult, if not impossible, to determine if the herbal product actually caused the reaction.

Unique to herbal products exist the issues of product quality and potential contamination or adulteration. If an herbal product is associated with a severe adverse reaction, it is important to determine what is actually contained in the product. If the product is contaminated with a prescription drug for instance, the adverse reaction may likely be due to that contaminant rather than the herbal product itself. However, when adverse reactions occur, it is very rare that investigators would conduct a laboratory assessment of the components of the herbal product to rule out contamination as a possible cause. Again, this limits our ability to adequately assess whether the herbal product itself is the causative factor of an adverse reaction.

Given this background, the following section will highlight some important or emerging adverse reaction issues that are related to commonly used herbal products.

Bitter Orange ⇔ Cardiac Toxicity

Bitter orange (*Citrus aurantium*) has largely replaced ephedra as the ingredient in herbal products used for weight loss and improving athletic performance. The fruit and peel of bitter orange contain the adrenergic agonists synephrine and octopamine. Synephrine is structurally similar to epinephrine and octopamine is similar to norepinephrine. Bitter orange fruit naturally contains approximately 0.02% synephrine. The dried fruit provides about 0.35% synephrine. Extracts of the dried fruit typically contain 3% synephrine. Commercially available bitter orange–containing herbal supplements typically provide between 1% and 6% synephrine (2).

Since bitter orange began to replace ephedra in many herbal products, the number of case reports of adverse reactions related to bitter orange has increased. In healthy adults, taking 900 mg of bitter orange extract, standardized to contain 6% synephrine, can increase diastolic and systolic blood pressure and heart rate for up to 5 hours (3, 4). Between 1998 and 2004, Health Canada received 16 reports of serious cardiovascular toxicity, including tachycardia, ventricular arrhythmia, cardiac arrest, blackouts, and death, in patients consuming bitter orange. In most of these cases, bitter orange had been combined with caffeine or another stimulant

(5). Several other cases have also been published linking bitter orange to reports of myocardial infarction, tachyarrythmia with QT-interval prolongation, angina, and ischemic stroke (6–10). In many of these cases, bitter orange has been identified as the probable cause of the adverse reaction.

Black Cohosh ⇔ Hepatotoxicity

Black cohosh (*Cimicifuga racemosa*) is most commonly used to reduce hot flashes in menopausal women (2). Concerns have developed over the last several years about its potential to cause hepatotoxicity. Although elevated liver enzyme levels have not been detected in clinical trials evaluating black cohosh, several cases have been reported describing liver damage, in many cases requiring liver transplant, in women taking various black cohosh products (11–15). Currently, more than 49 cases of hepatotoxicity have been reported in individuals taking black cohosh–containing products. Some of these reports have been published in the medical literature, but many remain unpublished and have been reported only via adverse event surveillance systems (16–18).

It remains unclear as to whether or not black cohosh was the actual cause of liver damage in these case reports. Many of these reports lack the critical details necessary to adequately assess causality. Reports have occurred with a variety of different formulations of black cohosh. In several cases, there are potential explanations for liver damage aside from the intake of black cohosh–containing products. Therefore, in most of these cases, while causality from black cohosh is possible, it may not be probable. Nonetheless, some countries require black cohosh products to carry warning labels indicating a risk for liver damage. Although such labeling is not currently required in the United States, the United States Pharmacopeia does recommend such labeling for black cohosh products.

Ginkgo ⇔ Spontaneous Bleeding

Ginkgo biloba is commonly used for memory enhancement and to reduce symptoms of dementia. Ginkgo is thought to have a variety of pharmacological effects including decreasing platelet aggregation (2).

Several published reports have linked ginkgo to spontaneous bleeding events ranging from minor to severe bleeding. There are several reports of intracerebral bleeding, which in some instances have led to neurological damage or death (19–24). Other bleeding events that have occurred in individuals who have taken ginkgo include ocular bleeding and excessive intra- and/or postoperative bleeding (27–30).

Interestingly, clinical trials evaluating ginkgo use have not detected a significantly increased risk of bleeding when compared to placebo (31, 32). This suggests that spontaneous bleeding may be a relatively uncommon event.

Ginkgo ⇔ Seizure

There are reports of seizure occurring in patients with or without a prior history of seizure following ingestion of ginkgo. In one reported case, a patient died after experiencing a seizure in a swimming pool. In these reports, it is unclear if ginkgo was the cause of seizure since other factors may have played a role (33–35).

It is important to note that ginkgo seed does contain a neurotoxin that could induce seizure. However, gingko products typically contain gingko leaf extracts. The ginkgo leaf also contains a very small amount of the neurotoxin, but it would not be expected to be enough to reduce the seizure threshold. Despite this, there is some concern that some gingko products may be contaminated with ginkgo seeds, thereby increasing the patient's exposure to higher concentrations of the neurotoxin (2). Standardized products based on ginkgo leaf are less likely to have potential contamination issues.

Until more is known, patients with epilepsy should avoid taking ginkgo-containing products.

Green Tea ⇔ Hepatotoxicity

There have been at least 30 reported cases of hepatotoxicity, primarily linked to ingestion of green tea extract products in pill form (36–39). In most cases, liver function returned to normal after discontinuation of the green tea product; however, a liver transplant was required in one report. The green tea product has been identified as the probable cause of the liver damage in many of the case reports.

The exact mechanism as to how green tea extracts potentially cause liver damage is unknown. It is possible that certain extraction processes, for example, those used for ethanolic extracts, produce hepatotoxic constituents. However, in most cases, green tea products were not assessed to determine if any contaminants were present. Finally, the traditional use of green tea as a beverage (i.e., free of special extracts or additives for specific indications) does not appear to be linked to hepatotoxicity.

Kava ⇔ Hepatotoxicity

Kava (*Piper methysticum*) is commonly used for reducing anxiety and feelings of stress. It is also used ceremonially by Pacific Islanders.

There are at least 68 reported cases of hepatotoxicity, following use of kava-containing products (40–43). Liver toxicity is more frequently associated with prolonged use of very high doses of kava. Symptoms seem to resolve spontaneously after discontinuation of kava. There is some concern that even short-term use of kava, in typical doses, might cause acute hepatitis including severe hepatocellular necrosis in some patients. A need for a liver transplant or death has been seen in some after as few as 1 to 3 months of kava use. Because of the risk of hepatotoxicity, kava supplements have been banned in Switzerland, Germany, and Canada. Several other countries are considering removing kava from the market (2).

It is important to note that kava tea used in the Pacific Islands as a ceremonial and social beverage has not been reported to cause hepatotoxicity (2). This suggests that the type of extraction method used could be responsible for liver damage. Alcohol and acetone extracts of kava have been linked to liver toxicity; water extracts have not. There is also speculation that "poor metabolizers," those patients with deficiency of the cytochrome P450 2D6 (CYP2D6) isoenzyme, may be at increased risk for hepatotoxic effects related to kava. It is estimated that up to 10% of people of European descent have a genetic deficiency of CYP2D6. This deficiency has not been found in Pacific Islanders.

Until more is known, patients should avoid kava supplements. Patients who continue to use kava should get routine liver function monitoring.

Red Yeast Rice ⇔ Myopathy

Red yeast rice is the product of rice fermented with *Monascus purpureus* yeast. This fermentation process naturally produces approximately 0.4% monacolins, including the drug lovastatin. Red yeast rice is traditionally consumed as a food. However, in North America, red yeast rice extracts are used in pill form to reduce cholesterol. The concentration of lovastatin and related compounds in these products ranges from about 0.4% to over 1%. As a result, a typical daily dose (1200–2400 mg) of a red yeast rice supplement may provide between 5 mg and 20 mg of lovastatin (2).

As such, it is not surprising that red yeast rice supplements improve cholesterol profiles. However, it also should not be surprising that red yeast rice can cause side effects similar to those seen in patients taking prescription "statin" (HMG-CoA reductase inhibitor) drugs. Red yeast rice products have been linked to reports of myopathy, rhabdomyolysis, and hepatotoxicity (44–46). Patients often do not realize that red yeast rice contains constituents similar to prescription statin drugs. These adverse reactions are more likely in patients who add red yeast rice to their existing statin drug.

HOW TO REPORT ADVERSE REACTIONS TO HERBALS PRODUCTS

Reporting potential adverse reactions caused by herbal products is a crucial step in identifying emerging safety concerns. Several systems exist for reporting adverse reactions on an institutional, local, national, and international level.

MedWatch

The U.S. Food and Drug Administration (FDA) has been operating a national adverse reaction reporting system since 1962. In 1993, this program became known as MedWatch. This system allows anyone, including health professionals and consumers, to voluntarily report suspected adverse reactions to prescription medications, over-the-counter medications, dietary supplements, herbal products, and medical products. Although reporting of adverse reactions is voluntary, the FDA highly encourages health professionals and consumers alike to report all suspected serious adverse reactions.

For drug manufacturers, including herbal product and dietary supplement manufacturers, reporting of adverse reactions to FDA is mandatory. If a manufacturer receives notification of an adverse reaction to one of its products, it is obligated to submit a report to the FDA describing the event.

Natural Medicines Watch™

Natural Medicines Watch™ is a new international program established in 2008 by Therapeutic Research Faculty. This program gives health professionals and consumers a simplified approach to reporting adverse reactions related to herbals products and dietary supplements. It allows reporting of adverse reactions at the point of care through the resource Natural Medicines Comprehensive Database (www.naturaldatabase.com). Therefore, clinicians are better able to pinpoint relevant product information and instantly develop an adverse reaction report using the same resource. Natural Medicines Watch™ was developed to work seamlessly with the FDA MedWatch reporting system. Therefore, reports originating in the United States submitted through Natural Medicines Watch™ are automatically shared with FDA.

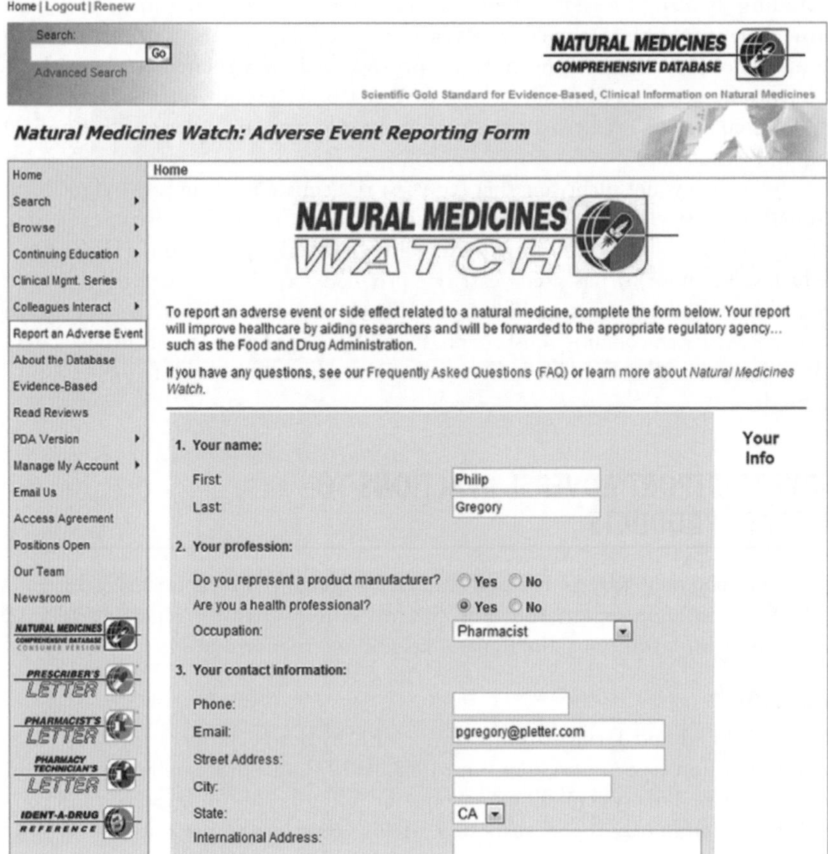

Figure 25.3 • Screenshots of how an adverse effect can be reported using Natural Medicines Watch™. *(continued)*

Figure 25.3 provides a screenshot of how an adverse effect can be reported using Natural Medicines Watch™.

CONCLUSION

High-quality information about the potential adverse reactions of herbal products remains very limited. Clinical trials alone often are not large enough to detect adverse reactions that might not be very common. As such, most available data about potentially severe adverse reactions come from case reports that may or may not be reliable. Assessing these reports to determine causality is a critical step in assessing the relevance of a potential adverse reaction. Reporting of suspected adverse reactions is crucially important to gain a better understanding of safety concerns related to herbal products. Serious reactions to herbal products should be reported via the FDA's MedWatch program or Natural Medicines Watch.

Patient Info

4. Patient Information if known:

To protect privacy, do NOT enter patient names or any other patient identifiers. A tracking number will be issued upon completion of this report that you can use for the patient's records, if necessary.

Did you personally experience this adverse event or side affect? ○ **Yes** ○ **No**

Gender: ○ **Male** ○ **Female**

Age: [ ] years

Race/Ethnicity:
○ **American Indian or Alaska native**
○ **Asian**
○ **Black or African American**
○ **Hispanic or Latino**
○ **Native Hawaiian or Other Pacific Islander**
○ **White**
○ **Other** [ ]

Weight [ ] ◉ **lbs** ○ **kg**

Height [ ]

Medicines & Conditions

5. Product(s) suspected to have caused adverse event or side effect:

Add suspected products

6. Other medications taken include:
Search for medications, select from a list, or enter the completed drug name below:

[ ]

7. Medical conditions include:
Search for conditions, select from a list, or enter the full condition name below:

[ ]

Figure 25.3 • (*Continued*)

References

1. Gregory PJ, Kier K. Medication misadventures. In: Malone P, Mosdell K, Kier K, et al., eds. *Drug Information: A Guide for Pharmacists*. McGraw-Hill: New York, 2001.
2. Jellin JM, Gregory PJ, eds. Natural Medicines Comprehensive Database. Available at: www.naturaldatabase.com. Accessed November 3, 2009.
3. Bui LT, Nguyen DT, Ambrose PJ. Blood pressure and heart rate effects following a single dose of bitter orange. *Ann Pharmacother* 2006;40:53–57.
4. Haller CA, Benowitz NL, Jacob P III. Hemodynamic effects of ephedra-free weight-loss supplements in humans. *Am J Med* 2005;118:998–1003.
5. Jordan S, Murty M, Pilon K. Products containing bitter orange or synephrine: suspected cardiovascular adverse reactions. *CMAJ* 2004;12:993–994.
6. Nykamp DL, Fackih MN, Compton AL. Possible association of acute lateral-wall myocardial infarction and bitter orange supplement. *Ann Pharmacother* 2004;38:812–816.
7. Firenzuoli F, Gori L, Galapai C. Adverse reaction to an adrenergic herbal extract (Citrus aurantium). *Phytomedicine* 2005;12:247–248.

8. Nasir JM, Durning SJ, Ferguson M, et al. Exercise-induced syncope associated with QT prolongation and ephedra-free Xenadrine. *Mayo Clin Proc* 2004;79:1059–1062.
9. Gange CA, Madias C, Felix-Getzik EM, et al. Variant angina associated with bitter orange in a dietary supplement. *Mayo Clin Proc* 2006;81:545–548.
10. Bouchard NC, Howland MA, Greller HA, et al. Ischemic stroke associated with use of an ephedra-free dietary supplement containing synephrine. *Mayo Clin Proc* 2005;80: 541–545.
11. Lontos S, Jones RM, Angus PW, et al. Acute liver failure associated with the use of herbal preparations containing black cohosh. *Med J Aust* 2003;179:390–391.
12. Vitetta L, Thomsen M, Sali A. Black cohosh and other herbal remedies associated with acute hepatitis. *Med J Aust* 2003;178:411–412.
13. Levitsky J, Alli TA, Wisecarver J, et al. Fulminant liver failure associated with the use of black cohosh. *Dig Dis Sci* 2005;50:538–539.
14. Lynch CR, Folkers ME, Hutson WR. Fulminant hepatic failure associated with the use of black cohosh: a case report. *Liver Transpl* 2006;12:989–992.
15. Chow ECY, Teo M, Ring JA, et al. Liver failure associated with the use of black cohosh for menopausal symptoms. *Med J Aust* 2008;188:420–422.
16. Mahady GB, Low Dog T, Barrett ML, et al. United States Pharmacopeia review of the black cohosh case reports of hepatotoxicity. *Menopause* 2008;15:628–638.
17. Adverse Drug Reactions Advisory Committee. Hepatotoxicity with black cohosh. *Aust Adverse Drug React Bull* 2006;25:6. Available at: www.tga.gov.au/adr/aadrb/aadr0604.htm#a1.
18. Adverse Drug Reactions Advisory Committee. Black cohosh and liver toxicity—an update. *Aust Adverse Drug React Bull* 2007;26:11.
19. Benjamin J, Muir T, Briggs K, et al. A case of cerebral haemorrhage—can Ginkgo biloba be implicated? *Postgrad Med J* 2001;77:112–113.
20. Rowin J, Lewis SL. Spontaneous bilateral subdural hemotomas with chronic Gingko biloba ingestion. *Neurology* 1996;46:1775–1776.
21. Miller LG, Freeman B. Possible subdural hematoma associated with Ginkgo biloba. *J Herb Pharmacother* 2002;2:57–63.
22. Bent S, Goldberg H, Padula A, et al. Spontaneous bleeding associated with Ginkgo biloba. A case report and systematic review of the literature. *J Gen Intern Med* 2005;20; 657–661.
23. Meisel C, Johne A, Roots I. Fatal intracerebral mass bleeding associated with Ginkgo biloba and ibuprofen. *Atherosclerosis* 2003;167:367.
24. Vale S. Subarachnoid haemorrhage associated with Ginkgo biloba. *Lancet* 1998;352:36.
25. Rosenblatt M, Mindel T. Spontaneous hyphema associated with ingestion of Gingko biloba extract. *N Engl J Med* 1997;336:1108.
26. Fong KC, Kinnear PE. Retrobulbar haemorrhage associated with chronic Ginkgo biloba ingestion. *Postgrad Med J* 2003;79:531–532.
27. Fessenden JM, Wittenborn W, Clarke L. Gingko biloba: a case report of herbal medicine and bleeding postoperatively from a laparoscopic cholecystectomy. *Am Surg* 2001;67:33–35.
28. Destro MW, Speranzini MB, Cavalheiro Filho C, et al. Bilateral haematoma after rhytidoplasty and blepharoplasty following chronic use of Ginkgo biloba. *Br J Plast Surg* 2005; 58:100–101.
29. Hauser D, Gayowski T, Singh N. Bleeding complications precipitated by unrecognized Gingko biloba use after liver transplantation. *Transpl Int* 2002;15:377–379.
30. Yagmur E, Piatkowski A, Groger A, et al. Bleeding complication under Gingko biloba medication. *Am J Hematol* 2005;79:343–344.
31. Dodge HH, Zitzelberger T, Oken BS, et al. A randomized placebo-controlled trial of ginkgo biloba for the prevention of cognitive decline. *Neurology* 2008;70(19, pt 2):1809–1817.
32. DeKosky ST, Williamson JD, Fitzpatrick AL, et al. Ginkgo biloba for prevention of dementia. *JAMA* 2008;300:2253–2262.

33. Gregory PJ. Seizure associated with Ginkgo biloba? *Ann Intern Med* 2001;134:344.
34. Granger AS. Ginkgo biloba precipitating epileptic seizures. *Age Ageing* 2001;30:523–525.
35. Kupiec T, Raj V. Fatal seizures due to potential herb-drug interactions with Ginkgo biloba. *J Anal Toxicol* 2005:755–758.
36. Bonkovsky HL. Hepatotoxicity associated with supplements containing Chinese green tea (Camellia sinensis). *Ann Intern Med* 2006;144:68–71.
37. Jimenez-Saenz M, Martinez-Sanchez, MDC. Acute hepatitis associated with the use of green tea infusions. *J Hepatol* 2006;44:616–619.
38. Gloro R, Hourmand-Ollivier I, Mosquet B, et al. Fulminant hepatitis during self-medication with hydroalcoholic extract of green tea. *Eur J Gastroenterol Hepatol* 2005;17: 1135–1137.
39. Sarma DN, Barrett ML, Chavez ML, et al. Safety of green tea extracts: a systematic review by the US Pharmacopeia. *Drug Saf* 2008;31:469–484.
40. Escher M, Desmeules J, Giostra E, et al. Drug points: hepatitis associated with kava, a herbal remedy for anxiety. *BMJ* 2001;322:139.
41. Russmann S, Lauterberg BH, Helbling A. Kava hepatotoxicity [letter]. *Ann Intern Med* 2001;135:68–69.
42. Gow PJ, Connelly NJ, Hill RL, et al. Fatal fulminant hepatic failure induced by a natural therapy containing kava. *Med J Aust* 2003;178:442–443.
43. Liver toxicity with kava. *Pharmacist's Letter/Prescriber's Letter* 2001;18(1):180115.
44. Prasad GV, Wong T, Meliton G, et al. Rhabdomyolysis due to red yeast rice (Monascus purpureus) in a renal transplant recipient. *Transplantation* 2002;74:1200–1201.
45. Mueller PS. Symptomatic myopathy due to red yeast rice. *Ann Intern Med* 2006;145: 474–475.
46. Roselle H, Ekatan A, Tzeng J, et al. Symptomatic hepatitis associated with the use of herbal red yeast rice. *Ann Intern Med* 2008;149:516–517.
47. Naranjo CA, Busto U, Sellers EM, et al. A method for estimating the probability of adverse drug reactions. *Clin Pharmacol Ther* 1981;30:239–245.

CHAPTER 26

Herb–Drug Interactions

Philip J. Gregory

INTRODUCTION

The elderly population in the United States is growing exponentially. This population represents the largest users of health care and medications in the United States. An estimated 21% to 40% of this population also takes at least one natural product such as an herbal supplement (1, 2). In addition, 20% to 60% of prescription medication users in the United States are taking their medication in combination with an herbal supplement (3–5). As a result, the potential for herb–drug interactions in this population is huge.

But how often do these interactions actually occur and result in a clinically significant adverse event? The answer to this question is not known. It is a question that may not even be knowable. Herb–drug interactions are not often recognized or reported by patients or health care providers. Because inconsistent or nonexistent reporting, true rates of herb–drug interactions in any population cannot be reliably estimated.

Some authors have attempted to assess the rate of clinically significant herb–drug interactions in specific populations with varying results. However, most of these assessments are similarly unreliable and incomplete.

FRAMEWORK FOR EVALUATING POTENTIAL INTERACTIONS

The research team at *Natural Medicines Comprehensive Database* has systematically reviewed evidence-related potential herb–drug interactions. More than 1,600 potential interactions between herbs or dietary supplements and conventional drugs have been identified. These potential interactions are based on pharmacokinetic research, pharmacodynamic research, case reports, animal model, and in vitro research. While some of these potential interactions have been documented to occur in humans, some are speculative based on very limited evidence.

To help clinicians determine which interactions are most likely to be clinically meaningful, these interactions are rated on the basis of the level of supporting evidence and the severity of the potential outcome. Based on these ratings, each potential interaction can be categorized as follows:

Major—Do not use the combination together: An herb–drug combination is contraindicated if it is likely to result in an interaction based on strong supporting evidence and that might reasonably cause a moderate to severe outcome.

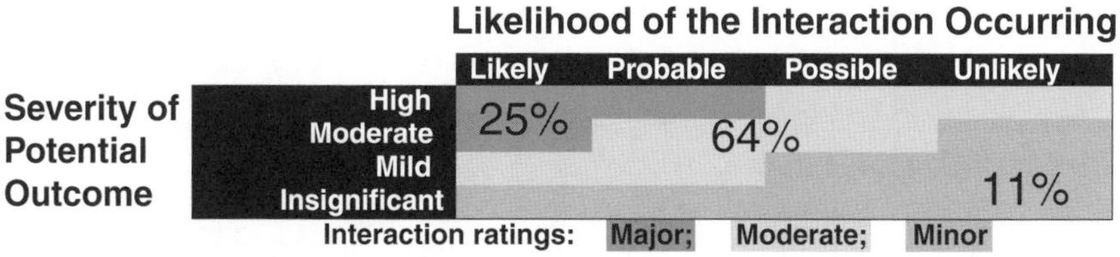

Likelihood of the Interaction Occurring
Likely Probable Possible Unlikely
Severity of Potential Outcome
High
Moderate
Mild
Insignificant
25%
64%
11%
Interaction ratings: Major; Moderate; Minor

Figure 26.1 • Distribution of herb–drug interaction ratings.

Moderate—Use with caution or avoid the combination: These are interactions that are less likely to occur and/or are less likely to result in a significant adverse outcome. However, if this level of interaction does occur it may cause significant discomfort and may require changes in therapy. An herb–drug combination that causes this level of interaction should be used cautiously, or avoided altogether, if reasonable to do so.

Minor—Be watchful with the combination: Interactions in this category are unlikely to occur or are likely to have only clinically insignificant outcomes in most people. However, patients should be monitored for the development of these interactions when suspected products are combined.

Based on this categorization, most potential herb–drug interactions, about 64%, fall in the middle and receive the "Moderate" rating. About 25% receive the "Major" rating and 11% receive the "Minor" rating (see Fig. 26.1).

TYPES OF HERB–DRUG INTERACTIONS

Herb–drug interactions can be broadly classified on the basis of the mechanism of the interaction. Interactions can be either pharmacokinetic or pharmacodynamic.

Pharmacokinetic interactions are those that physically affect the level of a substance in the body or at a site within the body. These interactions affect the absorption, distribution, metabolism, or elimination (ADME) of a substance. For example, when calcium binds ciprofloxacin in the gut and therefore reduces ciprofloxacin absorption, a pharmacokinetic interaction has occurred. When St. John's Wort induces a metabolic enzyme such as cytochrome P450 3A4 and increases metabolism and reduces levels of a protease inhibitor, a pharmacokinetic interaction has occurred.

Pharmacodynamic interactions pertain to the pharmacologic action of the two or more substances on the body. When two or more substances are combined, the effects can be additive or synergistic or antagonistic. For example, when two anticoagulant substances are used together, there is additive anticoagulation, which can result in excessive bleeding. When two antihypertensive agents are combined there can be excessive hypotension. These are pharmacodynamic interactions.

In general, pharmacokinetic interactions are better documented in the literature. These types of interactions can be objectively studied in animal models and humans by quantifying the serum levels of drugs or constituents following administration or potentially interacting substances.

However, pharmacodynamic interactions are much more difficult to measure objectively. These are usually documented by case reports. These types of interactions can also often be identified simply by recognizing the pharmacology of the substances involved. It is reasonable that additive effects are possible when two agents of a similar pharmacological class are combined (Table 26.1).

TABLE 26.1 Potential Herb–Drug Interactions Associated with Commonly Use Herbs[a,6]

Herb	Drug(s)	Rating	Mechanism of Interaction	Comments
American ginseng	Warfarin (Coumadin)	Major	American ginseng has been shown to decrease the effects of warfarin in healthy volunteers through an unknown mechanism.	It is not known whether Panax ginseng has a similar effect on warfarin.
Bitter orange	QT-interval prolonging drugs (e.g., amiodarone, dofetilide, sotalol)	Moderate	Bitter orange in combination with other stimulants such as caffeine can prolong the QT interval in some patients. Combining bitter orange could have an additive effect when used with other drugs that prolong the QT interval.	Bitter orange contains the stimulant synephrine, which has replaced ephedra in many weight loss and athletic performance products
Black cohosh	Hepatotoxic drugs	Moderate	Black cohosh products have been linked to several reports of hepatotoxicity via an unknown mechanism. Theoretically, combining black cohosh with other hepatotoxic agents might increase the risk of liver damage.	Case reports of hepatotoxicity associated with black cohosh do not prove that black cohosh is the cause. However, there is one report of increase in liver enzymes when black cohosh was combined with atorvastatin (Lipitor). Liver enzymes normalized when black cohosh was discontinued.

Garlic	Substrates of the Cytochrome P450 3A4 (CYP3A4) enzyme (e.g., oral contraceptives, some statins, some chemotherapy, many others)	Major	Some garlic extracts induce the drug metabolizing enzyme CYP3A4, which can increase metabolism and decrease levels of drugs metabolized by this enzyme. In one study, garlic reduced saquinavir levels by about 50%.	Some evidence is inconsistent, showing that some garlic products do not have this effect. There is speculation that extracts providing a high concentration of the allicin constituent are more likely to cause this interaction.
Ginkgo	Antiplatelet drugs	Major	Ginkgo leaf extract is thought to have antiplatelet activity. Ginkgo has been associated with several reports of spontaneous bleeding. Combining ginkgo with other antiplatelet or anticoagulant drugs might increase the risk of bleeding. There is a report of bleeding when ginkgo was combined with ibuprofen.	Some short-term studies have not demonstrated a consistent effect of ginkgo on platelet aggregation or bleeding time. However, it is thought that ginkgo may need to be taken for 2–3 wk to have a significant effect on platelets.
Ginkgo	Anticonvulsant therapy	Moderate	There are case reports of seizure occurring in patients with and without a history of seizure after taking ginkgo leaf products. Theoretically, ginkgo might reduce the seizure threshold and decrease the effectiveness of anticonvulsant drugs.	How ginkgo might cause seizure is not known. However, there is speculation that some ginkgo leaf products could be contaminated with ginkgo seed which contains a neurotoxin.

(continued)

TABLE 26.1 *(Continued)*

Herb	Drug(s)	Rating	Mechanism of Interaction	Comments
Kava	Hepatotoxic drugs	Moderate	Kava extracts have been linked to several reports of hepatotoxicity. Theoretically, combining kava with other hepatotoxic agents might increase the risk of liver damage.	Because of safety concerns kava has been banned in many countries; however it is still available in North America.
Red yeast rice	"Statins" (e.g., atorvastatin, simvastatin, lovastatin)	Moderate	Red yeast rice contains concentrations of lovastatin. Combining the statin from red yeast rice with prescription statins can increase the risk of myopathy and liver enzyme abnormalities.	Lovastatin content can range from about 2 mg to 10 mg per dose of red yeast rice.
St. John's Wort	Substrates of the Cytochrome P450 3A4 enzyme (e.g., oral contraceptives, some statins, some chemotherapy, many others)	Major	St. John's Wort has been shown in numerous studies to consistently induce the drug metabolizing enzyme CYP3A4, increase metabolism, and decrease levels of drugs metabolized by this enzyme.	Unplanned pregnancy has occurred in women taking oral contraceptives who have started St. John's Wort. Advise women who take St. John's Wort to use an alternative form of birth control.
Soy	Tamoxifen	Moderate	The estrogenic effects of soy isoflavones might antagonize the antitumor effect of tamoxifen; however, these effects may be dose dependent. Low doses might antagonize tamoxifen, whereas high doses might enhance tamoxifen.	This interaction is based on very preliminary research. Until more is known, patients taking tamoxifen should avoid taking soy extracts.

[a]Note a comprehensive list. For comprehensive information, evidence, and ratings, go to www.naturaldatabase.com.

Interactions with Drugs:

ALPRAZOLAM (Xanax) <<interacts with>> GINKGO
Interaction Rating = Moderate Be cautious with this combination
Severity = Mild • Occurrence = Probable • Level of Evidence = B

Ginkgo might decrease the effectiveness of alprazolam in some patients. Ginkgo extract 120 mg twice daily (Ginkgold), seems to decrease alprazolam levels by about 17%. However ginkgo doesn't appear to decrease the elimination half-life of alprazolam. This suggests ginkgo is more likely to decrease absorption of alprazolam rather than induce hepatic metabolism of alprazolam (11029).

ANTICOAGULANT/ANTIPLATELET DRUGS <<interacts with>> GINKGO
Interaction Rating = Major Do not use this combination
Severity = High • Occurrence = Probable • Level of Evidence = D

Ginkgo leaf has been shown to decrease platelet aggregation and might increase the risk of bleeding when combined with antiplatelet or anticoagulant drugs. It is thought that the ginkgo constituent, ginkgolide B, displaces platelet-activating factor (PAF) from its binding sites, decreasing blood coagulation (6048,9760). Short-term use of ginkgo leaf might not significantly reduce platelet aggregation and blood clotting. One study shows that healthy men who took a specific ginkgo leaf extract (EGb 761) 160 mg twice daily for 7 days did not have reduced prothrombin time (12114). Also, a single dose of ginkgo plus clopidogrel (Plavix) does not seem to significantly increase bleeding time (14811). However, single doses of ginkgo plus cilostazol (Pletal) does seem to prolong bleeding time. It has been suggested that ginkgo has to be taken for at least 2-3 weeks to have a significant effect on platelet aggregation (14811). Use ginkgo cautiously or avoid in patients who are taking antiplatelet or anticoagulant drugs. Some of these drugs include aspirin, clopidogrel (Plavix), dalteparin (Fragmin), enoxaparin (Lovenox), heparin, indomethacin (Indocin), ticlopidine (Ticlid), warfarin (Coumadin), and others.

ANTICONVULSANTS <<interacts with>> GINKGO
Interaction Rating = Moderate Be cautious with this combination
Severity = High • Occurrence = Possible • Level of Evidence = D

Consumption of ginkgo seeds can cause seizures due to ginkgotoxin contained in the seeds. Large amounts of ginkgotoxin can cause neurotoxicity and seizure. Ginkgotoxin is present in much larger amounts in ginkgo seeds than leaves (8232). Ginkgo leaf extract contains trace amounts of ginkgotoxin. The amount of ginkgotoxin in ginkgo leaf and leaf extract seems unlikely to cause toxicity (11298). However, there are anecdotal reports of seizure occurring after use of ginkgo leaf both in patients without a history of seizure disorder and in those with previously well-controlled epilepsy (7030,7090). Theoretically, taking ginkgo might reduce the effectiveness of anticonvulsants for preventing seizure. Some anti-epileptic drugs include phenobarbital, primidone (Mysoline), valproic acid (Depakene), gabapentin (Neurontin), carbamazepine (Tegretol), phenytoin (Dilantin), and others.

ANTIDIABETES DRUGS <<interacts with>> GINKGO
Interaction Rating = Moderate Be cautious with this combination
Severity = Moderate • Occurrence = Possible • Level of Evidence = B

Ginkgo leaf extract seems to alter insulin secretion and metabolism, and might affect blood glucose levels in people with type 2 diabetes (5719,14448). The effect of ginkgo seems to differ depending on the insulin and treatment status of the patient. In diet-controlled diabetes patients with hyperinsulinemia, taking ginkgo does not seem to significantly affect insulin or blood glucose levels. In patients with hyperinsulinemia who are treated with oral hypoglycemic agents, taking ginkgo seems to decrease insulin levels and increased blood glucose following an oral glucose tolerance test. Researchers speculate that this could be due to ginkgo-enhanced hepatic metabolism of insulin. In patients with pancreatic exhaustion, taking ginkgo seems to stimulate pancreatic beta-cells resulting in increased insulin and C-peptide levels, but no significant change in blood glucose levels in response to an oral glucose tolerance test (14448). Theoretically, taking ginkgo might alter the response to antidiabetes drugs. Advise patients with type 2 diabetes to use ginkgo cautiously. Some antidiabetes drugs include glimepiride (Amaryl), glyburide (DiaBeta, Glynase PresTab, Micronase), insulin, pioglitazone (Actos), rosiglitazone (Avandia), and others.

Figure 26.2 • Sample partial listing of potential interactions with drugs for *Ginkgo biloba* as described in *Natural Medicine Comprehensive Database* (www.naturaldatabase.com).

A large number of herbs are suspected to potentially interact with the anticoagulant drug warfarin (Coumadin) (see Fig. 26.2). In most cases, this is due to antiplatelet effects of the herb demonstrated in vitro or in animal models. It is theorized that combining these herbs with antiplatelet effects with warfarin could increase the risk of bleeding. However, there is little documentation to show that these interactions occur. Nonetheless, because the potential outcome can be severe if serious bleeding occurs, adding any new drug, supplement, or herbal product in a patient taking warfarin should be approached cautiously (Table 26.2).

CONCLUSION

The true incidence of herb–drug interactions is not known and may never be known due to poor understanding of potential interactions by practitioners and a general

TABLE 26.2 Select Herbs with Known or Suspected Antiplatelet Activity

Andrographis	Ginger
Bilberry	Ginkgo
Borage oil	Guggul
Capsicum	Horse chestnut
Danshen	Jiaogulan
Dong quai	Red clover
Evening primrose	Policosanol
Fenugreek	Turmeric
Feverfew	Willow bark
German chamomile	Winter green

lack of consistent and adequate reporting of these events. A better understanding of these events will develop when reports of adverse outcomes due to herb–drug interactions are better documented through published cases and reporting through surveillance systems such as the Food and Drug Administration's *MedWatch* and *Natural Medicines Watch* (see chapter 24). Very few resources exist that provide reliable and up-to-date information regarding adverse reactions and interactions. Table 26.3 lists some resources that are available that examine adverse reactions and interactions related to natural products.

It is clear that herb–drug interactions can occur and can result in significant adverse outcomes. However, simply because herbal products have the potential to cause interactions, does not mean that this is a contraindication to their use in patients who are taking conventional medications. Clinicians should not discourage use of any and all herbals products based on these potential safety issues. Patients interested in these products will simply stop asking if the answer is always "no."

Instead, clinicians should focus on providing the best, responsible advice to patients based on the likelihood of risks, such as herb–drug interactions, and the likelihood of benefit.

TABLE 26.3 Selected Resources That Collect and Evaluate Information About Adverse Reactions and Interactions Related to Natural Products

- Alternative and Allied Medicine Database (www.ovid.com/site/catalog/DataBase/12.jsp)
- Embase (www.embase.com/)
- International Bibliographic Information on Dietary Supplements (grande.nal.usda.gov/ibids/index.php)
- *Natural Medicines Comprehensive Database* (www.naturaldatabase.com)
- PubMed (www.ncbi.nlm.nih.gov/pubmed)
- Reactions Database (www.ovid.com/site/catalog/DataBase/141.jsp)

References

1. Astin JA, Pelletier KR, Marie A, Haskell WL. Complementary and alternative medicine use among elderly persons: one-year analysis of a Blue Shield Medicare supplement. *J Gerontol A Biol Sci Med Sci* 2000;55:M4–M9.
2. Marinac JS, Buchinger CL, Godfrey LA, et al. Herbal products and dietary supplements: a survey of use, attitudes, and knowledge among older adults. *JAOA* 2007;107:13–23.
3. Eisenberg DM, Davis RB, Ettner SL, et al. Trends in alternative medicine use in the United States, 1990–1997 results of a follow-up national survey. *JAMA* 1998;280:1569–1575.
4. Archer EL, Boyle DK. Herb and supplement use among the retail population of an independent, urban herb store. *J Holist Nurs* 2008;26:27–35.
5. Gardiner P, Graham RE, Legedza ATR, et al. Factors associated with dietary supplement use among prescription medication users. *Arch Intern Med* 2006;166:1968–1974.
6. Jellin JM, Gregory PJ, eds. *Natural Medicines Comprehensive Database*. www.naturaldatabase.com. Accessed March 10, 2009.

V

Efficacy

CHAPTER 27

Evaluating Dietary Supplements: Efficacy

Robert Alan Bonakdar

There are many ways to examine the efficacy of dietary supplements. Although as clinicians we are familiar with the use of randomized controlled trials as the "gold standard" in evaluating clinical efficacy, there are many important caveats to consider. First, the efficacy of supplements is often linked to regulation and quality control (section 3). A poorly regulated supplement with poor quality control at some step in the manufacturing process, even if found beneficial in traditional usage or previous clinical trials, may be found ineffective or unsafe in a particular trial.

Next, even if the quality of a preparation is adequate, the benefit of a supplement may change dramatically based on preparations and usage. This may explain the divergence of research results, such as with Echinacea, whereby very different plant parts, formulations, standardizations, dosages, and administration protocols are utilized. It is no wonder that studies can be intimidating and confusing at times with Drs. Hardy and Betz discussing strategies to critically evaluate the literature. Dr. Alberte discusses emerging techniques for the ongoing discovery and standardization of novel compounds in herbal supplements. Dr. Barrett goes on to focus on specific well-researched formulations that attempt to standardize what is being evaluated. In many cases, this parallels what clinicians are often looking for as far as a reliable, reproducible result when recommending supplements. Lastly, in the arena of clinical guidance, Dr. Costello discusses National Institutes of Health programs and resources, which attempt to link research support with clinical tools to facilitate evaluation of efficacy.

Lastly, and probably of foundation importance, is the concept of efficacy on an agricultural, ecological, and cultural perspective. Although we often discuss an herbal or dietary supplement as an entity utilized for a clinical endpoint, it is important to keep in mind that the plant or supplement provides "efficacy" to other systems besides the patient. Julian Duval of the San Diego Botanic Gardens provides an overview of the importance of plants as living entities that can provide education, sustainability, and healing from a community and global perspective. Thus, as we debate the evidence for efficacy in a clinical sense, it is important to balance this discussion with an understanding and appreciation of how the plant exists in and sustains the ecosystem.

CHAPTER 28

The Importance of Botanic Gardens

Julian Duval

The earliest known gardens date from thousands of years ago and are from Egypt and China. There are also records of early gardens from Europe and Mexico. While they all have clearly independent origins, these gardens have in common the culture of plants for economic and aesthetic purposes. The economic importance of plants covers a broad range; however, plants believed to have medicinal value were of primary interest from the beginning. Gardens specific to the cultivation and study of medicinal plants in Europe were called physic gardens and were created to support the medical schools starting in the 16th century (1).

The dominance of the pharmaceutical industry in present day Western medicine makes it difficult to imagine the health profession without it. However, for most of human existence the direct use of plants was fundamental to the practice of medicine. In fact, for most of Western medicine's history, a successful clinician had to be a studied herbalist.

The physic gardens insured a supply of plants of known origin and identification. The documented collections in modern botanic gardens still provide for this function. In the early European physic gardens, the propagation of plants saved the often-challenging need to recollect wild plants. They were practicing conservation of a valuable resource. Nearly all modern botanic gardens have conservation as a tenet of their mission.

The reason for conservation is much more fundamental in modern times. At present, transportation to remote areas of the world is easy compared to even 50 years ago. However, wild populations of so many plants are now so reduced or fragmented that depending on wild harvest conflicts with the preservation of many different species. Loss of habitat, invasive species, overharvesting, and global climate change all continue to bring more species of plants, including plants of known medicinal value and the many yet to be discovered, under threat of extinction.

Zoos often come to mind in saving endangered species from extinction. Yet, botanic gardens have for a much longer time been maintaining plants that would otherwise be extinct. The well-documented medicinal *Ginkgo biloba* or maidenhair tree, may no longer exist in its original range in China. But the source for this tree, which aside from its common medicinal use is now a very popular ornamental grown worldwide, came from plants preserved in Chinese and Japanese temple gardens (2).

As important as ex-situ conservation can be in creating a last stand against a species' extinction, all plants and animals are living functioning parts of complicated and little understood ecosystems—their conservation in habitat is of first order of importance. A commonly held belief that wild collected plants have more medicinal potency over cultivated plants may have some basis in fact and needs further study (3).

San Diego Botanic Garden (SDBG) has important collections of rare cycads, some of which are critically endangered in habitat in Africa. It also maintains one of the most diverse collections of bamboo that has proven important as a hedge against the extinction of certain taxa. Yet, of the 36.5 acre SDBG facility, 10 acres are a native preserve with a rich variety of the maritime chaparral and coastal sage scrub flora including the federally listed endangered Del Mar manzanita, *Arctostaphylos glandulosa* ssp. *crassifolia*. While small, this 10 acres has significant conservation value given that nearly all of this Southern California coastal habitat has succumbed to urbanization. The flora of this area is one of the most diverse in North America. Unfortunately, much of what was known to the indigenous people of its medicinal use has been lost as early Europeans had other priorities in their contact with native people.

The Missouri Botanic Garden (MBG) in St. Louis is renowned for its work in plant conservation. MBG employs dozens of plant researchers worldwide who are involved in a wide range of conservation biology from basic plant exploration in which floras are documented for the first time to working with native people to document cultural uses of plants. Preserving the knowledge extant in the many cultures of the world in which the direct use of plants is still a daily experience has become a race against time as these cultures are quickly disappearing. As important is their work with local agencies to promote the preservation of wild populations of plants. Scientists at MBG estimate that half of the world's vascular plants is under some degree of threat of extinction—a frightening statistic for many reasons including the approximation that only one out of six plants has been studied for its potential benefit to humans.

Another of the great botanic gardens is the New York Botanic Garden (NYBG). The Institute of Economic Botany is a division of NYBG and with support from Merck sampled hundreds of the nearly 4,000 taxa in the SDBG collection for their potential medicinal value. SDBG was selected for this bio-prospecting effort due to the high number of subtropical and Mediterranean climate plants in the collection. In 2006, NYBG opened the $23 million Pfizer Plant Research Laboratory. This ultramodern facility located at the botanic garden is designed for a wide range of plant-based investigation including biodiversity prospecting and NYBG's genomics program.

As mentioned earlier, there are many reasons that threaten the preservation of the earth's botanic diversity. Medicinal plants are of course impacted by all of these threats but in many cases are particularly threatened by overharvesting from the wild. The rapidly growing worldwide demand for medicinal plants, most of which are still wild harvested (2), has conservationists concerned over the continued existence of many. The Durban Botanic Gardens in Durban, South Africa, has raised alarm over the growing pressure on wild plant populations for plants used in traditional medicine in South Africa and is in the process of encouraging their cultivation. Given the high prices offered for American ginseng, *Panax quinquefolius*, certain populations have been severely impacted. Despite legal protection, poaching continues to be a significant problem. Botanic gardens around the world will increasingly play an important role insuring that plants with known and potential medicinal properties will continue to be available for both use and study.

James Duke writes in *The Green Pharmacy* (4) that there is benefit to the clinician or the end user of plants for medicinal purposes to know the living plant, know its environment, and be involved in its culture. SDBG has been fortunate enough to work with Dr. Duke in providing tours of the gardens of medicinal plants for several years as part of the Scripps Natural Supplements Conference. Many physicians comment that this is the first time they have appreciated the plant that creates the pill. Moreover, a spiritual relationship to plants used for medicinal purposes is common in cultures in which traditional medicine is practiced. While this may be hard to prove scientifically, connecting the mind and body in medicine is verifiably important.

One of the original reasons for the creation of botanic gardens was to have places for the culture of plants for aesthetic reasons. These were places where people could be in contact with the wonder and beauty of nature. This purpose continues to this day and may have even more significance as humans increasingly live in urbanized settings. In trying to understand what attracts us to nature and natural settings or why it is that we find beauty in these things, there are good arguments that we are genetically predisposed in this way (5). Realizing the potential for therapeutic effect, SDBG provided free admission to everyone for a month after the tragedy of September 11, 2001. SDBG staff noted more people visiting singly and their inclination to be stationary for periods of time in what seemed a more meditative state.

Clinicians should make visiting botanic gardens part of their own continuing education. Places like botanic gardens have a restorative effect on mind and body. When considering a therapy for a patient, do remember that a visit to a botanic garden can be a powerful tonic for good health and healing.

References

1. Everett TH. *The New York Botanical Garden Illustrated Encyclopedia of Horticulture*. Vol. 2. New York & London: Garland Publishing Inc; 1981.
2. Huxley A. *Green Inheritance: Saving the Plants of the World*. Berkeley and Los Angeles: University of California Press; 2005.
3. Canter PH, Thomas H, Ernst E. Bringing medicinal plants into cultivation: opportunities and challenges for biotechnology. *Trends Biotechnol* 2005;23(4):180–185.
4. Duke JA. *The Green Pharmacy*. Emmaus, PA: Rodale Press; 1997.
5. Wilson EO. *Biophilia*. Cambridge, MA: Harvard University Press; 1986.

CHAPTER 29

Dose-Reliable Botanic Extracts for Clinical Studies

Randall S. Alberte, Dan Li, Bill Roschek Jr., Sloan Ayers, Ryan C. Fink, Matthew McMichael, George Sypert, Robert D. Smith, and Robert T. Gow

INTRODUCTION AND OVERVIEW

Evidence-based and clinically proven botanic extracts will drive and accelerate the broader acceptance of complementary and alternative medicines to the medical community as well as the public. One of the significant factors that has limited progress on this front is the lack of available batch-to-batch and dose-reliable botanic extracts with which to conduct reproducible human clinical trials. It is not surprising to find contradictory studies on the same extract source supplier conducted at different times (1). For example, the recent Cochrane meta-analyses of cranberry on urinary tract infections (UTIs) (2) revealed significant benefits for control of UTIs; however, among the clinical studies evaluated, some showed statistically insignificant benefits even when study designs were the same. A recent clinical investigation on turmeric contradicted similar previous trials, yet efficacy for impairment of neurological function was shown (3).

The inherent medical value of botanics lies within the rich and diverse compounds present and the synergies that can be obtained from this bioactive complexity (4). In recent investigations it was found that key bioactives in nettle (*Urtica dioica*) inhibit multiple pathways that produce the symptoms of seasonal allergies (5); the key bioactives in turmeric block initial steps in amyloid plaque generation and aggregation, hallmarks of Alzheimer's disease (6); and bioactive compounds in rice bran inhibit multiple key proinflammatory pathways associated with arthritis (7). Collectively, these types of studies clearly demonstrate synergies among the key bioactives present in these extracts that contribute to the overall health benefits.

It is well known that the chemistry of a plant leaf, for example, changes in very dynamic ways on time scales from seconds to months (and even years depending on the botanic), from location of growth (climate), recent weather, and varietal differences (8–10). Even leaves collected from different locations on the same plant will show significant chemical variation. As a consequence of the significant variability induced by growth conditions alone, a harvest from the same production field of the same species can differ dramatically from year to year (8). Due to the chemical variability of the source material, clinical studies conducted at different times from different harvests are difficult if not impossible to reproduce placing botanic extract trials at a very strong disadvantage when compared to pharmaceutical drug trials (1, 11).

The challenges of dose- and batch-reliable botanic extracts have been addressed to not only cover standard marker bioactives, or a set of standards, but to yield extracts containing hundreds and thousands of chemical species found in a given botanic source with less than 5–10% variation in chemical composition and *in vitro* biological activities. Highly reproducible proprietary extraction technologies (12, 13) have been developed and coupled with Direct Analysis in Real Time with Time of Flight Mass spectrometry (DART TOF-MS), a powerful new mass spectrometry capability to validate the reproducibility across the chemical complexity in botanics. Using this approach, the dose-reliability (pill-to-pill) of extracts generated from over 20 different botanics (e.g., Echinacea, nettle, holy basil, turmeric, ginger, red sage, etc.) proved to be much less than 5% across hundreds of chemical species. Extracts prepared in this manner provide "reagent" grade botanic extracts that are suitable for research and fundamentally important for clinical investigations on the impacts and benefits of dietary supplements. The evidence base to demonstrate the dose-reliability is summarized here.

SUPPORTING SCIENCE-BASED DATA

Utilizing proprietary extraction technologies that included super critical carbon dioxide as a solvent for extraction under precise physical conditions (pressure, temperature and flow rates), affinity absorbent chromatography, and in combinations with other technologies, botanic source materials are extracted with high reproducibility (5–10%) to generate whole extracts with hundreds-to-thousands of compounds. For example, using these extraction technologies and DART TOF-MS, rice bran (*Oryza sativa*) revealed more than 2,600 compounds, elderberry fruits (*Sambucus nigra* L.) more than 1,000 compounds, and stinging nettle (*Urtica dioica* L.) leaves revealed more than 500 compounds (Table 29.1). Root-based and bark-based botanics also have a broad chemical diversity with turmeric root (*Curcuma longa* L.) and cinnamon bark (*Cinnamomum cassia* B.) possessing greater than 1,600 and 1,400 compounds, respectively (see Table 29.1). Table 29.1 provides a summary of chemical complexity for a range of botanics.

In Figure 29.1, DART fingerprints of three different elderberry extracts (Panels A, B, and C) obtained from three different production runs on the same feedstock are shown. The DART TOF-MS fingerprints show the numbers and masses of chemical species (X axis) and relative abundances (Y axis) of these masses. The fingerprints reveal a rich diversity of compounds, as defined by the vertical lines in the fingerprint, with exact masses between 100 and 1,000 atomic mass units (amu) on the X axis. The fingerprints in Figure 29.1 appear almost identical; however, mathematical analysis allows for the quantitative differences among the different production runs to be determined for both compound diversity (presence/absence) and relative abundance. The "difference analysis" (Fig. 29.2A) shows that the abundances of an overwhelming majority of chemical species in elderberry differed by less than ca. 2% while a couple differed up to ca. 5% (e.g., m/z = 162, 187, and 288). There were insignificant differences ($<$0.7%) in the presence/absence of chemical species among the extracts. Mathematical analysis of the abundances of the chemical species present in the elderberry extracts shown in Figure 29.1 panels A, B and C revealed that they have a similarly index (S_w) of 92.3 (S.E. = 2.8) which yields an overall difference of the three extracts of only 7.7% for $>$1000 chemical entities present. Based on HPLC analyses using 3 marker flavonoids (Rutin, cyanidin 3-glucoside,

TABLE 29.1 Summary of Compound Diversity in Terms of Numbers of Compounds Identified Using DART TOF-MS for 10 Different Botanics.[a]

Botanic	Number of Compounds	Dose-Reliability (% Difference Among Three Pills)
Elderberry fruits	>1,000	0.4
Holy basil leaves	>1,200	3.2
Turmeric root	>1,600	0.4
Nettle leaves	>500	0.2
Rice bran	>2,600	1.0
Lingzhi	>900	1.2
Red sage leaves	>1,500	0.3
Cranberry fruits	>1,900	0.7
Cinnamon bark	>1,400	0.4
Yerba mate leaves	>2,500	0.6

[a]Also shown are the dose-to-dose reliability of these same extracts expressed as percent differences in the chemical composition based on presence/absence of the diversity of chemistries.

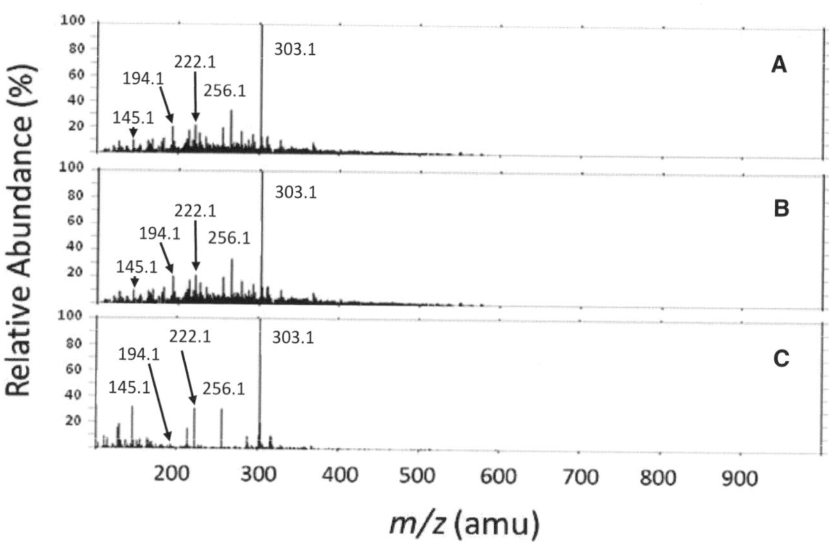

Figure 29.1 • DART TOF mass spectrometric fingerprints of three different production batches of elderberry showing the exact mass distribution (*X* axis) and relative abundances of each detected compound (*Y* axis). The high degree of similarity of the three fingerprints is visible.

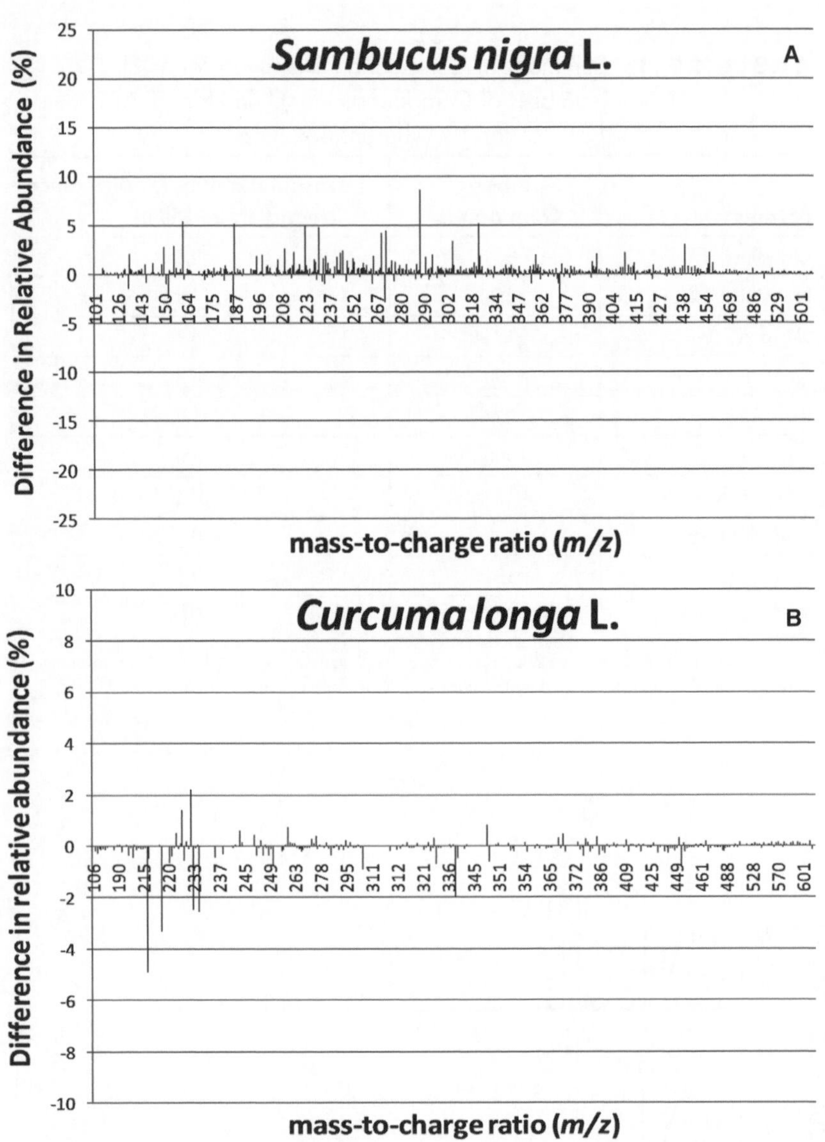

Figure 29.2 • The difference fingerprint of three randomly chosen pills from a 30-count bottle of elderberry (Panel A) and turmeric (Panel B) shows extremely low variability and high (>99%) dose-reliability of elderberry extract. Vertical lines (*Y* axis) represent positive and negative changes in specific compounds among the chemical complexity detected (*X* axis).

and cyanidin 3, 5-glucoside) and total anthocyanidins differences in the production batches were ca. 5%. The difference analysis of the turmeric extracts using DART TOF-MS and HPLC revealed <2% differences (Fig 29.2B).

This same approach was utilized to examine dose-to-dose reliability. Three pills from a 30-count bottle were selected blindly and at random (Fig. 29.2). Table 29.1 summarizes the pill-to-pill consistency of several different botanics. Except for the holy basil (*Ocimuntenuflorum*) extract which showed 3% variability, all other botanic extracts varied by less than 1.5% over the entire mass range of chemical constituents. Lastly, human pharmacokinetic studies on such extracts have revealed high bioavailability of the key functional bioactives (14, 15).

SIGNIFICANCE OF FINDINGS AND CONCLUSIONS

It is shown here that batch-to-batch and dose-to-dose reliable extracts with a full spectrum of compounds can be prepared on production scales using proprietary extraction technologies briefly described here. The dose-reliability of these extracts can be validated across the complex chemical diversity present, not just a single chemical standard or a class of compounds. This capability sets a new "standard" for botanic extracts for research and clinical investigations. The quantitative and validated approaches described here provide, for the first time, the ability to ensure the quality, reproducibility, and rich functional chemical diversity in botanics can be utilized in clinical investigations to rigorously demonstrate their health and wellness benefits. Further, the critical functional synergies that can only be realized from botanics can be validated and retained. This technology is suitable for the preparation of botanic extracts that can be delivered in the form of dietary supplements, functional foods medical foods and botanic drugs.

Clinical investigations on the health benefits of botanics have yielded highly variable results in many cases, and as such, many in the medical field do not accept, or minimally accept, the health value of botanics. Much of the cause for this variability in clinical outcomes arises from the highly dynamic properties of the chemical composition of botanics resulting in the evaluation of extracts with unreliable dosing. We believe that extracts prepared and characterized as described here can provide botanic extracts today, and into the future, that are assured to be dose-reliable. As such, these extracts, when used in clinical investigations, should dramatically improve reproducibility and statistical significance of the health benefits realized in clinical studies on botanics.

ACKNOWLEDGMENTS

The authors acknowledge the contributions of John McClelland, Maurie Romeo, Charles Henry, and Jin Gow to this work. Funding support was provided by HerbalScience Singapore Ltd. Pte.

References

1. Plant drugs and extracts in human and veterinary health promotion within Europe: benefits and risks. In: Watson RR, Preedy VR, eds. *Botanical Medicine in Clinical Practice*. London, UK: CAB International; 2008:64–70.
2. Jepson RG, Craig JC. Cranberries for preventing urinary tract infections. *Cochrane Database Syst Rev* 2008:1CD001321.
3. Grant KL, Schneider CD. Turmeric. *Am J Health Syst Pharm* 2000;57:1121–1122.
4. Schmidt BM, Ribnicky DM, Lipsky PE, et al. Revisiting the ancient concept of botanical therapeutics. *Nat Chem Biol* 2007;3:360–366.
5. Roschek B Jr, Fink RC, McMichael M, et al. Nettle extract (*Urtica dioica*) affects key receptors and enzymes associated with allergic rhinitis. *Phytother Res* 2009;23:920–926.

6. Shytle RD, Bickford PC, Rezai-zadeh K, et al. Optimized turmeric extracts have potent anti-amyloidogenic effects. *Curr Alzheimer Res* 2009;6:564–571.
7. Roschek B Jr, Fink R, Li D, et al. Pro-inflammatory enzymes, COX1, COX2, and 5LOX, inhibited by stabilized rice bran extracts. *J Med Food* 2009;12:615–623.
8. Augsburger LL, Hoag SW, eds. *Pharmaceutical Dosage Forms: Tablets* New York, NY: Informa Health Care; 2008.
9. Rezzi S, Cavaleiro C, Bighelli A, et al. Intraspecific chemical variability of the leaf essential oil of *Juniperus phoenicea* subsp. *turbinata* from Corsica. *Biochem Syst Ecol* 2001; 29:179–188.
10. Hartmann T. Diversity and variability of plant secondary metabolism: a mechanistic view. *Entomol Exp Appl* 1996;80:177–188.
11. Chen ST, Dou J, Temple R, et al. New therapies from old medicines. *Nat Biotechnol* 2008; 26:1077–1083.
12. Alberte RS, Gow RT, Sypert GW, et al. Extraction and methods comprising elder species. US patent application 11/687,897. October 25, 2007.
13. Gow R, Sypert G, Li D, et al. Extracts and methods comprising curcuma species. US patent application 11/725,140. March 17, 2007.
14. Ayers S, Roschek B Jr, Williams JM, et al. Pharmacokinetic analysis of anti-allergy and anti-inflammation bioactives in a nettle (*Urtica dioica*) extract. *Online J Pharmacol Pharmacokinetics* 2009;5:6–21.
15. Roschek B Jr, Alberte RS. Pharmacokinetics of cyanidin and anti-influenza phytonutrients in an elder berry extract determined by LC-MS and DART TOF-MS. *Online J Pharmacokinetics* 2008;4:1–17.

CHAPTER 30

Evaluating the Botanic Dietary Supplement Literature

Joseph M. Betz and Mary L. Hardy

INTRODUCTION

Clinical trials are conducted for several reasons, including determination of efficacy and safety. In many areas, health care providers seeking information will find little or no guidance, because of a lack of published human studies in the relevant area. In other cases, publications may exist but conclusions from apparently similar studies may be contradictory, making it difficult to provide informed recommendations to patients. Although many areas of medicine share these problems, the literature of complementary and integrative medicine is relatively young and may seem especially confusing. In addition, the peer-reviewed literature is not the only resource, and numerous books and the Internet provide access to an overwhelming volume of information. The problem for the practitioner is to separate fact from opinion and to make sense of areas where there are no facts, the facts are contradictory, or where opinion poses as fact.

Methodologists and meta-analysts have identified a number of criteria for evaluation of bodies of literature and for drawing conclusions from that literature. Over the past decade, several authors have published rating scales for evaluating the quality of published clinical trials, with an eye to assessing the reliability of the conclusions drawn from those trials so that evidence-based standards of medical care may be developed. These systems include the Jadad scale (1) and the Consolidated Standards of Reporting Trials Statement (CONSORT) (2). Although the raters agree that the most reliable evidence is provided by randomized, placebo controlled, double-blind clinical trials, variations among trial designs and their descriptions still allow for nominally similar designs to vary in quality. Elements of these systems allow readers to rate the strengths of individual trial designs based on variables such as sample size, intent to treat analysis, degree and adequacy of blinding (single blind, double blind), and randomization scheme. Linde et al (3) investigated trial design in the fields of homeopathy, herbal medicines, and acupuncture. They found the quality of the trials to be highly variable, with the majority having important shortcomings in reporting and/or methodology. Major problems in most trials were the description of allocation concealment and the reporting of dropouts and withdrawals. Unfortunately, the trial rating systems were designed with a narrow focus on the mechanics of the clinical trial itself and took for granted that the interventions used in the trials had been well characterized.

Three publications highlighted the importance of product quality determination and the necessity of defining and describing the nature of interventions to be used in biomedical research. In 2005, Gagnier et al (4) recognized that in the field of biomedical research on natural products, adequate characterization, and description of the intervention were not always provided in trial publications and proposed a revised CONSORT statement that includes scoring for the quality of the description of the intervention. As a result of the growing realization of the nature and extent of the problem, Wolsko et al (5) performed a systematic evaluation of the literature of herbal clinical trials with the intent of quantifying the reliability of the clinical botanic literature in terms of product quality. A review of 81 studies found that only 12 of the 81 (15%) reported having performed any kind of quantitative chemical analysis on the intervention. Of these, only eight studies reported results of the analyses. The authors also reported that only 40 of the 81 botanic studies (49%) identified the plant source of the intervention by Latin binomial name. Only 8 (10%) of the studies identified the plant part used in the study and only 23 (28%) of the studies described the extraction/processing method used to prepare the study intervention. In 2006, Gagnier et al (6) published an extensive review of 206 randomized controlled trials of herbal medicines and scored them against 42 separate CONSORT checklist items. A detailed description of the results is not within the scope of this discussion, but the finding that only 54% of the reviewed trials provided a precise description of the intervention confirmed the conclusions presented in the Wolsko (5) report. Investigators have thus far struggled to provide more complete descriptions of interventions, as they have discovered that there are few reliable published analytical methods and reference materials available for evaluating product composition.

READING THE LITERATURE

Editors and peer reviewers who are experts in clinical trials are aware of the Jadad scale and CONSORT checklist. However, few have been trained in pharmacognosy, botany, or phytochemistry. Although there is no such thing as a perfect trial, studies that are deeply flawed in the clinical area seldom make it through the peer review process. As pointed out by Wolsko et al (5) and Gagnier et al (6), many studies that are weak in nonclinical areas can and do reach the peer-reviewed literature.

As suggested by Swanson (7) and mandated by a policy set forth by the National Institutes of Health's National Center for Complementary and Alternative Medicine (8), all studies on natural products should share some common characteristics. First, there should be a detailed description of the nature of the test article. If the study is about a botanic intervention, the plant should be correctly named using the currently accepted Latin binomial. Correct Latin names are actually a phrase that consists of the name of the plant genus followed by the specific epithet and the designation of the botanist who is credited with naming the plant. The whole phrase identifies a particular plant species, for example, *Echinacea angustifolia* DC. A useful and easy to use resource for checking to see whether or not a plant has been correctly named is available at http://www.ars-grin.gov/cgi-bin/npgs/html/taxecon.pl (9). If the study has been performed on a material that is NOT a commercial product, it is usually helpful (and for some journals, mandatory) to include information about when and where the plant material was collected, by whom, and where a retained portion of the plant material is stored for future reference (10). If a reader cannot determine the plant used in the study, then neither will a future investigator trying to repeat it.

In addition to taxonomic information, the materials and methods section should indicate the part of the plant that was used to make the clinical material. The phytochemistry of different plant parts can vary dramatically and if the plant has been used in a traditional healing system, the part of the plant to be used for a particular indication is usually specified. For example, the German Commission E provides positive (i.e., approved) monographs for *Echinacea purpurea* (L.) Moench herb and *Echinacea pallida* (Nutt.) Nutt. root, whereas the *E. purpurea* **root** monograph is negative (unapproved) (11). Another important detail is the way in which the test article was processed before incorporating it into a dosage form. Over the past five decades or so, there has been an evolution in the production, sale, and use of botanic products. In the 1970s, these were largely sold as sifted, cut, or powdered plant material in the form of a tablet, capsule, tea bag, or tincture. Many modern botanic products are made using sophisticated plant extracts that have been spray dried onto a solid carrier and then formed into a hard or soft capsule or tablet. Traditional extracts were usually aqueous, but modern products are extracted with everything from acetone to isopropanol to supercritical carbon dioxide. The nature of the solvent can change the final chemistry of the product in ways that could affect safety and efficacy as compared to traditional preparations. There are a number of advantages to these new techniques, including savings in shipping costs as a result of reduced bulk, the ability to produce dosage forms that are more uniform in their composition, and the ability to concentrate preferentially the salubrious constituents of a plant while leaving behind undesirable constituents. Unfortunately, the ability to affirm identity and quality using simple and inexpensive techniques such as microscopy or chemical spot testing is lost when ingredients are processed and traded in this manner (12). In reading the herbal literature, it is important for the reader to note whether or not the investigators indicate the extraction solvent used in the production of the material, the solvent ratio (amount of herb/amount of solvent), and the carrier onto which the extract is spray-dried, along with the identities and amounts of other ingredients in the finished product. This information is important not only in evaluating the trial but also for ethical reasons. The presence of peanut oil, wheat gluten, soy, sulfites, lactose, or milk protein as "inert" component of a formulation is potentially dangerous to certain segments of the population.

Along the same lines, some commercial herbal preparations have been found over the years to be adulterated with prescription pharmaceuticals (13). Not all herbs are subject to such adulteration, but herbs intended for certain classes of claim (weight loss, male sexual enhancement, etc.) have been targets in the past. Investigators must be aware (and indicate that they are aware) of such possibilities and should if necessary identify steps taken to ensure that the clinical material is "clean." While on the topic of cleanliness, investigators should be aware that natural products are susceptible to contamination with pesticides, mycotoxins, toxic elements, or dangerous microorganisms. Details of testing protocols (including sampling plans) used and results of these determinations should be presented in studies. In some clinical trials, investigators acquire raw ingredients from a supplier and contract for the manufacture of custom dosage forms to provide a better match with placebo or to deliver a nonstandard dose. It is even more important to have such products evaluated for purity. Finally, the investigator should indicate in the publication whether or not the material used in the trial was standardized, and if so, to what? Standardization is a technical term of art that describes a process by which levels of certain phytochemical constituents are not only measured but also adjusted so that phytochemical content is consistent from batch to batch and falls within a certain predefined range (14, 15). Included in the information about standardization should be details about the analytical method(s) used to verify that the phytochemical contents are appropriate and that the method used to make the measurements is scientifically valid and fit for its purpose. In addition, analytical data generated during product evaluation and standardization should be provided along with the source and purity of chemical calibrants used in the analysis. It would also be useful to include information on the number of lots or batches of product used in the study, and information about whether or not phytochemical content was monitored throughout the study (some phytochemicals are unstable and some products have relatively short shelf-lives). If commercial products are used in trials, the same information is required. For the most part, such products must meet identity and purity standards mandated by regulators in the country of origin. However, regulatory requirements vary across nations and it would be prudent for investigators to indicate that they have confirmed product cleanliness along with the other specifications.

Additional information in the clinical area is usually necessary in herbal trials. For instance, justifications for the dose and dosage regimen used in the trial should be provided. Few dose-ranging studies have been performed on herbal products. Instead, investigators have often relied on information from "traditional use," where it exists. Even when such information does exist, it may be difficult to establish comparability of traditional and modern dosage forms. If a justification is made on the basis of traditional use, the traditional use should be noted. In traditional systems of healing, herbs were often used for a multitude of indications, with different doses and modes of preparation used for different indications.

Finally, adequacy of blinding and the selection of placebo must be evaluated. Herbs (including herbal extracts) generally have characteristic odors and tastes, and so-called "inert" botanics selected as placebo may not really be biologically inert. Investigators should explain and justify their reasons for choosing a particular placebo.

CASE STUDY: ECHINACEA

Background

Echinacea products and trials are confusing because the marketplace contains multiple species, multiple plant parts (root, aerial parts), and numerous preparations (tinctures, pressed fresh aerial parts, dried herb). The chemistry and means of standardization of all of these forms also vary considerably, so this genus provides a good case study for evaluating herbal trials in general.

According to Tyler (16), Echinacea was introduced to western medicine by H.C.F. Meyer, who had learned about it from Native Americans around 1871. The plant was commercialized by the Lloyd Brothers of Cincinnati around 1885, and it remained one of the most popular drugs in the United States until the 1930s, when the advent of the sulfa drugs pushed it to the side. The "Echinacea" monograph in the 20th edition of the United States Dispensatory (USD) (17) describes the properties and uses of *Brauneria pallida* (Nuttall) Britton (Sampson root, Pale Purple Coneflower) root and rhizome. The name *E. angustifolia* De Candolle is listed in the USD as a synonym, and this is the current accepted name for the species. *E. pallida* (Nutt.) Nutt. is now considered a separate species (9). This change in taxonomy was reflected in the 25th edition of the USD (18). According to the USD monographs, Echinacea was used to increase bodily resistance to infection and was used for boils, erysipelas, septicemia, cancer, syphilis, "other impurities of the blood," and as an aphrodisiac. More or less as an afterthought, the USD monograph describes the root and rhizomes of *Brauneria purpurea* DC Britton (*Rudbeckia purpurea* L., *E. purpurea* Moench) as having similar properties and uses (18). Both the 20th (1918) and 25th (1955) editions of the USD provide a description of the chemical composition of Echinacea, but the descriptions reflect the state of knowledge of organic chemistry at the time. Early attempts to discover a "physiologically active" substance were described as failures.

The reader will note several points in the above discussion. The first is that the modern use of Echinacea for the prevention and treatment of upper respiratory tract infections can be easily recognized in the phrase "Echinacea is used to increase bodily resistance to infection." The second is that botanic names are not static. What we now call *E. angustifolia* had a different official name in 1918 (*B. pallida*). What is more, the two names were used interchangeably at the time. Botanists subsequently determined that the two names (one of which was later changed to *E. pallida*) describe two different plant species, and the 1955 USD reflects this change. In conducting a literature search on a botanic, it can be useful to know the taxonomic history of the species. A third point is that the monograph identified the plant part used (root and rhizome). The monograph also provided the dosage form and dose. The dosage form is described as powdered root/rhizome or a fluid extract, and the daily dose was 1 g or 0.6 to 1.8 ml, respectively.[1]

When reading the description of a clinical trial in the literature, therefore, one can start by asking whether the author of the study got the name of the plant right. The next questions should be: did the author adequately describe the reason(s) for selecting a particular plant part, dosage form, and dose? It is not really important that the reader know the literature, although it would be nice. However, it would be inexcusable if the author of the paper was unfamiliar with the literature, and this can often be determined by the astute reader if there is no rationale for dose/dosage form presented or if the rationale is inconsistent with available sources of information. For example, a study that utilizes a supercritical fluid CO_2 extract of the aerial parts of *E. purpurea* is clearly not derived from the healing traditions of Native Americans or 19th century eclectic physicians, and justification for the dose/dosage form should in that case come from formal dose-ranging studies or some other scientific basis. Many of the more recent studies on Echinacea use products, doses, and dosage forms that stem from relatively recent European practice. The use of freshly pressed juice of the above ground parts of *E. purpurea* is a notable example. A trial on such a material is perfectly legitimate as long as the investigator recognizes and acknowledges that the pertinent literature includes the German Commission E monographs, the German or European Pharmacopeia, and previous clinical trials of the specific formulations and doses. When publishing their study results, clinical investigators who use commercial products that justify dosing on product label directions should demonstrate that there has been a dialog with the manufacturer, such that the manufacturer provides a rationale for the dose and dosage form.

A review of the peer-reviewed clinical literature surrounding Echinacea shows that many of the early published trials were "positive." In fact, a systematic review

---

[1]According to the 9th edition of the United States Pharmacopoeia (1910) "Fluidextracts are concentrated liquid preparations of vegetable drugs, containing alcohol either as a solvent or as a preservative, and bearing a uniform relation to the drug used so that *one mil* of the fluidextract closely represents the activity of *one gramme* of the air-dried and powdered drug of standard quality."

of 16 trials (3,396 participants) designed to evaluate Echinacea for the prevention and treatment of the common cold published by Melchart et al (19) in 2000 concluded that some preparations of Echinacea may be better than placebo. However, the authors also reported that variation in preparations studied and in methodological quality precluded quantitative meta-analysis of the studies and further stated that, although the majority of studies reported positive results, there was insufficient evidence to recommend a specific Echinacea product or preparation. A subsequent negative trial by Barrett et al (20) seemed to contradict the conclusion about efficacy drawn by Melchart et al (19), but a number of letters to the editor in response to the Barrett report as well as a commentary by Turner (21) pointed out the obstacles to designing definitive studies and performing systematic reviews for Echinacea. Among the difficulties noted were comparability of "1 g root/day" to 300 mg of an extract administered three times daily; timing of the intervention (continuous for prevention vs. at "first onset of symptoms," but before development of two identifiable symptoms); method of assessment (self-assessment, viral titer, parent-kept log for studies on children) (22, 23); adequacy of blinding (herbs have characteristic odors and tastes) (3); and nature of the test article (whether the product is standardized or not, nature of the phytochemical marker compounds). As noted by Wolsko et al (5) some authors fail to distinguish between species, and there are three commercially important species of Echinacea in the marketplace (*E. purpurea*, *E. angustifolia*, *and E. pallida*) (24). Although *the* biologically active constituent(s) of Echinacea remain unknown, the phytochemistry of the various species has been reasonably well described. The constituents identified to date fall into four distinct chemical classes: phenolic compounds related to caftaric acid (caftaric acid, chlorogenic acid, echinacoside, cynarin, cichoric acid), isobutylamides, polysaccharides, and glycoproteins (25). Different species and different plant parts are chemically distinct from one another, and some investigators use these variations as species identifiers. That level of detail is beyond the scope of this chapter. The more important concept to keep in mind is that failure to provide any details on the chemistry of the intervention means that the study is essentially irreproducible. Beyond that, the discerning reader can get a feel for the quality of the intervention (and therefore of the trial) by reading the description of the chemical content of the product. The least informative studies are those in which no chemical analysis was performed or reported. In such cases, it can be difficult to determine whether or not the test article contained Echinacea and, even if one were willing to give the investigator the benefit of the doubt, such a report provides no basis for evaluating the quality of the product. Low quality plant material and improper processing or storage can all contribute to a low-quality test material, and if the author provides no chemical information, it is difficult to say of a negative result whether the trial failed because Echinacea is not efficacious or because poor quality Echinacea is not efficacious.

There are competing hypotheses about which chemical constituents are most important for the biological activity of Echinacea and the levels at which they should occur, and individual experts may define "quality" in terms of those constituents (24). Informative studies are those that measure and report the full spectrum of constituents. Even better are those that use standardized extracts in which the chemical constituents are both measured and manipulated so that they are present at consistent levels from lot to lot and over time. Studies that do not report the full chemical spectrum are not easily interpreted or compared. If only a few of the many known constituents were reported or reported levels were very low (compared to previously published levels), this may indicate that low-quality study material was used. Finally, in practical terms there is no such thing as a generic "Echinacea trial." There are trials that evaluate specific Echinacea products for specific endpoints, but in the absence of detailed information on comparability of the products, it is impossible to make the blanket statement that Echinacea is or is not efficacious. Instead, one can point to individual studies or a body of studies and make the judgment that a specific Echinacea product(s) that has the described characteristics is or is not efficacious when evaluated under the conditions described in the trial.

Echinacea Summary

This discussion was not intended to be a systematic review, but in looking over the literature since 1998, it seems that the conclusions outlined in Melchart's (19) review of the Echinacea trial literature need not be changed very much. Although some poorly designed and described studies still manage to make it into the peer-reviewed literature, the biomedical research community has learned something over the past decade. This learning process and subsequent trials have led to several additional systematic reviews. In a 2006 review of the effects of Echinacea on the upper respiratory tract infection (URI) symptom severity and quality of life (QoL), Gillespie and Coleman (26) stated that studies depicting Echinacea's effect on URI symptoms and quality of life are contradictory but that further research is warranted. Another meta-analysis of studies on the effects of Echinacea in the prevention of induced rhinovirus colds reported that "...standardized extracts of Echinacea were effective in the prevention of symptoms of the common cold after clinical inoculation, compared with placebo, but noted that further prospective, appropriately powered clinical studies are required to confirm this finding" (27).

The two most recent meta-analyses, a Cochrane review by Linde et al (28) and an evaluation be Shah et al (29), refine the conclusions drawn by Melchart et al (19), Gillespie and Coleman (26), and Schoop et al (27) that "Echinacea seems like it might be better than placebo but more studies are needed" to draw conclusions about the nature and strength of the evidence. The Cochrane review by Linde and colleagues (28) concluded that "Echinacea preparations tested in clinical trials differ greatly. There is some evidence that preparations based on the aerial parts of *Echinacea purpurea* might be effective for the early treatment of colds in adults but results are not fully consistent. Beneficial effects of other Echinacea preparations and for preventative purposes might exist but have not been shown in independently replicated, rigorous randomized trials." The meta-analysis by Shah et al (29) reported that Echinacea decreased the odds of developing the common cold by 58% and the duration of the cold by 1 to 4 days. They also reported that significant reductions were maintained in subgroup analyses limited to use of a specific brand (which was named in the analysis), concomitant supplement use, method of cold exposure (natural or challenge), Jadad scores less than 3, or use of a fixed-effects model. The report concluded that an analysis of the current evidence in the literature suggests that Echinacea has a benefit in decreasing the incidence and duration of the common cold. A letter by von Maxen and Schoenhoefer (30) disagreed with the conclusions of Shah et al (29) concerning efficacy of Echinacea; however, the Shah report also highlighted the fact that large-scale randomized prospective studies that control variables such as species, quality of the Echinacea preparation, dose, method of cold induction, and objectivity of study endpoints evaluated are needed before Echinacea can become standard practice for preventing and treating the common cold.

CONCLUSIONS

Other authors have addressed adequacy of blinding, randomization, sample size, etc. in evaluating trial design (1–3). The examples provided in the preceding Echinacea case study are intended to emphasize the details of trial design that are taken for granted by investigators accustomed to the world of single-agent pharmaceuticals and can be applied to any herbal clinical trial. The elements that any natural product trial report (or grant application) should contain can be broken down into a series of specifications for identity, purity, composition, and strength. These are built into the conventional drug approval process and are generally in place long before humans are exposed to new single-entity drugs. Despite frequent claims to the contrary, specifications and tests for all of the quality elements noted do exist for a number of herbs in a number of pharmacopoeias, including but not limited to the United States Pharmacopeia, the European Pharmacopoeia, the Japanese Pharmacopoeia, the Pharmacopoeia of the People's Republic of China, the German Pharmacopoeia, and others. If specifications exist, investigators should, if applicable, use them to define their trial materials. If they do not use them, they should be able to provide a good justification for not doing so. If specifications do not exist, investigators may need to invent (and of course describe) them.

In evaluating a clinical trial report, readers should pay attention to the authors' documentation of the source of the specifications used, the tests used to identify whether or not specifications have been met, and the test results. Use of preexisting specifications is in the authors' interest in writing a paper, as details of testing, etc. can be provided by reference rather than by tediously describing the rationale for the specifications, the specifications themselves, the testing methods used, and results. While details of identity, purity, composition, and strength should be provided in all published natural product trials, the level of detail presented is especially important if the trial uses materials that are not from commercial sources (e.g., plant material collected or purchased by the investigator and then used in the trial with or without further processing). Information about the geographical origin of plant material and whether or not it was cultivated or wild-collected, and by whom, are important elements of identity. In addition, investigators should state whether or not voucher specimens were collected, and if so, where they are deposited (10). Other details, such as plant part, extract ratio, solvent composition, excipients used, chemical analysis, standardization details, and stability are all vital pieces of information necessary for evaluation of herbal clinical trial results. Because regulatory schemes are not uniform from country to country, an investigator who uses a commercial product should get as much of this information from the supplier/manufacturer as possible and include it in the manuscript. Other aspects of the trial such as adequacy of blinding, testing for impurities (e.g., microorganisms, pesticides), inertness of the placebo, reliability of the assessment tool, and rationale for dosing are also important, and readers who keep all of these elements in mind should have little difficulty sorting through the literature.

ACKNOWLEDGMENTS

The authors thank John H. Cardellina and Marguerite Klein for their editorial attentions.

References

1. Jadad AR, Moore RA, Carroll D, et al. Assessing the quality of reports of randomized clinical trials: is blinding necessary? *Control Clin Trials* 1996;17:1–12.
2. Moher D, Schulz KF, Altman DG. The CONSORT statement: revised recommendations for improving the quality of reports of parallel-group randomized trials. *Ann Int Med* 2001;134:657–662.
3. Linde K, Jonas WB, Melchart D, Willich S. The methodological quality of randomized controlled trials of homeopathy, herbal medicines and acupuncture. *Int J Epidemiol* 2001; 30:526–531.
4. Gagnier JJ, Boon H, Rochon P, Moher D, Barnes J, Bombardier C. Reporting randomized, controlled trials of herbal interventions: an elaborated CONSORT statement. *Ann Int Med* 2005;144:364–367.
5. Wolsko PM, Solondz DK, Phillips RS, Schachter SC, Eisenberg DM. Lack of herbal supplement characterization in published randomized controlled trials. *Am J Med* 2005;118: 1087–1093.
6. Gagnier JJ, DeMelo J, Boon H, Rochon P, Bombardier C. Quality of reporting of randomized controlled trials of herbal medicine interventions. *Am J Med* 2006;119:800. e1–e11.
7. Swanson CA. Suggested guidelines for articles about botanical dietary supplements. *Am J Clin Nutr* 2002;75:8–10.
8. Health and Human Services, National Institutes of Health. *Biologically Active Agents Used in CAM and Placebo Materials—Policy and Guidance*. Bethesda, MD: National Center for Complementary and Alternative Medicine. http://nccam.nih.gov/research/policies/bioactive.htm. Accessed March 4, 2009.
9. USDA, ARS, National Genetic Resources Program. *Germplasm Resources Information Network—(GRIN)* [Online Database]. Beltsville, MD: National Germplasm Resources Laboratory. http://www.ars-grin.gov/cgi-bin/npgs/html/index.pl?language=en. Accessed March 4, 2009.
10. Hildreth J, Hrabeta-Robinson E, Applequist W, Betz J, Miller J. Standard operating procedure for the collection and preparation of voucher plant specimens for use in the nutraceutical industry. *Anal Bioanal Chem* 2007;389:13–17.
11. Blumenthal M, Goldberg A, Brinckmann J, eds. *Herbal Medicine, Expanded Commission E Monographs*. Newton, MA: Integrative Medicine Communications; 2000.
12. Betz JM, Fisher KD, Saldanha LG, Coates PM. The NIH analytical methods and reference materials program for dietary supplements. *Anal Bioanal Chem* 2007;389:19–25.
13. Guns ES, Goldenberg SL, Brown PN. Mass spectral analysis of PC-SPES confirms the presence of diethylstilbestrol. *Can J Urol* 2002;9:1684–1688.
14. Busse W. The significance of quality for efficacy and safety of herbal medicinal products. *Drug Inf J* 2000;34:15–23.
15. Bauer R. Quality criteria and standardization of phytopharmaceuticals: can acceptable drug standards be achieved? *Drug Inf J* 1998;32:101–110.
16. Tyler VE. *Herbs of Choice—the Therapeutic Use of Phytomedicinals*. Binghamton, NY: Haworth Press; 1994.
17. Remington JP, Wood HC. *The Dispensatory of the United States of America*. 20th ed. Philadelphia, PA: JB Lippincott Company; 1918.
18. Osol A, Farrar GE. *The Dispensatory of the United States of America*. 25th ed. Philadelphia, PA: JB Lippincott Company; 1955.
19. Melchart D, Linde K, Fischer P, Kaesmayr J. Echinacea for preventing and treating the common cold. *Cochrane Database Syst Rev* 2000;2:CD000530.
20. Barrett BP, Brown RL, Locken K, Maberry R, Bobula JA, D'Alessio D. Treatment of the common cold with unrefined echinacea. A randomized, double-blind, placebo-controlled trial. *Ann Int Med* 2002;137:939–946.

21. Turner RB. Echinacea for the common cold: can alternative medicine be evidence-based medicine? *Ann Int Med* 2002;137:1001–1002.
22. Barrett B, Brown R, Voland R, Maberry R, Turner R. Relations among questionnaire and laboratory measures of rhinovirus infection. *Eur Respir J* 2006;28:358–363.
23. Whelan AM, Jurgens TM, Lord L. Evaluating the quality of randomized controlled trials that examine the efficacy of natural health products: a systematic review of critical appraisal instruments. *Evid Based Complement Alternat Med* 2008;5:nem186.
24. Bergeron C, Livesey JF, Awang DVC, et al. A quantitative HPLC method for the quality assurance of *Echinacea* products on the North American market. *Phytochem Anal* 2000;11:207–215.
25. Barnes J, Anderson LA, Gibbons S, Phillipson JD. Echinacea species (Echinacea angustifolia (DC.) Hell., Echinacea pallida (Nutt.) Nutt., Echinacea purpurea (L.) Moench): a review of their chemistry, pharmacology and clinical properties. *J Pharm Pharmacol* 2005;57:929–954.
26. Gillespie EL, Coleman CI. The effect of Echinacea on upper respiratory infection symptom severity and quality of life. *Conn Med* 2006;70:93–97.
27. Schoop R, Klein P, Suter A, Johnston SL. Echinacea in the prevention of induced rhinovirus colds: a meta-analysis. *Clin Ther* 2006;28:174–183.
28. Linde K, Barrett B, Wölkart K, Bauer R, Melchart D. Echinacea for preventing and treating the common cold. *Cochrane Database Syst Rev* 2006 Jan 25;(1):CD000530.
29. Shah SA, Sander S, White CM, Rinaldi M, Coleman CI. Evaluation of echinacea for the prevention and treatment of the common cold: a meta-analysis. *Lancet Infect Dis* 2007;7:473–480.
30. von Maxen A, Schoenhoefer PS. Benefit of echinacea for the prevention and treatment of the common cold? *Lancet Infect Dis* 2008;8:346–347.

CHAPTER 31

Supplements Evaluated in Clinical Trials: Why Specific Formulations Matter

Marilyn Barrett

The decision to take a botanic product or advise a patient to take a botanic substance is based on an expected therapeutic benefit. This expected benefit can be based upon traditional use and/or on the results of modern clinical or pharmacological studies. The assumption is that the product selected from the shelf will be similar enough to the reference product to have the same therapeutic effect. This assumption is based upon working with drugs that are mandated to conform to official specifications for generics.

Perhaps because of this, in the United States an herbal preparation is often not specified beyond the common name of the plant. Simply "valerian," "echinacea," or "garlic" is used to describe the preparation. That might suffice if all valerian, echinacea, or garlic products were equivalent. But they are not. For example, valerian root preparations are available as teas (aqueous extracts) and aqueous alcoholic extracts (70% ethanol with an herb to extract ratio of 4-7:1). As for echinacea products, three different species are used in commerce and the preparations are as diverse as the expressed juice of *Echinacea purpurea* flowering tops and an aqueous alcoholic extract of the roots of *Echinacea angustifolia* roots. Garlic is available raw, dried, aged (aqueous alcoholic extract), and as an oil. None of these preparations can be assumed to chemically and therapeutically equivalent.

For products sold as dietary supplements in the United States, there are suggested guidelines on establishing bioequivalence. However, there are no mandated criteria to use to compare products which might be considered equivalent. The Federal Trade Commission, in its advertising guide for the dietary supplement industry, states that "...advertisers should examine the underlying research to confirm that it is relevant to the advertiser's product..., ...dosage and formulation are comparable..., ...an advertiser should not rely on studies where ... the advertisers product is made using a different extraction method..." (1).

In contrast, for drugs there are established mandated criteria to define a generic product. Generic drugs are pharmaceutically and therapeutically equivalent to the reference product as established by United States Food and Drug Administration mandates (2). A substance is considered pharmaceutically equivalent if it contains the same active pharmaceutical ingredient (API), same chemical composition, same strength, same dosage form, same route of administration, and labeled for the same condition of use. Therapeutic equivalency is established by measuring disintegration (the ability of the capsule or tablet to dissolve), dissolution (release of active components), and bioavailability (metabolism, distribution, and excretion). Often, bioequivalence is established with a clinical study that includes a time course of plasma concentrations after single administration of the original and test products. The study is usually a two-way, crossover study with 24 to 36 healthy volunteers that demonstrates identical plasma exposure over time. Critical parameters are the extent of absorption of the active constituent, measured as the area under the plasma concentration time curve (AUC) and the rate of absorption as measured by maximum plasma concentration (C_{max}).

The challenge with defining a generic botanic product lies in establishing the API. Is the API the whole plant, an extract, an extract of selected groups of compounds, or a specific chemical constituent? What about a multicomponent mixture? This question can be addressed by referring to the original material that delivered the specific benefit. As an example, there is a "nerve tea" formula in the German Pharmacopoeia 7 that is based upon traditional use. The formula includes valerian root, balm leaves, and peppermint leaves in a ratio of 2:1:1 (3). In this example, the whole formula is the API. As another example, most of the clinical and pharmacological data for ginkgo leaf extracts is based upon a proprietary extract (EGb 761) that is a 50:1 concentrate (4). In this example, the specialized concentrated ginkgo extract is the API. Although preparations of ginkgo-powdered leaf are offered for sale in the United States, it is highly improbable that this preparation will offer the same benefits. A third example is the sennosides, found in senna leaves and pods. The sennosides are purgative laxatives and these specific compounds, which can be purified from the plant, are the API (3).

A more subtle distinction in establishing the API is the type of extract prepared from the plant material. Different solvents can pull different chemical compounds from the plant and this may affect the therapeutic efficacy of the preparation. As an illustration, an experiment was conducted to determine the effects of different extraction solvents on hawthorn preparations. Extracts were prepared using aqueous ethanol (40% to 70% volume/volume), aqueous methanol (40% to 70%), and water. Chemical characterization determined that the contents (procyanidin, flavonoid, total vitexin, and total phenolic) were qualitatively and quantitatively different in the water extract compared with the aqueous alcoholic extracts. In addition, the ability of the water extract to have a relaxant effect on aortic tissue in vitro was reduced by more than half compared with the aqueous alcoholic extracts (5). This data suggest that the tea would be less effective than the tincture or dried aqueous alcoholic extract in treating cardiac insufficiency.

A rational approach to evaluating the APIs and phytoequivalence of herbal products was developed by an international group, the Herbal Medicinal Products Working Group of the International Pharmaceutical Federation (FIP). This group produced three categories of products according to the extent of information on APIs (6).

In the first category (A) are extracts containing constituents (single compounds or families of compounds) with known and acknowledged therapeutic activity deemed solely responsible for the clinical efficacy. In this category, the API can be established chemically. Tests for pharmaceutical equivalency and bioavailability can be conducted in the same way as they are for drugs. Examples of category (A) botanics in the European Pharmacopeia are aloe dry extract, buckthorn bark dry extract, senna leaf dry extract, and belladonna leaf dry extract. Examples in the German Pharmacopoeia are ipecacuanha dry extract, rhubarb dry extract, milk thistle fruit dry extract, and horse chestnut seed dry extract (6).

In the second category (B) are extracts containing chemically defined constituents (single or groups) possessing relevant pharmacological properties that are likely to contribute to the clinical efficacy. However, proof that they are solely responsible for the clinical efficacy has not been provided. The API is the whole extract and there is a need for product manufacturing details as well as chemical markers. In some cases, biological activity testing may replace chemical assays. Examples of category (B) botanics are ginkgo leaf dry extract and St. John's wort dry extract, listed in the German and European Pharmacopoeia, respectively (6).

Extracts that do not contain any constituents that are regarded as being responsible for the therapeutic activity are placed in category (C). For these botanics, chemically defined constituents (markers) may be used for quality control purposes to monitor Good Manufacturing Practices or to determine the contents in the product. Establishment of bioequivalency requires specification of the species, the plant part (root, rhizome, leaf, seed, etc.), and manufacturing processes (e.g., the solvent, the extraction conditions, the ratio of plant material to solvent, and final ratio of staring material to final product). An example of a category (C) botanic in the German Pharmacopoeia is valerian root dry extract (6).

Once chemical equivalency has been established, then bioavailability is the next step in establishing therapeutic equivalency. The biological effect of any substance is dependent upon the extent to which it is absorbed by the body. An array of factors influences bioavailability including the route of administration (oral, intravenous, topical) and the formulation of the product. Formulation in liquid or solid form along with the specifics of the excipients will influence the absorption of the product.

The importance of formulation in bioavailability was demonstrated in a study comparing two ginkgo products. Both preparations contained extracts characterized as containing 24% flavone glycosides and 6% terpene lactones. The reference product was Ginkgold, containing the EGb 761 extract which is the basis for the Commission E monograph (7). Dissolution studies, which are designed to detect the presence and quantity of the API in simulated digestive fluid, were conducted on Ginkgold and the test product. The assay indicated that Ginkgold released more than 99% of its terpene lactone content in 15 minutes, whereas the test product released less than 33% in 60 minutes. These two products were then alternately given to 12 healthy volunteers using a crossover trial design. After administration the plasma concentrations of ginkgolides A, B, and bilobalide were determined. The result of the study was that EGb 761 caused statistically significant greater C_{max} and AUC for ginkgolides A, B, and bilobalide compared to the test product. Statistical analysis, using 90% confidence intervals, showed that these two products were not bioequivalent (8). As with drugs, information on chemical characterization, as well as bioavailability, is required to establish therapeutic equivalency.

Product characterization can also influence the safety of a product. Experimental evidence with St. John's wort extract suggests that two different types of preparations might be effective in treating mild depression, although one type of preparation may be less safe than the other due to drug–herb interactions. Previous to 1998 it was thought that hypericin was the chemical constituent in St. John's wort that was largely responsible for the antidepressant effect. At that time, research by a group of scientists demonstrated evidence that another compound, hyperforin, was more active than hypericin in treating depression (9). However, a St. John's wort extract that did not contain any significantly amounts of hyperforin was also clinically active (10). It was soon established that St John's wort extracts interacted with specific drugs via the induction of cytochrome P450 enzymes (particularly CYP3A4) and/or P-glycoprotein (11). Further studies determined that the degree of enzyme induction correlated with the amount of hyperforin in the extract. Thus, St. John's wort extracts that did not contain substantial amounts of hyperforin (<1%) do not appear to produce clinically relevant enzyme induction (12–15). Thus, there are St. John's wort extracts with different chemical profiles that have demonstrated clinical efficacy in treating mild to moderate depression. Depending of the chemical profile of the extract, St. John's wort products may or may not interact with certain drugs.

Guidance on the characterization of botanic products comes from sources such as pharmacopoeias, government guidelines, and journal editors. Pharmacopoeial monographs specify the identity of the plant material, the plant part, and chemical composition. As an example, goldenseal is defined in the United States Pharmacopoeia (USP) as the dried roots and rhizomes of *Hydrastis canadensis* L that contain not less than 2% hydrastine and not less than 2.5% berberine (16). The goldenseal extract is defined as having a ratio of staring crude plant material to powdered extract of 2:1.

Pharmacopoeial monographs can also specify tests for disintegration and dissolution of capsules and tablets. As an example, the USP monograph for milk thistle capsules specifies that, using the described method, not less than 75% of the labeled amount of silymarin as silybin is dissolved in 45 minutes (17). Compliance with the USP specifications on dietary supplement ingredients is not mandatory in the United States. In contrast, compliance is mandatory for drugs sold in the United States. Botanic products are regulated differently in other countries. For example, Canada and Germany require either compliance with a monograph or individualized approval before marketing.

Guidelines for botanic characterization are given on the Web site for the National Center for Complementary and Alternative Medicine (NCCAM) of the US National Institutes of Health. In its guidelines for clinical trial grant applications, NCCAM suggests that when plant material is used in a trial, it be accompanied by a botanic description, extraction procedure, the quantity of any known active constituent(s), as well as identity and stability tests. When a product is used, information about the manufacturing process, analysis for impurities, and quality controls for manufacturing must be included. In addition, where appropriate, disintegration/dissolution rates are required to estimate bioavailability (http://grants.nih.gov/grants/guide/notice-files/NOT-AT-05-004.html).

Some journals give precise details on the information needed to characterize botanic products. The *Journal of Natural Products*, published by the American Chemical Society and the American Society of Pharmacognosy, provides such guidance to its authors. The journal requires that experimental biological material be authenticated as to its identity and that the herbarium that holds the voucher specimen be given along with the voucher number. It further requires that the scientific name (genus, species, authority citation, and family) be given. It also requires authors who purchase dried "herbal remedies" or other materials from companies to deposit a specimen in an herbarium for future access. It requires that the extraction procedure be specified when studying a commercially available extract and that the identification of the extract be supported by an HPLC trace of known secondary metabolite constituents (http://pubs.acs.org/page/jnprdf/submission/authors.html).

In summary, therapeutic efficacy cannot be assumed when substituting one botanic product for another. Regulatory guidance on establishing bioequivalence (generics) in dietary supplements is suggested but not specified or mandated. The risks associated with assumption of generic status include efficacy different from expected, unknown safety status, and uninformed /misleading decisions made by health care providers, consumers, and policy makers.

Practical steps that can be taken to move toward identifying botanic products with therapeutic equivalency are listed below. In addition, Table 31.1 lists select

TABLE 31.1 Select Proprietary Products That Have Been Clinically Tested[a]

Indication	Botanic	Product; Manufacturer	Characteristics	Daily Dose in Trials
Benign prostatic hyperplasia	Grass Pollen (Flower Pollen)	Cernilton; AB Cernelle, Sweden; Graminex, USA	Pollen; water and acetone extracts (Cernitin)	180–360 mg
Benign prostatic hyperplasia	Pygeum	Tadenan; Lab. Fournier, France	Bark; lipophilic extract	100–200 mg
Benign prostatic hyperplasia	Saw palmetto	Permixon; Pierre Fabre, France	Berries; hexane extract (PA 109)	320 mg
Cardiovascular risk	Garlic	Kwai; Lichtwer Pharma, Germany	Dried bulb; standardized to 1.3% alliin, 0.6% allicin (LI 111)	900 mg
Chronic heart failure	Hawthorn	Crataegutt, HeartCare; Schwabe, Germany	Leaves and flowers; hydroalcoholic extract (WS1442)	160–180 mg
Chronic venous insufficiency	Grape seed	Leukoselect; Indena, Italy	Seed; extract standardized to 80%–85% oligomeric proantho-cyanidins	100–300 mg
Chronic venous insufficiency	Horse chestnut	Venastat, Venostasin; Pharmaton, Switzerland	Seed; extract standardized to 16% aescin	600 mg; 100 mg aescin
Cognitive function	Ginkgo	Ginkoba, Gingold, Schwabe, Germany	Leaf; 50:1 extract standardized to 24% flavonoids, 6% terpenes (EGb 761)	120–240 mg, up to 600 mg
Depression	St John's wort	Kira, Jarsin; Lichtwer, Germany; Indena, Italy	Flowers; extract standardized to 0.3% hypericin, >3% hyperforin (LI 160)	900 mg
Insomnia	Valerian	Sedonium; Lichtwer, Germany	Root/rhizome; ethanolic extract (LI 156)	600 mg before bed
Liver disease/ alcoholic cirrhosis	Milk thistle	Legalon; Madaus, Germany	Seeds; extract standardized to 80% silymarin	210–800 mg

(continued)

TABLE 31.1 *(Continued)*

Indication	Botanic	Product; Manufacturer	Characteristics	Daily Dose in Trials
Menopause symptoms	Black cohosh	Remifemin; Schaper & Brummer, Germany	Root/rhizome; isopropanolic extract	2 or 4 tablets – equivalent to 40 mg root/day
Physical performance	Ginseng (Asian)	Ginsana; Pharmaton, Switzerland	Root/rhizome; extract standardized to 4% ginsenosides (G115)	200–600 mg

[a] Information in this table is excerpted from Barrett, 2004 (18).

proprietary products that have been tested clinically for various indications. This information is excerpted from The Handbook of Clinically Tested Herbal Remedies (18).

PRACTICAL STEPS TOWARD BIOEQUIVALENCE

1. Identify the source of the information on expected efficacy. For example, is the source of information on efficacy a book on traditional Chinese medicine or clinical studies conducted on a specific product?
2. Look at the source for information of the characteristics of the product. Note the scientific name of the plant, the plant part and any information on the way it is prepared (dried, heated, extracted, etc), as well as any available information on chemical constituents.
3. Identify sources for products that look like they might be similar to the original preparation. Ask pharmacies that specialize in dietary supplements or search the Web. Look for information on the label of the new product that correlates with the information you gathered above. The Handbook of Clinically Tested Herbal Remedies (Barrett, 2004) lists proprietary products that have been tested clinically and possible sources of these products in the United States (18).

References

1. Federal Trade Commission. *Dietary Supplements: An Advertising Guide for Industry*. Federal Trade Commission Bureau of Consumer Protection; 1998.
2. Food and Drug Administration. *FDA Generic Drugs Final Rule and Initiative*. US Food and Drug Administration; 2003.
3. Schulz V, Hänsel R, Blumenthal M, Tyler V. *Rational Phytotherapy: A Reference Guide for Physicians and Pharmacists*. 5th ed. Berlin: Springer-Verlag; 2004.
4. Birks J, Grimley EJ. Ginkgo biloba for cognitive impairment and dementia. *Cochrane Database Syst Rev* 2009;(1):CD003120.
5. Vierling W, Brand N, Gaedcke F, Sensch KH, Schneider E, Scholz M. Investigation of the pharmaceutical and pharmacological equivalence of different Hawthorn extracts. *Phytomedicine* 2003;10(1):8–16.

6. Lang F, Keller K, Ihrig M, et al. Biopharmaceutical characterization of herbal medicinal products. *Pharmacopeial Forum* 2003;29(4):1337–1346.
7. Blumenthal M, Busse W, Hall T, et al. *The Complete German Commission E Monographs: Therapeutic Guide to Herbal Medicines*. Austin, TX: American Botanical Council; 1998.
8. Kressmann S, Biber A, Wonnemann M, Schug B, Blume HH, Muller WE. Influence of pharmaceutical quality on the bioavailability of active components from Ginkgo biloba preparations. *J Pharm Pharmacol* 2002;54(11):1507–1514.
9. Muller WE. Current St John's wort research from mode of action to clinical efficacy. *Pharmacol Res* 2003;47(2):101–109.
10. Woelk H. Comparison of St John's wort and imipramine for treating depression: randomised controlled trial. *BMJ* 2000;321(7260):536–539.
11. Kober M, Pohl K, Efferth T. Molecular mechanisms underlying St. John's wort drug interactions. *Curr Drug Metab* 2008;9(10):1026–1036.
12. Will-Shahab L, Bauer S, Kunter U, Roots I, Brattstrom A. St John's wort extract (Ze 117) does not alter the pharmacokinetics of a low-dose oral contraceptive. *Eur J Clin Pharmacol* 2009;65(3):287–294.
13. Whitten DL, Myers SP, Hawrelak JA, Wohlmuth H. The effect of St John's wort extracts on CYP3A: a systematic review of prospective clinical trials. *Br J Clin Pharmacol* 2006;62(5):512–526.
14. Madabushi R, Frank B, Drewelow B, Derendorf H, Butterweck V. Hyperforin in St. John's wort drug interactions. *Eur J Clin Pharmacol* 2006;62(3):225–233.
15. Mueller SC, Majcher-Peszynska J, Mundkowski RG, et al. No clinically relevant CYP3A induction after St. John's wort with low hyperforin content in healthy volunteers. *Eur J Clin Pharmacol* 2009;65(1):81–87.
16. *Goldenseal. United States Pharmacopeia 32/National Formulary 27*. Rockville, MD: United States Pharmacopeial Convention; 2009: 1033.
17. *Milk Thistle Capsules. United States Pharmacopeia 32/National Formulary 27*. Rockville, MD: The United States Pharmacopeial Convention; 2009: 1056.
18. *The Handbook of Clinically Tested Herbal Remedies*. London: Haworth Press, now owned by Taylor & Francis Group, LLC; 2004.

CHAPTER 32

The Role and Programs of the NIH Office of Dietary Supplements

Rebecca B. Costello

BACKGROUND

The mission of the Office of Dietary Supplements (ODS) is to strengthen knowledge and understanding of dietary supplements by evaluating scientific information, stimulating and supporting research, disseminating research results, and educating the public to foster an enhanced quality of life and health for the US population.

On the last day, in the last hours, the 103rd Congress passed the Dietary Supplement Health and Education Act (DSHEA) of 1994 (Public Law 103-417) (1) and opened the marketplace to an array of dietary supplement products. DSHEA also authorized the establishment of the ODS at the National Institutes of Health (NIH). The ODS was created shortly thereafter within the Office of Disease Prevention, Office of the Director, NIH. DSHEA defined the purpose and responsibilities of ODS as follows:

- To explore more fully the potential role of dietary supplements as a significant part of the efforts of the United States to improve health care.
- To promote scientific study of the benefits of dietary supplements in maintaining health and preventing chronic disease and other health-related conditions.
- To conduct and coordinate scientific research within NIH relating to dietary supplements.
- To collect and compile the results of scientific research relating to dietary supplements, including scientific data from foreign sources.
- To serve as the principal advisor to the Secretary and to the Assistant Secretary for Health and provide advice to the Director of NIH, the Director of the Centers for Disease Control and Prevention, and the Commissioner of the Food and Drug Administration (FDA) on issues relating to dietary supplements.

When DSHEA became law in 1994, there were an estimated 600 US dietary supplement manufacturers producing about 4,000 products (2). According to FDA estimates there were more than 29,000 different dietary supplement products on the market by the year 2,000, with an average of 1,000 new products added annually. Sarubin (3) projected that 40,000 supplement products would be on the US market by 2010, although other sources report estimates as high as 75,000 dietary supplement products were available to consumers in 2008 (4).

Dietary supplements can have an impact on the prevention of disease and on the maintenance of health. In the United States, these ingredients are usually defined as including plant extracts, enzymes, vitamins, minerals, amino acids, and hormonal products that are available without prescription and are consumed in addition to the regular diet. Although vitamin and mineral supplements have been available for decades, their specific health effects have been the subject of detailed scientific research only within the last 20 to 25 years. Currently, this research has expanded to include the health effects of other bioactive factors consumed as supplements to promote health and prevent disease. Considerable research on the effects of botanic and herbal dietary supplements has been conducted in Asia and Europe where plant products have a long tradition of use. However, the overwhelming majority of these supplements have not been studied using modern scientific techniques, nor have they been extensively studied in population groups that may be at risk for chronic diseases. For many reasons, therefore, it is important to enhance research efforts to determine the benefits and risks of dietary supplements.

Since its inception in 1995, ODS has grown and expanded its programs. In the early years, ODS focused attention on supporting the needs of academic and industry researchers. As the office expanded, ODS designed and developed programs to reach out to an array of interested constituents to include consumers, clinicians and public health officials, and policy makers. Today, ODS supports several programs to increase the public awareness of the benefits and risks of dietary supplements and stimulate research and development programs in the public and private sector.

METHODS DEVELOPMENT PROGRAM

The rapid expansion of the dietary supplement marketplace has resulted in a proliferation of ingredients and products and outstripped the pace of development of reliable analytical methods. Precise, accurate, and rugged analytical methods and reference materials are essential for verification of ingredient identity, for identifying and measuring contaminants, and for measuring the amounts of declared ingredients in raw materials and finished products.

The Dietary Supplements Methods and Reference Materials Program was created in 2002 in response to direction from the US Congress. It is a broad-based initiative that supports the technical aspects of methods development as well as the administrative and consensus building foundation necessary for advancing the field. The Program supports critical laboratory research and the infrastructure necessary for evaluation and dissemination of new methods and reference materials. Continued expansion of this program is anticipated as emerging science identifies new needs and opportunities (5).

While clinicians may not be immediately impacted by the ODS Methods Development Program, it will over time help address the notable lack of well-characterized herbal supplements being utilized in randomized controlled trials (6) and markedly reduce the variability of products in the marketplace (7–9). The Methods Development Program is based on the premise that clinical trials of phytomedicines should follow good clinical practice guidelines, include positive and negative control arms, use careful documentation procedures, employ rigorous statistical design and analyses, and be conducted for a sufficient period of time for the chosen study design (10). To improve the design and reporting of randomized controlled trials using phytomedicine interventions, members of the Consolidated Standards of Reporting Trials (CONSORT) group have developed a checklist to assist investigators and clinicians (11). For those dietary supplement products in the marketplace that have not benefited from clinical studies, clinicians should ascertain the following information before prescribing the product:

- Conformance to FDA labeling regulations for dietary supplements:
  - a descriptive name of the product stating that it is a "supplement"; the name and place of business of the manufacturer, packer, or distributor; a complete list of ingredients; and the net contents of the product;
  - nutrition labeling must be in the form of a "Supplement Facts" panel. This label must identify each dietary ingredient contained in the product.

In addition, clinicians should remain alert to gender-based and genotypic/phenotypic differences in pharmacological and toxicological responses to dietary supplements (12).

Recent Approved Standard Reference Materials of Interest to Clinicians

- *Ginkgo biloba* as extract, leaves, or Ginkgo containing tablets
- *Serenoa repens* (saw palmetto) as extract or fruit
- Omega-3- and 6-containing oils (flax, borage, evening primrose, Perilla)
- Multivitamin/multielement tablets
- Vitamin D in human serum

For more information, visit http://www.nist.gov/srm.

OFFICE OF DIETARY SUPPLEMENTS EVIDENCE-BASED PROGRAM

In FY 2001, ODS received a Congressional mandate to review the current scientific evidence on the efficacy and safety of dietary supplements and identify research needs. ODS responded by developing an evidence-based review program using the Evidence-based Practice Centers Program established by the Agency for Healthcare Research and Quality (AHRQ) and others to conduct systematic reviews of the scientific literature and prepare reports of their findings. These reports are invaluable in presenting what is and is not known in a research area as well as communicating information on the efficacy and safety of supplements under study that clinicians will find helpful.

Completed Reports

- Glucose and Insulin Responses to Dietary Chromium Supplements: A Meta-Analysis
- Ephedra and Ephedrine for Weight Loss and Athletic Performance Enhancement: Clinical Efficacy and Side Effects
- A series of reports on omega-3 fatty acids and a variety of health conditions including cardiovascular disease, asthma, cancer, eye health, cognitive function, and organ transplantation
- Effect of Soy on Health Outcomes
- B Vitamins and Berries and Age-Related Neurodegenerative Disorders
- Multivitamin/Mineral Supplements and Prevention of Chronic Disease
- Effectiveness and Safety of Vitamin D in Relation to Bone Health
- Vitamin D and Calcium: A Systematic Review of Health Outcomes

These reports have resulted in the publication of a number of articles in the peer-reviewed literature (a list is available on the ODS Web site at http://ods.od.nih.gov).

OFFICE OF DIETARY SUPPLEMENTS COMMUNICATIONS PROGRAM

The goals of the program are to promote the public's understanding of the role of nutrition and dietary supplements in maintaining health; to oversee outreach activities that inform and educate the public, health care providers, and scientists about the benefits and risks of dietary supplements; and to develop, maintain, and update the information products disseminated by ODS. Science-based information and products for the clinician available via the ODS Web site include the following:

- ODS Fact Sheets and links to other useful information on dietary supplement (vitamins, minerals, and botanics) use, research findings, nutrient recommendations, database, and other research resources
- News, events and media resources that present up-to-date details on conferences and workshops, announcements, and news releases
- Links to AHRQ Evidence-Based Reports
- Link to a brochure for consumers, *What Dietary Supplements Are You Taking? Does Your Health Care Provider Know? It Matters and Here's Why*, designed to stimulate communication between patient and clinician. Includes tear-out medication and dietary supplements record.
- Link to a minitutorial on *How to Evaluate Health Information on the Internet: Questions and Answers.*

ODS Resources for Clinicians and Consumers

- ODS Fact Sheets—Professional and Consumer versions
- Links to AHRQ Evidenced-Based Reports
- Links to Consumer Brochures

Visit http://www.ods.od.nih.gov.

INTERNATIONAL BIBLIOGRAPHIC INFORMATION ON DIETARY SUPPLEMENTS DATABASE

The International Bibliographic Information on Dietary Supplements (IBIDS) database provides access to bibliographic citations and abstracts from published, international, and scientific literature on dietary supplements. IBIDS is collaboration between two government agencies, the ODS at the NIH, and the Food and Nutrition Information Center at the National Agricultural Library and the Agricultural Research Service at the United States Department of Agriculture.

IBIDS contains more than 750,000 citations, most with abstracts, from 1986 to the present on the topic of dietary supplements from four major bibliographic databases: MEDLINE, for biomedical literature; AGRICOLA and AGRIS for botanic and agricultural literature; and the Commonwealth Agricultural Bureau International's CAB Abstracts and CAB Global Health for selected nutrition journals. IBIDS permits seamless searching across records from all these sources simultaneously.

IBIDS includes bibliographic records on

- the use and function of vitamin, mineral, phytochemical, botanic, and herbal supplements in human nutrition;

- the role of nutrient supplementation in metabolism in normal nutrition and disease states;
- animal studies that relate to the function of dietary supplements in human nutrition;
- chemical composition, biochemical roles, and antioxidant activity of botanic and nutrient supplements;
- fortification of foods with supplemental nutrients and health-related effects;
- nutrient composition of herbal and botanic products;
- surveys on dietary supplement use by various populations; and
- the growth and production of herbal and botanic products used as dietary supplements.

Clinicians can search the IBIDS database in several ways. Users can access the **Full Database** that contains all citations in the peer-reviewed and consumer databases as well as citations from other sources; **Peer-Reviewed Citations Only; Consumer IBIDS, or IBIDS Clinical,** a specialized subset of IBIDS geared to those involved in clinical practice or clinical research. In addition to records on published clinical studies, IBIDS Clinical also contains records on organizational statements, such as practice guidelines, consensus statements, and position papers released by authoritative organizations and professional scientific societies. Coverage includes materials published since 1994 and the database is updated quarterly. IBIDS is free to the public and can be accessed at http://www.ods.od.nih.gov. Plans are underway to enhance the features of IBIDS.

OFFICE OF DIETARY SUPPLEMENTS BOTANIC RESEARCH CENTERS PROGRAMS

The ODS, in collaboration with the National Center for Complementary and Alternative Medicine funds six Dietary Supplement Research Centers focused on botanics, collectively referred to as the NIH Botanic Research Centers Program. The Centers identify and characterize botanics, assess bioavailability and bioactivity, explore mechanisms of action, conduct preclinical and clinical evaluations, help select botanics to be tested in clinical trials, and provide a rich environment for training and career development. The Centers are expected to advance the scientific base of knowledge about botanics, including issues of their safety, efficacy, and biological action. The Botanic Research Centers Program for 2005–2009 includes the following grantee institutions:

University of Illinois at Chicago for Women's Health

Research Focus: Botanic ingredients used in herbal supplements that have potential benefits for women's health, particularly therapies for symptoms of menopause.

Research Projects:

- Standardization
- Mechanisms of Action
- In Vitro and In Vivo Studies of Metabolism, Bioavailability and Toxicity

Purdue University and the University of Alabama at Birmingham

Research Focus: Study of botanics as dietary supplements with an emphasis on polyphenols for age-related diseases.

Research Projects:

- Isoflavones: metabolism and bone health
- Kudzu (*Pueraria lobata*) polyphenols: cardiovascular and cognitive function
- Polyphenol Antioxidants and eye health

Iowa State University and the University of Iowa

Research Focus: Two widely used botanics, Echinacea and *Hypericum perforatum* (St. John's Wort); and on Prunella (commonly known as self-heal).

Research Projects:

- Studies of diversity in Echinacea, Hypericum, and Prunella in relation to antiviral activities
- Studies of diversity in Echinacea, Hypericum and Prunella in relation to anti-inflammatory activities
- Pain receptor mediated anti-inflammatory activity of Echinacea and Hypericum species

Pennington Biomedical Research Center of the Louisiana State University

Research Focus: Basic and clinical studies to determine how selected botanics may influence molecular, cellular, and physiological mechanisms by which these botanics may prevent or reverse the development of insulin resistance.

Research Projects:

- Actions of Russian tarragon (*Artemisia dracunculus*) on insulin action
- Antiobesity potential of Shilianhua (*Sinocrassula indica*)
- Grape anthocyanins and insulin sensitivity

Wake Forest University and Brigham and Women's Center for Botanic Lipids

Research Focus: Studies on specific fatty acids derived from a single biochemical pathway involving the elongation and desaturation of n-3 and n-6 fatty acids.

Research Projects:

- Mechanisms of atherosclerosis prevention by flaxseed oil
- Echium oil triglyceride metabolism and atherosclerosis
- Mechanism of leukotriene inhibition by botanic oils
- Treatment of bronchial asthma with borage seed oil

Memorial Sloan Kettering Research Center for Botanic Immunomodulators

Research Focus: Studies on botanic immunomodulators relevant to the treatment of cancer and infectious disease.

Research Projects:

- Botanics as adjuvants or immunomodulators with vaccines against cancer
- Modulation of antibody-based cancer immunotherapy by botanics
- Regulation of pathogen-specific immune defense by botanics
- Development of biomarkers for study of botanic immunomodulators in humans

CONCLUDING REMARKS

Clinicians and consumers are reminded that dietary supplements can have not only beneficial but also adverse effects on the prevention of disease and on the maintenance of health. They are neither over-the-counter drugs nor prescription drugs and are not intended to treat, diagnose, mitigate, or cure disease, or replace a variety of foods important to a healthful diet. It will take many groups working together such as industry, government, researchers, health care providers, and policy makers many more years to provide open access to safe, reliable, and suitably tested dietary supplement products for the American public. Until that time, clinicians should utilize evidence-based resources to seek answers to their questions and patients' concerns on dietary supplements, which have been provided in this chapter and throughout the book.

References

1. *Dietary Supplement Health and Education Act of 1994 (United States Public Law 103-417; 103rd Cong., 25 October 1994)*. Washington, DC: Food and Drug Administration, Department of Health and Human Services; 1994.
2. Commission on Dietary Supplement Labels. *Report of the Commission on Dietary Supplement Labels*. Washington, DC: US Government Printing Office; 1997:17.
3. Sarubin A. *The Health Professional's Guide to Popular Dietary Supplements*. Chicago, IL: The American Dietetic Association; 2000: 3.
4. *Government Accountability Office. Dietary Supplements. FDA Should Take Further Actions to Improve Oversight and Consumer Understanding. GAO-09-250*. Washington, DC: 2009.
5. Betz JM, Fisher KD, Saldanha LG, Coates PM. The NIH analytical methods and reference materials program for dietary supplements. *Anal Bioanal Chem* 2007;389:19–25.
6. Wolsko PM, Solondz DK, Phillips RS, Schachter SC, Eisenberg DM. Lack of herbal supplement characterization in published randomized controlled trials. *Am J Med* 2005;118: 1087–1093.
7. Foreman J. St John's wort: less than meets the eye, globe analysis shows popular herbal antidepressant varies widely in Content, Quality. *Boston Globe*. January 10, 2002:C1.
8. Harkey MR, Henderson GL, Gershwin ME, Stern JS, Hackman RM. Variability in commercial ginseng products: an analysis of 25 preparations. *Am J Clin Nutr* 2001;73: 1101–1106.
9. Draves AH, Walker SE. Analysis of the hypericin and pseudohypericin content of commercially available St John's Wort preparations. *Can J Clin Pharmacol* 2003;10:114–118.
10. Piersen CE, Booth NL, Sun Y, et al. Chemical and biological characterization and clinical evaluation of botanical dietary supplements: a phase I red clover extract as a model. *Current Medicinal Chemistry* 2004;11:1361–1374.
11. Gagnier JJ, Boon H, Rochon P, Moher D, Barnes J, Bombardier C. Reporting randomized controlled trials of herbal interventions: an elaborated CONSORT statement. *Ann Intern Med* 2006;144:364–367.
12. Christian MS. Introduction/overview: gender-based differences in pharmacologic and toxicologic responses. *Int J Toxicol* 2001;20:145–148.

VI

Clinical Management

CHAPTER 33

Dietary Supplement Management: A Clinical Team Approach

Robert Alan Bonakdar

The management of dietary supplements in clinical practice is a rapidly evolving phenomenon that can be challenging for any one clinician to fully grasp or manage. Keeping up with increasing number of supplements contained in various formulations from differing treatment paradigms can be overwhelming. One of the tools I have found most helpful in dealing with the process is to think of supplement management from a team approach. Just as clinical reference tools are important, so too are community and provider references to help with management. The first reason this approach is helpful is simply that by working as a team we often make the job easier. By understanding that the nurse, pharmacist, dietician, or other provider working with the patient may have already obtained and reviewed some of the supplements the patient is taking we can often delve into new areas of the supplement discussion during our particular visit.

Other reasons, beyond information gathering, for a team approach come from a practical and philosophical perspective. Of note, patients do not pursue health care in a vacuum. They are typically *integrating* various treatments in an attempt to arrive at a comprehensive approach to their health care. By not being aware of other clinicians patients are consulting and/or receiving dietary supplement recommendations from, we may be missing vital information that is affecting patients' health and our treatment plans. Moreover, by knowing the other team members we begin to understand the perspective of the patient in how they view their status and choices for prevention and treatment. It is often comforting to realize during a patient visit that the burden is not just on oneself, but that other members of the team are available to provide input and expertise when making care decisions. From an integrative perspective, as health care continues to move in this direction, it is also imperative that discussion between health care providers parallels the health care choices the patient is pursuing.

This section starts with an overview that is helpful in understanding how herbal medicine has evolved over time as well as the place of the traditional herbalist. Other chapters discuss the role of physician, pharmacist, dietician, nurse, naturopath, and Traditional Chinese Medicine practitioner as part of the dietary supplement team. There are certainly many other potential members of the team based on one's particular practice and demographics. However, this list will hopefully begin to demonstrate how understanding the perspective, training, and strengths of various health care providers involved in dietary supplement management can help create a team approach.

CHAPTER 34

Herbalism and the Role of the Herbalist: Past, Present, and Future

Amanda McQuade Crawford

The role of the herbalist is to restore wholeness to systems, whether those systems function within our bodies or are the larger ecosystems from which we take our medicines. As explorers of the natural world of medicinal botany, herbalists are bio-prospectors. To define an herbalist requires patience, for a complex list of roles exists. An herbalist is usually considered to be a practitioner or contributor to the field of herbal medicine.

One accepted term among professionals for herbal medicine is Phytotherapy, from the Greek *phyton*, or "plant," plus *therapeia*. The less preferred Herbology is a neologism mixing a Latin prefix, *herba* or "grass," with a Greek suffix, *logos*, or "study of." Other commonly accepted definitions of herbalist include indigenous healers worldwide, acupuncturists who use herbs, Ayurvedic physicians, some naturopaths or other clinicians trained in medical herb use, and holistic medical physicians who integrate herbs into allopathic practice. Related to the practice of herbal medicine are roles of herb specialists: dealers in herb products ranging from tea blends to standardized extracts, plant researchers in phyotchemistry or other disciplines, herb growers, ethnobotanists, collectors, conservationists, and educators. The answer to what an herbalist does changes in response to contemporary social and environmental pressures.

In times long past, the role of the herbalist was also characterized by diversity. In prehistory, people observed the natural world such as animal use of plants, and made use of instinct and inspiration. A common modern belief about how herbs were discovered as useful medicines centers on the notion of prehistoric experimentation, or trial and error. Anthropological study examines herb use in ancient cultures, such as marshmallow root found with yarrow and ephedra in a Middle Paleolithic grave in Iraq. Those three herbs are still in use by herbalists today.

There is a consensus in related fields of study that 14,000 years ago the growing of cereal, legume, and other food crops fell mainly to women who stayed close to home with children in their care. Women developed this aspect of herbal medicine, food growing or agriculture, in a shift from nomadic hunter-gatherer societies to settled civilization in different eras across Mesopotamia, Asia, Africa, China, and the Americas. Archeological digs lead some researchers to estimate that ancient women domesticated 250 species of plants, while developing tools for cultivation and preparation. The oldest systems of herbal medicine acknowledged a powerful earth as Mother, again reflective of women's role as provider of new life, food, and medicine. This may be seen as a distant echo of contemporary interest in reconciling hard bioscience with humanity's yearning for meaning and connection with Nature. Ancient civilizations circa 3000 BCE began to systematize knowledge of healing foods and curative properties of plants. There are chemistry writings on tablets of Tapputi-Belatekallim, one of many women chemists in Babylon and Sumer. In India, 750 plants used in Ayurveda were described in the *Rig Veda*. The *Pen T'so* in China described 366 plants. The Egyptian *Papyri Antiquarium*, 22 yards long, presents some evidence of how the use of surgery and herbal medicine was taught.

Far from trial and error in prehistory, Egyptian medical schools were established at Sais and Heliopolis where the *Kahun* medical papyrus (2500 BCE) and other records show that general medicine, and especially obstetrics, were taught by women, primarily to women students, for about a thousand years (Wynn, 2000). In the 18th Dynasty (15th century BCE) Queen Hatshepsut, who was possibly trained as a physician, sent out a botanic expedition to eastern Africa in search of new medicinal plants such as myrrh and live Boswellia trees (frankincense). The great civilizations of Africa did not leave written records. Centuries of competing empires disrupted oral traditions and environmental resources. In some African civilizations, the credentials of an herbalist came through the family tree, the knowledge passed down over generations.

Today, studies seem to corroborate the common experience of teachers and providers that it is primarily women who use complementary and alternative medicine (CAM), while women who undertake medical training today are slightly more likely than male medical students to express an interest in learning about CAM therapies. Patient surveys suggest that the renewed use of CAM springs from a reverence across gender lines for the power of Nature, whether perceived as Mother Earth or nurturing biosphere.

During the medieval era throughout Europe and the expansive civilizations of the Holy Roman Empire, herbalists were outlawed by University physicians, yet were used by the poor. During the 19th century, the vanguard of medicine moved away from the liberal use of mercury and bleeding, catering instead to the elite with homeopathy, herbs, and increasingly conservative use of chemical drugs. Even surgery had its place in the Eclectic herbal system of medicine as defined by Wooster Beach, MD. During the years following the American Civil War, the tension between philosophies of medicine escalated as a positivist scientific method gained ascendancy. Except for tens of thousands of westward pioneers whose only choice was herbal doctoring with or without speculation as to ultimate causes of disease, the growing North American population chose health care in ways that reflected economic status. Standard practice medicine increasingly became the most common type of care and thus the refuge of the poor. The American Medical Association (AMA) launched its professional journal in the 1880s. At this same period, as Coca-Cola was introduced as medicine for gastrointestinal and nervous disorders including spasm and pain, it seemed desirable to purify herbs into drugs. At the beginning of the 21st century, Coca-Cola is developing Chinese herbal medicine drinks in Beijing. The Western discovery of Asian *materia medica* is experiencing a cycle in which it becomes institutionalized for the masses, a centuries-old business strategy for marketing herbal medicine, as opposed to practicing it.

At the close of the 19th century in the West, there was a large market for herbs. Father Kneipp, the herbalist and Swiss pastor who considered the scent of St. Johns Wort's "the perfume of God," sold herbal remedies. The less medical of his formulas are still available as herbal bath products in drugstore chains across Europe and North America. In 1899, Bayer made aspirin and physicians used this new wonder drug empirically since salicylate effects on inflammatory prostaglandins (named in the 1930s) were not understood until several decades later. Around the turn of the 20th century in North America, records show 115,000 Irregular Doctors were in practice versus 60,000 Regular Doctors. Between the middle of the 19th century through to the end of the 1800s, women were admitted to medical schools, with 7,000 in practice by 1899. In 1901, the AMA invited all sects, including herbal "irregular" physicians, to join their association. The following year, a council was established to judge all medical schools. In 1905, the Eclectic Medical Institute flourished. In 1906, the AMA Journal accepted paid advertising from drug companies, the Food and Drug Administration was formed, and the Pure Food and Drug Act passed. Within a year, the Carnegie endowment for AMA evaluation of all medical training schools began. The results of the 1911 Flexner Report in the United States closed most herbal medicine schools. Across the ocean in England, the National Insurance Act excluded herbalists regardless, they and the Eclectics, using mainly herbs but also homeopathy along with a judiciously small application of the new chemical drugs, became the health care providers to the wealthy. Oscillating cycles of fashion in medicine altered the social status of herbalists rather than their role, while epidemics showed that no school of medicine had a monopoly on guaranteed survival of their patients.

In the mid-20th century, herbs as medicine in North America and Europe were again dismissed in the face of antibiotics and vaccines developed through two world wars and great scientific progress. Yet, the use of herbs among those without access to modern drugs persisted. In England, the Pharmacy and Medicines Act of 1941 banning herbalists was dropped because of public reaction. The role of herbalists was primary, affordable health care. As a professional group, British herbalists chose not to repeat history when their organization, The National Institute of Medical Herbalists, founded in 1861, rejected the place offered to it by the National Health Service in 1946, preferring to practice within the traditional philosophical context of "wholesome" herbal medicine. In contemporary debates within the European Union, "harmonization" of laws affecting herb use and medicine remains elusive.

In the United States, the Food and Drug Administration spent decades consolidating an unwieldy field of health care. In 1962, the Safe and Effective Act was passed, mirrored by a similar law in England, while in 1972 the Over-the-Counter labeling law was put into effect. The surge in regulation overlapped with a late 20th century renaissance of widespread interest in rediscovering natural solutions in preference over drugs and surgery. This occurred throughout the northern hemisphere. Herbal medicine flourished outside the purview of standardized medicine until the herbal renaissance coincided with more mainstream concerns for the environment and media attention on unforeseen limitations of standard practice medicine. In 1979, the World Health Organization began to call for an international policy favoring the return of traditional medicines, citing herbal safety, efficacy, and cost for the majority of the world's human population. As herbs moved from the margins of society to the masses, England was among the first western nations to establish standards for herb use with the Council for Complementary and Alternative Medicine in 1985, now superseded by innumerable bodies governing the role of herbalists, the use of herbs, and allied natural health care.

WHAT ARE THE WORLD'S HERBAL TRADITIONS TODAY?

Every traditional society has its own herbal medicine. The best known are not static relics of a bygone age but have evolved over time. Among these are Traditional

Chinese Medicine, Traditional Ayurvedic Medicine, Phytotherapy, Naturopathy, Eclectic Medicine, Native American Medicine, Arabic medicine including Unani Tibb, Tibetan Medicine, and African Traditional Medicine as well as many others. These major systems became legitimate learned professions at some point in time, producing healers acknowledged by their communities, often after years of arduous apprenticeship. As a group herbalists are characterized by a lack of uniform standards of self-identification. What herbalists usually agree upon is that, despite different paths of training and even creeds, we have systems for practicing herbal medicine. These are based on theories, experience, standards of practice, and results. Evidence builds and amends these living systems as they evolve and adapt to the needs of today.

Qualified medical herbalists are professionals from any of the major traditions who are trained in diagnosis and prescription of herbal medicines. At the time of this writing, there is a shortage of trained herbalists from any philosophical or medical background in the United States. In modern western culture, including postcolonial Australia, New Zealand, South Africa, North and South America, as well as Europe, herbalists differ from "regular" medical practitioners not only in their *materia medica* but also in their philosophies. As we see CAM integrated with standard practice medicine, it is this different *vitalist* philosophy that herbalists still emphasize. Though countless unallied practitioners defy a single umbrella categorization except as herbalists, there are few who do not dedicate themselves to years of study and practice in order to continue self-identifying as herbalists. The common denominator of most herbal schools of healing is respect for the earth and the herbal remedies available.

Health consumers are able to overcome uncertainty in choosing an herbalist by seeking out those who have had valid training, or belong to organizations requiring members to adhere to standards of care sought by the patient, and/or inform prospective clients of their treatment and rationale satisfactorily. Although no foolproof way has been legislated to prevent harm, those who hold licenses are not automatically qualified to give herbs to the ill. Community-based recognition of skill still determines who succeeds in practice. Most contemporary herbalists in North America chose *not* to first learn a system of standard practice medicine that differs in paradigm so profoundly. Instead, 21st century herbalists have learned from a range of domestic educational centers or foreign degree programs, or by apprenticeship, and there are also a select few self-taught iconoclasts.

The American Herbalists Guild

There are hundreds of national and international associations promoting the use of herbs, but only one in North America represents a majority of herbalists in practice. The American Herbalists Guild is an organization linking and listing herbalists from different traditions to help the public identify qualified practitioners. According to their Web site, "The American Herbalists Guild (AHG) was founded in 1989 as a non-profit, educational organization to represent the goals and voices of herbalists. It is the only peer-review organization for professional herbalists specializing in the medicinal use of plants." Herbalists from any tradition with sufficient education and at least 4 years of clinical experience, and who pass the AHG admissions process, receive professional status and the title RH (Registered Herbalist, AHG). With professional ties to European and Australasian, Asian, African, and South American organizations, guild members agree to a code of ethics and abide by the concept of accountability to those receiving herbal medicine.

A qualified herbalist has more identifying characteristic qualities than simply knowing about plants and diagnostics, as important as these are. To evoke compliance with patients requiring holistic health care, he or she must also be able to move beyond barriers of culture, language, and emotion to achieve deep emotional, physical, and spiritual connections and understanding with patient and remedy. The role of the herbalist includes a responsibility to the best interests of each patient and the biosystem providing the specific herbs required. This integrity guides herbalists in touch with tradition to refer people whenever necessary to other professionals so that the person finds the providers best qualified to earn that patient's trust by restoring complete health.

To do this, there must be an underlying philosophy and reverence for life and for Nature. This is the common link shared by herbalists from around the world. It allows them to identify each other. Although this idea is often mentioned in the field of holistic health, it loses something when we try to put it in writing. One has to feel it personally perhaps on a walk alone in the woods, in clinic, or in starting an organic bed of herbs in the backyard. Most of the herbalists known to the medical community and the public started this way.

WHAT WILL THE ROLE OF THE HERBALIST BE NEXT?

It will be what it has always been, though in response to a changing culture. Our role is to discover plants that restore wholeness and new uses of familiar botanic medicines, while reminding those who develop drugs that there is a vital energy that is inseparable from the other values of herbal medicine. "Quality control" to an herbalist is more than label claims for purity and efficacy to match the material so labeled. The role of the herbalist has become that of the conservationist because we see that global marketing trends may cause us to lose our *materia medica*.

Biodiversity is measured at three levels: number of species (2 million on earth cataloged, estimated at 13 million and up), genetic variations within species, and different ecosystems that support species. However defined or measured, biodiversity is threatened by habitat destruction directly tied to human population pressures. It is estimated the pharmaceutical industry earns US $32 billion each year from products developed from natural resources. The World Bank estimates the global herb trade at US $65 billion annually. As an example, Pygeum bark for prostatic hypertrophy is endangered in its native central African highlands.

Herbalists share a commitment to all sectors of our society, maintaining or awakening awareness regarding the end results of our discoveries. It is not that the herbal drugstore will be "closed for the holidays" but that the plants are disappearing. In a 100 years what will herbalists care which Echinacea species had more cichoric acid on analysis if there is only one species of immunomodulating Aster that is available then? Organic farms and wild plant gathering do not meet market demands for raw bulk resources that can be harvested at a large profit. It may become part of our evolving role to teach our patients to plant seeds, to pick flowers, and dig roots. The push for evidence (in 2003 at US $1.7 million per new drug) and quality control (patented isolated compounds recoup investments) may have the unintended effect of forcing a dramatic change in supply and demand. Evidence of efficacy and safety is paramount, but the way to know what is true has not been well protected by the current system of designing, funding, or publishing research. Thus, the herbalist's new role also includes participating in collecting and assessing herbal medicine evidence.

The herbalist's mission is still to unify medical need with sustainability, in turn pursued with awareness of the spirit that causes a Hawthorn tree to thrive. Herbalists understand that in times of crisis and adaptation, plant medicines can be taken as part of a change of life every bit as inspiring as the technological miracles of biomedicine. There is enough suffering so that we need not be concerned with physicians and herbalists having enough work to go around.

What emerges out of this complexity is that herbalists of the future will not be defined by initials after one's name, number of product outlets in malls, household public recognition, units of herb product sold, or even the number of satisfied patients. The role of the herbalist is, as ever, to return our attention to the Earth. The herbalist is a living reminder of our right and humble place in a magnificent Nature.

Suggested Readings

Leveaga GS. Uncommon trajectories: steroid hormones, Mexican peasants, and the search for a wild yam. *Stud Hist Philos Biol Biomed Sci.* 2005;36(4):743–760.

Wynn R. Saints and sinners: women and the practice of medicine throughout the ages. *JAMA* 2000;283:668–669.

CHAPTER 35

The Role of the Physician

Robert Alan Bonakdar

WHY CONSIDER DIETARY SUPPLEMENTS AS A PHYSICIAN

There are few topics that appear to create more discomfort for physicians than a complementary and alternative medicine (CAM) or dietary supplement discussion. Corbin and colleagues confirmed this in a survey of more than 700 physicians in which 84% felt uncomfortable with the discussion. The authors noted that the physicians wanted to "*to learn more about CAM to adequately address patient concerns*" and concluded "*Education may help alleviate the discomfort physicians have when answering patients' questions about CAM*" (1).

There are many reasons for physicians' discomfort which can lead to potentially NOT considering/discussing dietary supplements. Some of the comments I have heard from physicians include the following:

- *I don't have enough education or training in dietary supplements*
- *There are too many supplements to keep up with*
- *Discussing supplements opens you up to increased liability*
- *Supplement are not (well) regulated*
- *Supplements are not evidence-based*
- *Supplement are too costly*
- *I don't have enough time to discuss supplements*
- *Patients aren't going to listen anyway*

I understand the frustration behind these statements and have felt many of these myself at one time. Hopefully, the contributors' chapters will help clarify the above scenarios and provide the needed education to allow comfort and confidence in venturing into this important dialogue. With the appropriate education, the role of the physician in the arena of dietary becomes very similar to that utilized with other areas of lifestyle counseling, that is, open discussion, guidance, and monitoring of the interventions reviewed.

To capture the specific steps of counseling in relation to dietary supplements, the H.E.R.B.A.L. Mnemonic was created (Table 35.1). By starting with openly asking and educating our patients on the importance of discussing dietary supplements we overcome the most common reasons for nondisclosure ("Doctor didn't ask" and "Didn't know it was important for me to mention"). Further, by recording the details of the supplement discussion and reviewing the supplements' appropriateness for the patient we ensure ongoing safe use and dialogue. By agreeing to discuss further

TABLE 35.1 The H.E.R.B.A.L. Mnemonic

HEAR THE PATIENT OUT
EDUCATE
RECORD
BE AWARE OF REACTIONS/INTERACTIONS
AGREE TO DISCUSS
LEARN

dietary supplement considerations we build on the idea that supplements, like any intervention, are worth discussing and reviewing with a health care advocate to assess their outcome. Lastly, as we learn about supplements using our favorite resources, the physician has a powerful ability to reset the health care button in regard to dietary supplements. What was previously a "don't ask, don't tell" scenario becomes an opportunity for important dialogue that can influence health care decisions.

Beyond the obstacles noted in the comments, as a physician I like to look at the best-case scenario for discussing dietary supplements. Basically stated, the reasons to consider dietary supplement discussion and management as outlined below far outweigh the reasons to wait on the sidelines. The majority of your patients have jumped into the game and eagerly await your unique individual guidance as part of their health care team. The following is an outline of the reasons I consider the discussion of dietary supplements an essential part of my practice.

REASONS FOR PHYSICIANS TO CONSIDER DIETARY SUPPLEMENTS IN CLINICAL CARE

Steering Toward Safety

As section 4 on reactions and interactions notes the typical scenario in which a potential reaction or interaction can occur is typically predictable. There is potentially no better health care provider than the physician (hopefully with a long-term relationship with a patient and access to the total health care picture of the patient) to provide guidance. With the appropriate education and ongoing learning, the beginning step of "first, doing no harm" can be met in a partnership with a patient to help make the safest initial choice.

Balancing the Information

Once safety is discussed, many clinicians are also needed to balance the information patients are often receiving. This can be both extensive and biased in a worst case. The physician can be helpful in reviewing with the patient the sources of information and why or why not a particular supplement is a wise choice in their particular scenario. This exercise is also empowering for the patient and a preventative strategy for the physician. In future interactions patients will appreciate the new sources of balanced information provided as well as the higher-level dialogue that they can create.

New Options in the Refractory State (Or, *What Else Do You Have for Me, Doc*?)

In many cases, the treatment or "cure" of a condition is not so clear. Prevention may be even more difficult a task to consider. As we attempt to be evidence-based in our practice we quickly realize that in many ways the statistical improbability that the complex patient in front of us will match the guidelines for a particular condition in the research study we are trying to follow. In addition to this factor you have the importance of patient preference. They may have had previous positive or negative experiences which may place them in a very different trajectory than the conventional guidelines. Thus, a patient with rheumatoid arthritis who has failed or maximized current best practices and continues to have symptoms may have mild to moderate benefit from the incorporation of omega-3 oils which also go beyond the condition. As one review points out: "*n-3 fatty acids provides modest symptomatic benefit in groups of patients with RA . . . Epidemiological studies and RCTs show cardiovascular benefits in the broader population & patients with ischemic heart disease . . . Dietary manipulation provides a means by which patients can a regain a sense of control over their disease*" (2).

The Patient with a Borderline State

There are a number of conditions which may benefit from the use of dietary supplements before the initiation of prescription medications. One example is the National Cholesterol Education Program Adult Treatment Panel III (NCEP ATPIII) Guidelines for therapeutic lifestyle changes for reaching goals in patients with elevated cholesterol levels(3). In this guideline patients who have borderline cholesterol are encouraged to initiate lifestyle changes which, in addition to exercise and dietary modification, can include supplementation with plant sterols and fiber. (This is elaborated in section 8.)

New Options in Prevention

As clinicians, especially primary care physicians, we are always looking for ways to incorporate prevention, whether it is dietary, exercise, behavioral, or other options. Dietary supplements have some history in this arena but are often overlooked. A classic example is the use of folic acid in pregnancy to reduce neural tube defects. However, there are a number of scenarios in which dietary supplement should be considered in daily practice from a prevention standpoint. One example is the use of probiotics to prevent antibiotic associated diarrhea. Several studies and reviews have noted this potential benefit. One study examining the consumption of a probiotic drink containing *Lactobacillus casei*, *Lactobacillus bulgaricus*, and *Streptococcus thermophilus* in the reduction of *Clostridium difficile* and other antibiotic associated diarrhea. The analysis found 17% to 21% absolute risk reduction with a number needed to treat of 5 to 6 to derive benefit, respectively (4).

Decrease Deficiency

As chapter 13 on the dietary supplement user points out, certain segments of the population suffer from nutrient deficiency (Coenzyme Q10 in pediatric headache, vitamin D in certain rheumatological conditions, etc). Replacement of the nutrient by food and dietary supplementation may help the underlying condition as well as reduce risk of other negative outcomes. As an example, a patient with fibromyalgia whose vitamin D level (25 OH) is very low (<17.8 ng/ml) may not only have more sequelae of his/her condition but may also be at increased risk for hypertension, diabetes mellitus, obesity, and all-cause mortality (5–7).

Cost Benefit

Several dietary supplements have shown cost savings benefit under different circumstances including reduction of negative outcomes as well as reduction of other, typically more costly, interventions. Examples include the following:

- *Probiotics in prevention of diarrhea*: The probiotic intervention in the above example cost an average of $20 per patient. With the number needed to treat of 5 to 6, the cost to prevent one case of antibiotic associated diarrhea and *C. difficile* associated diarrhea was between $100 and $120. This is compared to the estimated $3669 for the cost of treating one case of *C. difficile* associated diarrhea based on increased hospital stay and use of medications such as vancomycin. As the authors conclude: "Clearly substantial savings could be made by the routine use of probiotics" (4).
- *Glucosamine sulphate in knee replacement*: An analysis found that at 5 years after discontinuation of glucosamine in knee osteoarthritis, previous use of glucosamine for 12 to 36 months provided a 57% decrease in the need for total joint replacement as compared to placebo. In addition, there was a decrease in symptomatic medications and use of other health resources as compared to the placebo group during the last year of follow-up (8).

Integrative Approach to the Patient

As previous chapters have noted, patients are increasingly interested in integrative approaches to their health care. There are many potential reasons why patients and physicians are looking at this approach.

Additional Benefit in the Well-Controlled Patient

- *Fish oils (eicosapentaenoic acid) added to statins*: Adding eicosapentaenoic acid at 1.8 g a day for patients with coronary artery disease already taking a statin reduced major coronary events by an additional 19% after 4+ of follow-up (9).
- *Plant sterols added to statins*: Adding up to 2 g of plant sterols can additionally reduce total cholesterol by 3% to 11% and LDL cholesterol by 7% to 16% (10, 11).

Medication Sparing and Reduced Side Effect Profile

- *Blond psyllium added to statins or bile acid sequestrants (e.g., Cholestyramine, Colestipol)*: Adding blond psyllium (Metamucil) 15 g daily to statins appears to have similar cholesterol lowering effects as doubling the dose of the statins (12). A combination of blond psyllium 2.5 g added to colestipol 2.5 g was better tolerated and as effective as 5 g of colestipol or 5 g blond psyllium and reduced the side effects of bile acid sequestrants such as constipation and abdominal pain (13, 14).

Cross Condition Benefit and Protection

As noted above, there are many examples of dietary supplements which may provide benefit or protection beyond their primary indication. For example, the use of fish oils in the setting of hypertriglyceridemia may have additional benefit in the setting of joint pain (15); Coenzyme Q10 taken for migraine headache may have benefit in certain cases of heart failure associated with CoQ10 deficiency (16). One of the best examples may be the use of vitamin D in the setting of postfracture care. Those with deficiency not only appear to have worse outcomes as far as fracture healing, fall rates, and balance but may also have increased risk for cardiovascular mortality (6, 7, 17).

SUMMARY

The discussion of dietary supplements by physicians is often seen as a negative from various perspectives. Fortunately, when the proper resources and tools are incorporated to allow the discussion to take place in a productive manner, hopefully the physician can see the benefit. These benefits start from a patient protection, trust, and guidance standpoint, which are reason enough to consider discussion. Beyond these, I find a host of reasons that can make the rationale, evidence-based incorporation of dietary supplements a positive both for the patient and the physician. In many cases, the patient appreciates the additional novel care choices considered for his or her care. From a clinician standpoint, I find the incorporation of dietary supplements a prime example of the art of medicine in action whereby we are often placed in a difficult scenario requiring additional tools to improve a refractory clinical state or minimize side effects. When the discussion is properly supported, the example above hopefully demonstrates the positive potential and satisfaction that incorporation of dietary supplements can provide for physicians and their patients.

References

1. Corbin WL, Shapiro H. Physicians want education about complementary and alternative medicine to enhance communication with their patients. *Arch Intern Med* 2002;162(10):1176–1181.
2. Stamp LK, James MJ, Cleland LG. Diet and rheumatoid arthritis: a review of the literature. *Semin Arthritis Rheum* 2005;35(2):77–94.
3. Grundy SM, Cleeman JI, Merz CN, et al. Implications of recent clinical trials for the National Cholesterol Education Program Adult Treatment Panel III Guidelines. *J Am Coll Cardiol* 2004;44(3):720–732.
4. Hickson M, D'Souza AL, Muthu N, et al. Use of probiotic Lactobacillus preparation to prevent diarrhoea associated with antibiotics: randomised double blind placebo controlled trial. *BMJ* 2007;335(7610):80.
5. Armstrong DJ, Meenagh GK, Bickle I, et al. Vitamin D deficiency is associated with anxiety and depression in fibromyalgia. *Clin Rheumatol* 2007;26(4):551–554.
6. Martins D, Wolf M, Pan D, et al. Prevalence of cardiovascular risk factors and the serum levels of 25-hydroxyvitamin D in the United States: data from Third National Health and Nutrition Examination Survey. *Arch Intern Med* 2007;167(11):1159–1165.
7. Melamed ML, Michos ED, Post W, Astor B. 25-hydroxyvitamin D levels and the risk of mortality in the general population. *Arch Intern Med* 2008;168(15):1629–1637.
8. Bruyere O, Pavelka K, Rovati LC, et al. Total joint replacement after glucosamine sulphate treatment in knee osteoarthritis: results of a mean 8-year observation of patients from two previous 3-year, randomised, placebo-controlled trials. *Osteoarthritis Cartilage* 2008;16(2):254–260.
9. Yokoyama M, Origasa H, Matsuzaki M, et al. Effects of eicosapentaenoic acid on major coronary events in hypercholesterolaemic patients (JELIS): a randomised open-label, blinded endpoint analysis. *Lancet* 2007;369(9567):1090–1098.
10. Gylling H, Radhakrishnan R, Miettinen TA. Reduction of serum cholesterol in postmenopausal women with previous myocardial infarction and cholesterol malabsorption induced by dietary sitostanol ester margarine: women and dietary sitostanol. *Circulation* 1997;96(12):4226–4231.
11. Gylling H, Miettinen TA. Effects of inhibiting cholesterol absorption and synthesis on cholesterol and lipoprotein metabolism in hypercholesterolemic non-insulin-dependent diabetic men. *J Lipid Res* 1996;37(8):1776–1785.
12. Moreyra AE, Wilson AC, Koraym A. Effect of combining psyllium fiber with simvastatin in lowering cholesterol. *Arch Intern Med* 2005;165(10):1161–1166.
13. Spence JD, Huff MW, Heidenheim P, et al. Combination therapy with colestipol and psyllium mucilloid in patients with hyperlipidemia. *Ann Intern Med* 1995;123(7):493–499.

14. Maciejko JJ, Brazg R, Shah A, et al. Psyllium for the reduction of cholestyramine-associated gastrointestinal symptoms in the treatment of primary hypercholesterolemia. *Arch Fam Med* 1994;3(11):955–960.
15. Goldberg RJ, Katz J. A meta-analysis of the analgesic effects of omega-3 polyunsaturated fatty acid supplementation for inflammatory joint pain. *Pain* 2007;129(1–2):210–223.
16. Molyneux SL, Florkowski CM, George PM, et al. Coenzyme Q10: an independent predictor of mortality in chronic heart failure. *J Am Coll Cardiol* 2008;52(18):1435–1441.
17. LeBoff MS, Hawkes WG, Glowacki J, et al. Vitamin D-deficiency and post-fracture changes in lower extremity function and falls in women with hip fractures. *Osteoporos Int* 2008;19(9):1283–1290.

CHAPTER 36

The Role of the Pharmacist

Cydney E. McQueen and Celtina K. Reinert

PHARMACISTS—GENERAL

The duty of a pharmacist is to provide pharmaceutical care, defined as "the direct, responsible provision of medication-related care for the purpose of achieving definite outcomes that improve a patient's quality of life" (1). What does this mean in relation to dietary supplements? In addition to having pharmacologic action themselves, dietary supplements can also interact with a patient's prescription and nonprescription drug therapies. Because health care providers do not control access to a patient's use of supplements, it is necessary for pharmacists to have at least a basic knowledge of supplements simply in order to provide full and complete pharmaceutical care regarding prescription medications. This is true even for pharmacists who do not believe that dietary supplements should ever be used therapeutically. Pharmacists must also be aware that not all supplements are equal in safety or efficacy. The evidence for use is much stronger for some supplements than others. These differences mean that pharmacists must determine the appropriateness of dietary supplement use for each patient individually.

All of the general concepts of the pharmaceutical care definition are relevant to dietary supplements and should be applied in the same manner. However, the unique circumstances and legal position of dietary supplements place some additional requirements on pharmacists when managing patients using these products. It is vital that each pharmacist understand the basic issues that must be addressed with supplements so that good judgments can be made about when to offer advice, when to seek out more information, and when to refer patients.

Resources/Knowledge

The pharmacist must recognize that self-learning is vitally important, since there is generally not extensive education in this area in most pharmacy schools (2). Each pharmacist should be able to evaluate his or her own knowledge and access to knowledge through reliable information resources, to be able to determine, "am I going to be able to make a valid judgment in this situation or is more help needed?" Resources are further discussed in chapter 42. In addition to print or electronic information resources, pharmacists should identify other resources available in their communities, such as physicians and other practitioners working in integrative health centers or drug information centers serving that region.

Regulations/Legality of Dietary Supplements

Regulations for dietary supplements are vastly different than for prescription and nonprescription drugs. A discussion of the regulations is provided in chapter 16. Pharmacists should be aware of the regulations and able to explain the broad issues to patients. Moreover, if a community pharmacist has control over or a voice in what products are stocked in the store, then ethically, only products that adhere to the government regulations should be sold. Unfortunately, many community pharmacists do not have control over what is stocked in the stores in which their pharmacies are located, but even in these cases, pharmacists can direct patients to products that do adhere to regulations and/or have been tested for product quality as well as studied for safety and efficacy. An overview of these supplements can be found in chapter 31.

Product Quality

For most prescription and nonprescription drugs, quality is typically not a concern because the regulations regarding production and quality control are more clearly defined and enforced. Even in this scenario, there are occasional cases of poor quality and regulation, but in far smaller proportion than occur with dietary supplements (3, 4). Such production and quality regulations did not exist for dietary supplements until 2007—and enforcement of the requirements is not immediate. Beginning in 2008, required adherence to the regulations will be slowly phased in, dependent on the size of the manufacturer, over the course of a few years (5). For now and some time into the future, various problems with strength and quality of products, contamination, adulteration, and misidentification will continue to be a major concern. This requires pharmacists to be continually aware of supplement regulation and quality issues, such as through regular updates from the Food and Drug Administration/Center for Food Safety and Nutrition (FDA/CFSAN) site on dietary supplement Warnings and Safety Information (6).

Product quality concerns can be associated with several issues. Obviously, the first is that a product may not work because it does not contain the proper ingredient as labeled. Second, it may cause harm if it is contaminated with pathogenic bacteria, adulterated with unlabeled prescription drugs, or contains a poisonous plant that was misidentified as a healthful one. Third, if a product causes an adverse event, and yet does not contain the labeled ingredient, this can muddy the waters of scientific knowledge, as a negative pharmacologic action is misattributed to the substance. Unfortunately, the general public does not generally consider the issue of product quality or mistakenly believes that the products are more regulated than they are—this is a vital area of patient education in which all pharmacists should engage. This also speaks to the reasons for recommending and stocking dietary supplements of known and high quality from reputable manufacturers.

Adverse Drug Reactions, Interactions, and Contraindications

Many patients are surprised to learn that supplements may be associated with adverse reactions, interactions with prescription and nonprescription drugs, or be dangerous when used in certain medical conditions. Perhaps this could be because there is such a strong feeling that "natural" means safe and that the advantage of a supplement therapy is that it has no side effects or problems (reactions and adverse events are discussed further in chapter 25). Because this is such a widespread misconception with the general public, this may be one of the most important areas in which a pharmacist can provide guidance and information to patients.

INPATIENT

Mr. Smith is a 62-year-old male with chronic atrial fibrillation whose medication regimen includes warfarin 10 mg/d, a beta-blocker, and a statin for cholesterol. He takes a daily multivitamin and St. John's wort and has been stable on all his medications for several months. Mr. Smith enters Memorial Hospital because of an acute kidney stone. His prescription medications and multivitamin are continued upon admission, but the St. John's wort is stopped, per hospital policy to discontinue all dietary supplements. Within 48 hours, although the kidney problem seems to be under control, Mr. Smith's International Normalized Ratio (INR) has risen sharply, to almost 8, and he is experiencing excessive bruising and increased bleeding time.

This incident illustrates what can go wrong with patient care without the participation of pharmacists with dietary supplement knowledge. St. John's wort is an inducer of the CYP450 3A4 enzyme that metabolizes warfarin, meaning that it causes swifter degradation of the drug (7). Mr. Smith had been stable for some time on both medications, but when the St. John's wort was stopped, he became overly anticoagulated because his warfarin blood levels increased. The problem could have been avoided by a variety of actions, such as allowing Mr. Smith to continue taking the St. John's wort, or stopping it and holding or reducing his warfarin dose from the day he entered the hospital. Unfortunately, many hospitals do not have a formal policy regarding dietary supplements management during an acute care stay (8, 9).

In hospitals, pharmacists are often not as visible to patients as members of the health care team as nurses and physicians; however, pharmacists do provide pharmaceutical care throughout patients' hospital stays. There are multiple opportunities to have an impact on dietary supplement use and safety. During a patient's visit, a pharmacist's knowledge of supplements is vital in several areas as follows:

- Recognizing the importance of obtaining during the admission process full and complete information on all products a patient is taking
- Assessing possible drug interactions and the impact of starting or stopping a supplement
- Assessing the risks of a patient's supplements for either elective or emergency surgical procedures
- Educating other members of the health care team on supplements in relation to a specific patient
- Educating patients on discharge to help them avoid harm and gain maximum benefit from products they are using with their other medications

Even before a patient's visit, a pharmacist's knowledge of dietary supplements is vital to aid in:

- Stressing the importance of hospital personnel obtaining upon admission full and complete information on all products all patients are taking
- Educating other members of the health care team on general knowledge of supplements
- Helping the institution create and implement formal policy and guidance regarding dietary supplement management

In many cases, like that of Memorial Hospital in the example above, the policy is that no dietary supplements are permitted to be used by inpatients. This is generally appropriate, as long as there are safeguards in place to prevent endangering patients like Mr. Smith. The pharmacist can play an essential role in helping other health care practitioners in the institution understand what impact discontinuing supplements may have on their patients—whether a change in a prescription medication or management of a withdrawal syndrome may be necessary. Education of patients on discharge may help them avoid supplement-related interactions and problems and avoid readmission.

COMMUNITY/RETAIL

When patients think of pharmacists they often think of those working in retail settings—these are the most accessible and most visible pharmacists to patients. Because of their visibility and accessibility, pharmacists can be a great resource to patients for drug and dietary supplement information as well as information on potential interactions and adverse events. A pharmacist providing dietary supplement information allows a patient to have a health care provider within proximity of supplements on the shelf and allows a patient to ask questions with relative ease.

As previously discussed, a pharmacist must recognize that dietary supplements have pharmacologic action and therefore have the potential to interact with medications, increase risks of some side effects, cause a decreased need for a particular medication, or duplicate the actions of a medication. Retail pharmacists are well-positioned to ask patients about supplements they are taking, screen for potential interactions, and encourage patients to inform other practitioners of the supplements they are using. Each patient's needs, disease states, and other medications must be individually evaluated to determine the risks and benefits for that patient when he/she approaches the pharmacy counter looking for a supplement recommendation. That recommendation must be based on safety, efficacy, and product quality, and take into account respect for patient choice as much as possible.

In regard to dietary supplements, a retail pharmacist's most valuable role is providing quality information. Pharmacists are accustomed to regularly providing drug information as drug experts. Dietary supplements, due to the pharmacologic actions, also fall under information a pharmacist should be able to offer to patients. The key to being able to offer this information revolves around the pharmacist's access to good dietary supplement resources and being able to appropriately use these resources. A pharmacist should be able to provide information on the supplement regarding the appropriateness for the patient, appropriateness of the product for what the patient wants to treat, most appropriate dose and product formulation, and be able to evaluate the product for any interactions with the patient's available medication list. One's access to quality resources is imperative to determine the benefit and harm of a particular supplement to a particular patient. An overview of dietary supplement resources for health care providers is provided in chapter 42.

A pharmacist also must be a continual learner, focusing on the dietary supplements patients are asking about on a daily basis, especially when one is unfamiliar with a particular supplement. Research may need to be done by the pharmacist either in response to a single patient's question or to have knowledge to answer many patients' questions revolving around a particular theme or type of question. Quality supplements are another offering retail pharmacists can provide to patients. As mentioned earlier in this chapter, pharmacists need to do everything possible to provide patients access to quality products—those that meet government regulations or that have been independently tested for purity and contamination. Pharmacists can also be familiar with quality brands, regardless of whether they are stocked in the store, and refer patients to appropriate brands whenever possible.

Pharmacists have a role to promote and provide general dietary supplement knowledge, both on a daily basis and in the community. This can be accomplished through flyers posted in the pharmacy or at the pharmacy counter, through community presentations, or by making sure the questions of the patients they pass in the supplement aisle with a bottle in hand have been answered.

Since a pharmacist usually is not the only person working in a pharmacy, educating the other pharmacy personnel as to the importance of supplement awareness is critical. Many times, especially in busier pharmacies, the pharmacy technicians conduct many of the transactions patients have with pharmacy personnel. The entire pharmacy team must be aware that dietary supplements have pharmacologic action and pose a potential for duplicate therapies or interactions. Even without specific, advanced knowledge of dietary supplements, all pharmacy personnel can help make patients aware of these potential risks. Pharmacists can also strongly encourage patients to keep all practitioners up-to-date on both medications and dietary supplements by sharing the importance of this with patients. A pharmacist's knowledge of a particular patient's supplements can also help screen for therapeutic duplications and interactions, thereby allowing the pharmacist to alert a prescriber when a new medication or supplement is added to the regimen that poses a potential problem. This communication will allow the pharmacist and prescriber to evaluate together the risks and benefits the new therapy may have.

A pharmacist, in addition to informing prescribers of potential duplications or interactions, also must have the ability to refer patients to other health care practitioners as appropriate, when necessary. This requires recognizing the roles of other practitioners, including herbalists, acupuncturists, and naturopaths. The quality of each practitioner a pharmacist recommends to a patient must also be ascertained as much as possible. A pharmacist must recognize the patient's needs and the potential therapies and practitioners likely to be of benefit for an individual patient, as well as a patient's receptivity to a particular therapy.

OUTPATIENT/CONSULTING

Some pharmacists may greatly expand upon the quality and quantity of knowledge of dietary supplements and the ability to provide this knowledge to patients. This can be done through consulting services. Pharmacists with a greater interest in dietary supplements, either through extended training or personal study, may offer private consultations to patients with questions regarding dietary supplements within the pharmacy or in another location, such as a medical office, as a fee-based service. Ideally, these consultations are provided in a private, comfortable location.

Consultations can vary depending on the pharmacist's expertise and style as well as the patient's needs. A patient may need information on a particular supplement or on a particular type of supplement. Patients may want the pharmacist to check their supplements for interactions and duplicate therapies and provide advice on which therapies would be beneficial to add and which may be unnecessary. Other patients may desire recommendations for a particular disease state or general health maintenance. Some may want to decrease the number of prescription medications they are on or may want to decrease the number of supplements they are taking and are seeking advice on the best way to accomplish this.

Consultation services can vary on the basis of the pharmacist and the information desired by the patient. Some pharmacists may offer longer consultations but allow for as much patient follow-up as needed with no extra charge. Others can feel drained from long appointments, so instead choose to limit appointments to short amounts of time but may need to see patients more frequently, with or without follow-up fees. Patients may be charged on the basis of the length of appointment and the preparation required by the pharmacist.

Pharmacists trained in dietary supplements have a special ability to be able to partner drug expertise with dietary supplement expertise to develop the most appropriate recommendations for a patient's drug and supplement regimen to meet the needs of that individual. Because these pharmacists practice in a specialized area, pharmacists providing dietary supplement consultations may be a better resource for patients with many questions or many concerns regarding individual supplements or in-depth information on supplements in general. Pharmacists providing dietary supplement consultations are able to sit down with patients and discuss issues regarding supplements whereas pharmacists in other settings may not have the time, resources, or expertise to provide such a service. A knowledgeable pharmacist is a good choice of practitioner to see a patient with supplement questions and also has the ability to tie in information with the patient's prescription and nonprescription medication regimen. When referring patients to a pharmacist who provides dietary supplement consultations, practitioners must exercise caution in the same way a pharmacist must exercise caution when referring patients to other practitioners. Reputation, education, skill set, and compatibility with a patient should be taken into consideration by practitioners when referring patients to, and patients when seeking, a pharmacist who specializes in dietary supplement consultations.

Drawbacks to pharmacists providing dietary supplement consultations include the lack of standardization of training, focus, and the information provided. One pharmacist may have training in nutrition or homeopathy, whereas another may have a strong personal interest and completed informal training. This variance in training may alter the focus of information a patient receives from this pharmacist. These variances do not preclude any one pharmacist from providing valid dietary supplement information but should be taken into consideration by the patients who see these pharmacists and the practitioners who refer to them. Pharmacists who provide dietary supplement consultations are few in number. Pharmacists in typical community settings do not charge patients for the information and expertise they provide but rather charge for the product (i.e., prescription or nonprescription medication). Having a pharmacist charge a fee for dietary supplement information is different from the typical outpatient pharmacy business model. To be able to provide quality information to patients and receive compensation for knowledge rather than just a product are only two of the challenges that this change to the typical model creates. This may be the future of pharmacy consultations with medication therapy management and reimbursement to pharmacists for their knowledge, not just their products.

CONCLUSION

Pharmacists work in many different settings and fill various roles in these settings. However, whether inpatient or outpatient, a pharmacist has a vital role to fill regarding dietary supplements. This includes providing thorough and quality information, providing access to quality supplements, being aware of potential interactions and adverse events and informing patients of these whenever possible, sharing knowledge on dietary supplements with patients and practitioners whenever pertinent, as well as aiding patients and other health care practitioners to assess the risks and benefits of a particular supplement or therapy.

References

1. American Society of Health-System Pharmacists. ASHP statement on pharmaceutical care. http://www.ashp.org/s_ashp/bin.asp?CID=6&DID=5400&DOC=FILE.PDF. Accessed March 2008.
2. Dutta A, Shields KM, McQueen CE, Bryant PJ. Natural product and CAM education in U.S. pharmacy schools. *J Pharm Teach* 2004;11(2):1–12.
3. FDA Public Health Update. Recall of heparin sodium injection and heparin lock flush solution (Baxter). http://www.fda.gov/cder/drug/infopage/heparin/public_health_update.htm. Accessed May 24, 2008.
4. United States Food and Drug Administration. Recalls, market withdrawals and safety alerts. www.fda.gov/opacom/7alerts.html. Accessed June 4, 2008.
5. United States Food and Drug Administration. Dietary supplement current good manufacturing practices (CGMPs) and interim final rule (IFR) facts./www.cfsan.fda.gov/~dms/dscgmps6.html. Accessed June 4, 2008.
6. Food and Drug Administration/Center for Food Safety and Nutrition (FDA/CFSAN) Dietary Supplement Warnings and Safety Information. www.cfsan.fda.gov/~dms/ds-warn.html. Accessed May 24, 2008.
7. Jiang X, Williams KM, Liauw WS, et al. Effect of St John's wort and ginseng on the pharmacokinetics and pharmacodynamics of warfarin in healthy subjects. *Br J Clin Pharmacol* 2004;57:592–599.
8. Bazzie KL, Witmer DR, Pinto B, et al. National survey of dietary supplement policies in acute care facilities. *Am J Health Syst Pharm* 2006;63(1):65–70.
9. Gardiner P, Phillips RS, Kemper KJ, et al. Dietary supplements: inpatient policies in US children's hospitals. *Pediatrics* 2008;121(4):e775–e781.

CHAPTER 37

The Role of the Dietitian

Cathy-Ann Garvey

GENERAL INFORMATION

Registered dietitians (RDs) are experts in the knowledge of and application of food and nutritional science. RDs are responsible for providing nutrition education as well as medical nutrition therapy, defined as "nutritional diagnostic, therapy, and counseling services for the purpose of disease management which are furnished by a registered dietitian or nutrition professional..." (1). As the nutrition expert, it is essential that the RD is also an expert in questions regarding the use and safety of dietary supplements.

RDs focus on recommending food first to overcome nutritional deficiencies, prevent disease, and promote optimal health. However, food alone may not always be sufficient. It may be necessary to incorporate dietary supplements to maximize the nutritional outcome. It may be difficult to obtain the recommended amount of a particular supplement through addition of food alone. For example, if a patient was recommended to add 1,000 IU of vitamin D to correct a vitamin deficiency, the patient would need to add roughly 10 cups of vitamin D—fortified milk daily to achieve that goal. Obviously, that may not be realistic or desired by the patient. In this case, a dietary supplement would be more appropriate and helpful in promoting long-term compliance.

In addition, there are certain populations that may be at risk for development of nutritional deficiencies. Patients who are infants, adolescents, or elderly; have chronic health conditions; malabsorption issues; alcohol-dependency; practice certain restricted diets (vegans); or belong to certain ethnic populations may be more at risk for inadequate diet (2) and require dietary supplements to ensure optimal health.

Nutritionally compromised patients are not the only populations using dietary supplements. The results of the 2000 National Health Interview Survey indicate that the use of dietary supplements in the United States has increased from 23.2% in 1987 to 23.7% in 1992 to 33.9% in 2000 (3). Clearly, it is vital that the RD is a resource to the community. RDs must be able to use an evidence-based approach to evaluate supplement data, identify risks and benefits to the patient, effectively educate patients regarding use of the supplement, communicate with others on the health care team, and document clinical response and any adverse reactions.

DEFINITIONS AND REGULATIONS

As defined in the Dietary Supplement Health and Education Act (DSHEA) in 1994, a "dietary supplement" is a product taken by mouth that contains a dietary ingredient that is intended to supplement the diet (4). This includes not only vitamins and minerals but also herbs, botanics, amino acids, and other substances. Every supplement is required to be clearly labeled as a dietary supplement and not to be confused with a drug. DSHEA also requires that it is up to the manufacturer to provide a supplement that is safe and does not indicate any false or misleading claims about the supplement treating disease. Simply, the supplement cannot state that it prevents or cures a disease, as it would then fall under the drug definition and not the dietary supplement definition. Manufacturers are allowed to use three types of claims on dietary supplement packaging: health claims, including qualified health claims, structure/function claims, and nutrient content claims (5). RDs must be knowledgeable about these different classifications of claims and able to educate their patients on not only what these claims mean but also on what they do not mean in order for the patient to be an informed consumer. Many times a patient may come to RDs for their opinion of a supplement that has been advertised on the Internet, in the media, or from word of mouth. It may be a dietary supplement that is part of a multilevel marketing program. As the nutrition expert, the RD must feel comfortable reviewing the dietary supplement and educating the patient. The RD is the nutrition resource to help guide the patient's decision. (For further information on dietary supplement regulation, refer to chapter 16.)

Safety of the dietary supplement is an important concern and a focus of the Food and Drug Administration (FDA). The FDA has established a system to document adverse effects of supplements, called the Adverse Event Reporting System. RDs should be familiar with this Web site and review it periodically to assess safety issues. In addition, RDs should be familiar with resources including Web sites that provide evidence-based information and/or reliable independent review and certification of dietary supplements. Several recommended resources are noted below. (A full list of resources can be found in chapter 42.)

Suggested Resources for the Dietitian

- American Botanic Council, www.herbalgram.org
- U.S. Food and Drug Administration, Center for Food Safety and Applied Nutrition, www.cfsan.fda.gov
- ConsumerLab.com, www.consumerlab.com
- Natural Medicines Comprehensive Database, www.naturaldatabase.com
- National Center for Complementary and Alternative Medicine, www.ncca.nih.gov
- Natural Standard, www.naturalstandard.com
- Supplement Watch, www.supplementwatch.com
- United States Pharmacopoeia, www.usp.org

THE REGISTERED DIETITIAN AS A RESOURCE

Dietary supplement use in the United States continues to grow and it is necessary for the RD to be an expert resource for his/her patients and community. In order for the RD to be that resource, the American Dietetic Associations' practice paper on dietary supplements recommends that the RD must become competent in the following areas (6):

Recommendations for Dietitians Based on the Practice Paper of the American Dietetic Association: Dietary Supplements (6).

- Identification of the supplement and its usage patterns in the patient
- Evaluation of the proposed benefits of the supplement
- Evaluation of the safety of the supplement
- Assessment of the supplement quality
- Educate patients on "food first" along with appropriate dietary supplementation
- Monitor the patient's clinical response over time
- Evaluate the research critically
- Educate other health care professionals regarding dietary supplementation and health
- Become knowledgeable about the regulatory issues regarding supplement labels
- Become knowledgeable about the legal and ethical issues related to recommending or selling supplements

RDs must also be aware of new developments in dietary supplement research and recommendations. One challenge can be that new research may contradict older research. Unfortunately, the media often does not provide a complete analysis of the research, minimizing the research to "sound bites," which may be confusing messages for the public. Dietitians must know where to access reliable information and verify claims that may be stated and expounded upon in the media. RDs use an evidence-based approach to assessing the data. The Centre for Evidence-Based Medicine has defined five steps to the evidence-based approach (7):

- Ask answerable questions
- Find the best evidence
- Critically appraise the evidence
- Act on the evidence
- Evaluate the performance

The American Dietetic Association's Evidence Analysis Library is a valuable resource for RDs as it uses an evidence-based approach to evaluating the research, rating the strength of the evidence and summarizing the research for nutrients and health conditions (8). The American Dietetic Association also features a dietetic practice group, Dietitians in Integrative and Functional Medicine, for health care professionals who have an interest in dietary supplements and alternative therapies in health and disease prevention (9). The Dietitians in Integrative and Functional Medicine practice group provides frequent updates regarding research in dietary supplements, professional conferences, and news updates. It provides a community for health care professionals to connect and share ideas, challenging patient situations, and network.

While it is essential for the RD to use an evidence-based approach and evaluate scientific studies on dietary supplements, it is also important to recognize that there may not be the gold standard randomized, controlled clinical trials on traditional botanics or herbs. When assessing the safety and efficacy of traditional botanics or herbs that do not have substantial peer-reviewed journal research, it may be helpful for the RD to consult with traditional healers for additional information as well as reviewing the literature on the long-term safety and/or efficacy of the product in question (6).

PRACTICE GUIDELINES

Application of dietary supplement knowledge is critical in the dietitian—patient interaction. Once the RD has the foundation of supplement knowledge, skills, references, and reference materials, the next steps are imparting this information to the patient and educating the patient on the dietary supplement in question. Clearly, RDs should review diet and supplement use in the context of food choices and dietary reference intakes (DRIs). When DRIs have not been established, such as for botanics or herbs, there are often different approaches on how to handle these instances. Some dietitians may argue that it is important to understand the usage of the botanic in question as it may interact with medications and/or harm the patient. It is important to inform the patient of such concerns, and to avoid doing so would be ethically wrong. Other dietitians may not feel comfortable providing recommendations and guidance, as there may not be evidence-based information to draw from. As a result, the dietitian may prefer to refer the patient to another health care professional to serve as a resource. Regardless of the RD's personal opinion, the RD should document all supplements that the patient is taking because certain dietary supplements have been shown to interact with certain medications.

In order to provide structure to the patient consultation when evaluating dietary supplements, the RD should use a systematic approach such as the H.E.R.B.A.L. mnemonic as outlined in chapter 1. Another approach is outlined in the American Dietetic Association (ADA) practice paper on dietary supplements: ask, evaluate, educate, and document (6). Open the conversation by asking patients what type of dietary supplements or other over-the-counter medications they are taking, the dosages, the length of time they have been taking them, why they are taking them, and who recommended the supplements. Where did the patient receive the information and what is goal to be achieved by taking the dietary supplement?

Next, examine the patient. Review the patient's diet intake, including foods, beverages, and fortified foods; current health status; health history; laboratory values; clinical response to the dietary supplement; and any possible side effects or adverse reactions. Also review any prescribed or over-the-counter medications in the context of the patient's overall situation.

Once the RD has completed questioning and evaluating the diet and supplements, the dietitian can begin the patient education. Patient education should be presented in a factual, nonbiased fashion. The dietitian should draw from the knowledge base of the DRIs and evidence-based recommendations. The dietitian should discuss with the patient the possible benefits, side effects, interactions with other medications or other dietary supplements, mechanism of action, length of time used, and how to administer the supplement. Is the supplement to be stored in the refrigerator? Should the supplement be stored out of direct light? The dietitian should also be knowledgeable about reputable manufacturers that produce quality dietary supplements. The dietitian should always emphasize with the patient that the dietary supplement should be used to supplement the diet, not to be used in place of food choices. The dietitian should document in the patient chart the complete list of dietary supplements including dosages, manufacturer name and batch number in case an adverse event occurs, medication—supplement interactions, and time line for follow-up. It is also helpful to note the patient perception and expected level of compliance.

SUMMARY

Dietary supplement use continues to grow in the United States, as individuals are trying not only to correct deficiencies but also, more important, to promote optimal health. The current American diet sadly is one that is promoting obesity and nutritional deficiencies, while still resulting in caloric excess. As Americans try to promote optimal health, they often turn to dietary supplements as the answer.

RDs, with their comprehensive training in nutritional science, behavior modification, and motivational interviewing, are a critical part of the health care team and essential dietary supplement resources. Improvement in food choices and maximizing the quality of the diet are primary goals of the dietitian. By understanding dietary supplement research, critical thinking and assessment, and patient counseling skills, the dietitian can confidently serve as the resource for patients and the community when choosing dietary supplements.

References

1. Medicare MNT Legislation, 2000. http://www.eatright.org/ada/files/chart_of_mnt_vs_nut_ed_revised_short_version_8_06.pdf. Accessed September 2008.
2. Fairfield KM, Fletch RH. Vitamins for chronic disease prevention in adults: scientific review. *JAMA* 2002;287:3116–3126.
3. Millen AE, Dodd KW, Subar AF. Use of vitamin, mineral, nonvitamin, and nonmineral supplements in the United States: The 1987, 1992, and 2000 National Health Interview Survey Results. *J Am Diet Assoc* 2004;104:942–950.
4. Dietary Supplement Health and Education Act of 1994. Pub L No. 10S-417 (codified at 42 USC 287C-11).
5. US Food and Drug Administration. Food labeling and nutrition. http://www.cfsan.fda.gov/label.html. Accessed September 2008.
6. ADA Reports. Practice paper of the American Dietetic Association: dietary supplements. *J Am Diet Assoc* 2005;105:460–470.
7. Centre for Evidence-Based Medicine. Learning EBM. http://www.cebm.net. Accessed September 2008.
8. ADA Evidence Analysis Library. http://www.adaevidencelibrary.com/default.cfm. Accessed September 2008.
9. Dietitians in Integrative and Functional Medicine. A dietetic practice group of the American Dietetic Association. http://www.complementarynutrition.org/. Accessed September 2008.

CHAPTER 38

The Role of the Nurse in Dietary Supplement Management

Margie Moore and Robert Alan Bonakdar

Nurses are a diverse group of health care providers who are in an ideal role to be involved in the discussion, counseling, and comanagement of dietary supplementation. Starting from the standpoint of the workforce, nurses represent the highest number of health care professionals (more than 2.9 million registered nurses) employed in the most diverse of clinical, research, and educational settings. From a philosophical perspective, nurses are often regarded as the most holistic members of the health care team based on their existing training perspective. Several surveys have pointed out that nearly half to 84% of nursing schools provide some levels of complementary and alternative medicine (CAM) education in their curriculum. This appears to be higher than most other graduate level medical education programs and may better prepare nurses to be comfortable and educated regarding discussion and management of dietary supplements (1, 2). In addition, nurses are often regarded as the bridge, both in discussion and in clinical interventions, between patients, their families, and other health care providers. Thus, nurses are pivotally situated to initiate, record, and advance the dialogue and management that surrounds dietary supplement for the good of their patients and other members of the health care team. The following chapter will attempt to provide the current status, recommendations, and resources regarding the role of nurses on the dietary supplement management team.

WHAT IS A NURSE AND NURSING

According to the American Nurses Association, to become a registered nurse:

> *...an individual must graduate from a state-approved school of nursing—either a four-year university program, a two-year associate degree program, or a three-year diploma program—and pass a state RN licensing.*

Once credentialed the role of nursing is broadly defined in several ways including:

> *the protection, promotion, and optimization of health and abilities, prevention of illness and injury, alleviation of suffering through the diagnosis and treatment of human response, and advocacy in the care of individuals, families, communities, and populations.* (3)

Similarly, the Royal College of Nursing defines nursing as:

> *The use of clinical judgment in the provision of care to enable people to improve, maintain, or recover health, to cope with health problems, and to achieve the best possible quality of life, whatever their disease or disability, until death.* (4)

In a more detailed fashion, the American Nurses Association has provided a revised Code of Ethics for Nurses, which provides guidance on principles that clearly intersect with those needed to properly address the use of dietary supplements. These principles include protecting health and safety, respecting patient treatment preferences, and collaborating with other health care providers. The code is provided in Table 38.1.

ROLE OF THE NURSE IN COMPLEMENTARY AND ALTERNATIVE MEDICINE: SCOPE OF PRACTICE

More than half of the State boards of nursing have taken positions that permitted nurses to practice a range of complementary therapies (6). Several guidelines from state and national associations are available such as those endorsed by the

TABLE 38.1 Code of Ethics for Nurses from the American Nurses Association (5)

1. The nurse, in all professional relationships, practices with compassion and respect for the inherent dignity, worth, and uniqueness of every individual, unrestricted by considerations of social or economic status, personal attributes, or the nature of health problems.
2. The nurse's primary commitment is to the patient, whether an individual, family, group, or community.
3. The nurse promotes, advocates for, and strives to protect the health, safety, and rights of the patient.
4. The nurse is responsible and accountable for individual nursing practice and determines the appropriate delegation of tasks consistent with the nurse's obligation to provide optimum patient care.
5. The nurse owes the same duties to self as to others, including the responsibility to preserve integrity and safety, to maintain competence, and to continue personal and professional growth.
6. The nurse participates in establishing, maintaining, and improving health care environments and conditions of employment conducive to the provision of quality health care and consistent with the values of the profession through individual and collective action.
7. The nurse participates in the advancement of the profession through contributions to practice, education, administration, and knowledge development.
8. The nurse collaborates with other health care professionals and the public in promoting community, national, and international efforts to meet health needs.
9. The profession of nursing, as represented by associations and their members, is responsible for articulating nursing values, for maintaining the integrity of the profession and its practice, and for shaping social policy.

TABLE 38.2 New York State Nurses Association Position Statement: Use of Complementary and Alternative Therapies (CAT) in the Practice of Nursing

1. Provide full disclosure when offering CAT to patients, including discussing the pros and cons of all therapeutic options available to the patient.
2. Be cognizant of the ethical and cultural issues and considerations surrounding CAT to fully function as an advocate for quality, comprehensive care of patients.
3. Discuss with the patient, and family when appropriate, available options regarding CAT and support the patient's choice.
4. Incorporate the American Holistic Nurses' Association's *Standards of Holistic Nursing Practice* and the American Nurses Association's *Code of Ethics for Nursing* into their practice.
5. Continually seek avenues to raise community awareness about the benefits of CAT in wellness and preventative medicine.
6. Conduct, support, and/or participate in research to study the effectiveness of CAT as nursing interventions.
7. Support continued funding of the federal Office of Alternative Medicine and urge professional nursing organizations to work collaboratively with that office.
8. Advocate for the adequate coverage and access of CAT by federal, state, and insurance programs.
9. Advocate that health care practitioners and health care facilities provide the patient with the opportunity to obtain conventional and CAT by accepting and integrating the availability of such therapies into the health care delivery system.
10. Advocate that nursing programs integrate CAT concepts and information into their existing curricula (7).

New York State Nurses Association (Table 38.2) and the American Holistic Nurses' Association Position Statement on the Role of Nurses in the Practice of Complementary and Alternative Therapies (resources, Table 38.3). Nurses should become familiar with their individual state's position on CAM; specifically, what

TABLE 38.3 Dietary Supplement Resources for the Nurse

- The American Holistic Nurses' Association Position Statement: Role of Nurses in the Practice of Complementary and Alternative Therapies:
  - http://www.ahna.org/Resources/Publications/PositionStatements/tabid/1926/Default.aspx#P1
- Fitzgerald A. Herbal facts, herbal fallacies. American Nurse Today. December 2007.
  - http://nursingworld.org/MODS/mod454/Herbalarticle.pdf
- Frisch N. Standards for holistic nursing practice: a way to think about our care that includes complementary and alternative modalities. *Online J Issues Nurs* 2001;6(2): Manuscript 4.
  - www.nursingworld.org/MainMenuCategories/ANAMarketplace/ANAPeriodicals/OJIN/TableofContents/Volume62001/No2May01/HolisticNursingPractice.aspx
- Heltemes L. The root of the matter: herbs and anesthesia. *OR Nurse* 2007;1(3):20–22.

is allowed in the recommendation and monitoring of CAM, including dietary supplements.

ROLE OF NURSE IN COMPLEMENTARY AND ALTERNATIVE MEDICINE: FILLING THE DISCUSSION AND EDUCATIONAL GAP

Numerous surveys have documented the poor level of communication regarding dietary supplement between patients and physicians. In several surveys the disclosure and discussion rate has been approximately 50% (8, 9). This discussion gap happens for several reasons. Up to 60% of patients have noted in previous surveys that they did not discuss supplement use because they were not asked nor did they think it was important for them to let their clinicians know. The nurse can be an important part of the clinical team in clarifying these common obstacles. Simply asking in the usual setting of nondiscussion can prompt new and important information. Moreover, nurses can be in the forefront of reducing the second misconception by educating patients during encounters on the importance of discussing dietary supplement from the standpoint of optimized care with full disclosure as well as prevention of potential interactions. Simply by engaging patients in this discussion, educating them on the importance of the discussion, and recording this information both for documentation purposes and as a lead-in to other providers, the nurse can be a most valuable member of the health care team. A stepwise approach to patient care in this area is reviewed using the H.E.R.B.A.L. Mnemonic in Table 38.4.

ROLE OF NURSES IN DIETARY SUPPLEMENTS

Although the role of nurses in the field of CAM has been discussed by many state organizations, the specific use of dietary supplement often borders on the recommendation of medications and most state organizations discuss supplement in conjunction with safe medication practices. In this scenario nurses are expected to ask about, discuss indications, record, and educate patients on safe utilization in the same way they would for prescriptions medication. As an example, the Minnesota Nurses Association Position Statement on the *Role of the Registered Nurse in Safe Administration of Medications* notes in the section on Best Practice Recommendations to Improve Patient/Client Safety the following two recommendations in regard to dietary supplements.

- Inquire about herbal medications and dietary supplements. Know the implications of any of these substances being administered.
- Ascertain that the users of medication administration devices are knowledgeable about the functions and limitations (10).

TABLE 38.4 Recommendation for Nurses Based on the H.E.R.B.A.L. Mnemonic

- Hear the patient out with respect
  - Much research has pointed out the communication gap, especially between patient and physicians, in the area of CAM and dietary supplements. Nurses are often the first to have the conversation about dietary supplement and more likely to garner a discussion which can be beneficial for the patient and care team.
- Educate
  - Nurses play a vital role in many aspects of patient education and dietary supplements are no different. Patients should be made aware of both the supplements they are considering, including the risk, benefits, and alternatives for their use, and resources for ongoing learning.
- Record
  - Nurses are often the first to be able to record dietary supplements in the medical chart (progress note, medication section). This can set both a powerful example as well as provide information, that is often missed, which can significantly impact patient care.
- Be aware of reactions and interaction
  - When patients have potential adverse effects, nurses are often the first to receive this information and are also on the frontlines in reaction and interaction prevention. By taking an active role in discussing the appropriateness of dietary supplement in the context of patient medical history as well as documented allergies and contraindication to certain therapies, nurses can play a leading role in education patients regarding optimal dietary supplement use.
- Agree to discus
  - After leaving the office, patients often have questions regarding existing recommendations for dietary supplements as well as consideration regarding additional choices. In many cases, nurses can provide timely patient education regarding utilization of current supplements as well as counseling regarding other supplement considerations between clinic visits. By discussing supplement considerations, nurses can often balance the information and resources the patient is utilizing on dietary supplements to help the patient come up with the best choice for ongoing care.
- Learn
  - Nurses should learn about their state board's position regarding nursing scope of practice in regard to complementary therapies including dietary supplements. These positions can be used to inform local practice policies to educate nursing staff on maximizing their role in dietary supplement management.
  - A number of point of care and continuing education resources are available for nurses to stay updated on dietary supplements. These are noted in Table 38.3 as well as in chapter 42.

CONCLUSIONS

Nurses are well-known for their holistic and patient-centered clinical care. Their diverse practice settings as well as training, education, and philosophy are perfectly suited to broadly improve the typical dietary supplement scenario that is unfortunately lacking in discussion, charting, and counseling. Nurses have the ability to transform their current best practice tools of open dialogue and patient advocacy/education into the expanding realm of dietary supplementation. By doing so and involving other members of the health care team, nurses can play a leading role in optimizing dietary supplement management.

References

1. Dutta AP, Dutta AP, Bwayo S, et al. Complementary and alternative medicine instruction in nursing curricula. *J Natl Black Nurses Assoc* 2003;14(2):30–33.
2. Fenton MV, Morris DL. The integration of holistic nursing practices and complementary and alternative modalities into curricula of schools of nursing. *Altern Ther Health Med* 2003;9(4):62–67.
3. http://www.nursingworld.org/EspeciallyForYou/StudentNurses.aspx.
4. Royal College of Nursing. Defining nursing. http://www.rcn.org.uk/__data/assets/pdf_file/0003/78564/001983.pdf. Published April 2003. Publication code 001 983. Accessed April 21, 2009.
5. American Nurses Association, *Code of Ethics for Nurses with Interpretive Statements*. Silver Spring, MD: American Nurses Publishing; 2001. http://www.nursingworld.org/MainMenuCategories/ThePracticeofProfessionalNursing/EthicsStandards/CodeofEthics/2110Provisions.aspx. Accessed April 21, 2009.
6. Sparber A. State boards of nursing and scope of practice of registered nurses performing complementary therapies. *Online J Issues Nurs* 2001;6(3):10.
7. New York State Nurses Association. POSITION STATEMENT. Use of Complementary and alternative therapies in the practice of nursing. Approved by the NYSNA Board of Directors on August 08, 2007. This position statement was developed under the direction of NYSNA's Council on Nursing Practice. http://www.nysna.org/practice/positions/position14.htm. Accessed April 21, 2009.
8. Cheung CK, Wyman JF, Halcon LL. Use of complementary and alternative therapies in community-dwelling older adults. *J Altern Complement Med* 2007;13(9):997–1006.
9. Brunelli B, Gorson KC. The use of complementary and alternative medicines by patients with peripheral neuropathy. *J Neurol Sci* 2004;218(1–2):59–66.
10. Role of the registered nurse in safe administration of medications. Adopted by MNA Commission on Nursing Practice July 10, 2001. http://nursesrev.advocateoffice.com/. Accessed April 21, 2009.

CHAPTER 39

The Role of the Naturopathic Physician

Michael Traub

The first two sections are significantly excerpted, with permission from the *Clinicians and Educators Desk Reference on the Complementary and Alternative Healthcare Professions*, published by the Academic Consortium for Complementary and Alternative Health Care (1) the authors of which are Paul Mittman, ND, DHANP, Pat Wolfe, and Michael Traub, ND, DHANP, FABNO.

PHILOSOPHY

First conceived in 1902, naturopathic medicine is a holistic, coordinated approach to health care that respects the unique individuality of each person and that integrates modern biomedical sciences with a wide array of natural and conventional therapies. It is a comprehensive system of health care that incorporates many modalities including clinical nutrition, botanic medicine, behavioral medicine, homeopathy, physical medicine consisting of hydrotherapy, physiotherapy and manipulation, as well as clinical practices such as minor surgery, pharmacology, and obstetrics (2). In addition, naturopathic physicians (NDs) respect and apply the principles of a variety of traditional world medicines such as Ayurvedic medicine, aboriginal medicines, and Oriental medicine. NDs encourage the inherent self-healing abilities of the individual through lifestyle education and the application of nonsuppressive therapeutic methods and modalities.

Currently, an estimated 5,000 NDs are licensed/regulated in 14 states (Alaska, Arizona, California, Connecticut, Idaho, Hawaii, Kansas, Maine, Montana, New Hampshire, Oregon, Utah, Vermont, and Washington), the District of Columbia, Puerto Rico, and the Virgin Islands, with an estimated growth to 6,000 by 2010. In these states, NDs are able to practice independently as primary care physicians. Prescribing privileges for each state vary greatly. A brief summary is given below.

Arizona has the broadest prescribing privileges for NDs in the nation. Arizona NDs are allowed to independently prescribe all classes of prescription drugs, with four exceptions (IV medicines except vitamins, minerals, and emergency resuscitation medications), chemotherapy drugs, and antipsychotics.

California currently allows NDs to prescribe drugs under the supervision of a medical doctor (MD) or a doctor of osteopathy (DO) and to prescribe hormones and epinephrine independently.

Hawaii state law authorizes NDs to prescribe vitamins, minerals, amino acids, and fatty acids.

Idaho passed a bill in 2005 authorizing licensure of NDs. The bill creates a formulary council to establish a formulary for use by NDs that is consistent with the training and education of NDs. The formulary will be reviewed on an annual basis. To date, the formulary has not been completed.

Kansas passed an ND licensing law in 2003. It authorizes an intravenous and intramuscular formulary which must be under the supervision of a physician. Kansas is the only state, other than California, which requires continuous MD supervision for prescribing.

Maine NDs are allowed to independently prescribe noncontrolled legend drugs after completing a 12-month collaborative relationship with a licensed allopathic or osteopathic physician to review the NDs prescribing practices.

Montana law requires a five-member formulary committee to establish a natural substance formulary list and review the list on an annual basis. Among other items, the approved list of natural substances contains antibiotics and hormones.

Oregon NDs have wide prescribing authority. All substances on the formulary are recommended by the formulary council and approved by the State Board of Naturopathic Examiners.

Utah NDs are allowed to prescribe noncontrolled drugs that are consistent with competent practice of naturopathic medicine and are approved in collaboration with the Naturopathic Formulary Advisory Peer Committee.

Vermont law authorizes the Commissioner of Health to establish the formulary with the advice of advisory appointees. The formulary lists the substances that are authorized as well as their route of administration, and in some instances even the specific dose and length of treatment.

Washington state law was recently amended to allow NDs a broader formulary. House Bill 1546 of 2005 defined naturopathic medicines to mean "vitamins; minerals; botanic medicines; homeopathic medicines; hormones; and those legend drugs and controlled substances consistent with naturopathic medical practice in accordance with rules established by the secretary." There are currently five schools of naturopathic medicine in the United States that are accredited or in candidacy status for accreditation, and two in Canada. For an updated listing of training and licensure, please refer to www.aanmc.org.

The American Association of Naturopathic Physicians defines naturopathic medicine as: "a distinct system of primary health care—an art, science, philosophy and practice of diagnosis, treatment and prevention of illness. Naturopathic medicine is distinguished by the principles upon which its practice is based. These principles are continually reexamined in the light of scientific advances. The techniques of naturopathic medicine include modern and traditional, scientific and empirical methods" (3).

The philosophy of naturopathic medicine is embodied by the six principles of naturopathic practice that date back to the time of Hippocrates (4):

The Healing Power of Nature

NDs recognize an inherent ability of the body to heal itself. It is the role of the ND to identify and remove obstacles to healing and recovery and facilitate and enhance this self-healing process.

Identify and Treat the Causes

NDs seek to remove the underlying causes of disease rather than merely eliminating or suppressing symptoms.

First Do No Harm

NDs strive to (i) use methods that minimize harmful side effects, using the least force necessary to diagnose and treat, (ii) prevent suppression of symptoms, and (iii) acknowledge, respect and work with each individual's self-healing process.

Doctor as Teacher

A primary role of the ND is to educate and encourage individuals to take responsibility for their own health. They also recognize the therapeutic potential of the physician/patient relationship.

Treat the Whole Person

NDs recognize that total health includes physical, mental, emotional, genetic, environmental, social, spiritual, and other factors. They encourage patients to pursue personal spiritual development.

Prevention

NDs encourage and emphasize disease prevention, that is, assessing risk factors, heredity and susceptibility to disease, and making appropriate interventions in partnership with patients to prevent illness. Naturopathic medicine is committed to creating a healthy world for humanity (5).

APPROACH TO PATIENT CARE

Using the six principles outlined above, NDs seek to understand the underlying and contributing factors in a patient's condition, remove obstacles to healing, strengthen or support the inherent healing ability, and teach the patient how to prevent recurrence of the condition. For example, a child with recurrent otitis media is conventionally treated with repeated courses of antibiotics, and in some cases tympanostomy and ear tubes. An ND would use the history, physical examination and, in some cases, laboratory tests to diagnose conditions that increase the child's susceptibility to becoming sick. These could include environmental allergies (dust mites, dander, etc.), food sensitivities (dairy, wheat, eggs are often implicated), a diet high in simple carbohydrates (processed sugars), mechanical misalignments of the cervical spine or cranial bones, and sometimes, emotional stress. Children routinely improve by addressing these factors, together with nutritional support and other naturopathic therapies.

In striving to attain an in-depth understanding of the patient's health, NDs consider the combination of genetic predispositions with superimposed factors such as nutritional status, work and emotional stress, environmental allergens and toxins, and biomechanical data such as gait and posture.

Essential to a comprehensive evaluation is the extended interview, which ranges from 60 to 90 minutes for new patients. Typical follow-up visits range between 30 and 60 minutes. A standard review of systems is supplemented with patient-generated reports of daily activities, such as dietary habits, physical activity, and psychological issues. NDs perform physical examinations appropriate to the patient's presenting complaint and health history and employ conventional laboratory and diagnostic imaging services as needed. Clinical evaluation is patient-centered and addresses a full range of factors that influence health as well as illness, generating a problem-oriented patient record (6).

With many treatment options at their disposal, NDs follow a distinct clinical thought process to individualize patient care according to naturopathic principles. In 1997, "The Process of Healing, a Unifying Theory of Naturopathic Medicine" was published in the *Journal of Naturopathic Medicine* (Zeff). The article presented three principles underlying the practice of naturopathic medicine. The first of these is the characterization of disease as a *process* rather than a *pathologic entity.* The second is the focus on the determinants of health rather than on pathology. The third is the concept of a therapeutic hierarchy. As taught in naturopathic medical schools, the therapeutic hierarchy is a guideline to applying the modalities of naturopathic medicine according to the unique needs of an individual patient. The therapeutic hierarchy proposed is as follows:

- Establish the conditions for health.
- Stimulate the self-healing mechanisms (*vis medicatrix naturae*).
- Support weakened or damaged systems or organs.
- Address structural integrity.
- Address pathology using specific natural substances, modalities, or interventions.
- Address pathology using specific pharmacologic or synthetic substances.
- Suppress pathology.

Let us return to our example of a child with recurrent otitis media, a common reason for seeking naturopathic care. Using the hierarchy above, a typical naturopathic approach to care would follow this protocol:

- Look for and remove or address obstacles to health, such as allergies, environmental irritants (e.g., secondhand cigarette smoke), diet high in simple sugars, and so forth.
- Stimulate the healing power of nature with therapies like homeopathy and hydrotherapy.
- Strengthen affected systems by providing immune support with vitamins C and A, and oligopolysaccharides.
- Address structural factors with soft tissue manual therapy like lymphatic drainage.
- Treat the pathology with specific natural therapies such as topical garlic and/or Hypericum oil.
- Typically, children respond well to the naturopathic approach outlined above, experiencing fewer infections with faster recovery. However, should a child experience a particularly severe ear infection, or if there are other compromising factors, it may be necessary to prescribe a course of antibiotics.
- If the infection still does not subside, referral to a MD may be necessary.

The therapeutic hierarchy creates a guideline for prescribing (or referring for) therapeutic life changes, homeopathic and botanic medicines, nutritional supplements, manipulative therapy, and prescription drugs by naturopathic physicians that is both consistent with the profession's principles and addresses the patient's dynamic needs (7).

NATUROPATHIC PHYSICIANS—EXPERTS IN NATURAL MEDICINE

NDs are, by their education and training, experts in natural medicine. No other health care professional has undergone a 4-year medical program which emphasizes the use of nutrition, nutritional supplements, botanic and homeopathic medicines, and lifestyle counseling in the treatment of disease and the promotion of health. The naturopathic approach generally starts with the use of these modalities. These modalities are viewed by the ND not as adjuncts to conventional treatment but as foundational underpinnings of patient care. In certain cases, for example, cancer therapy or other serious, advanced degenerative disease states, naturopathic treatment may be used to complement conventional treatment.

The naturopathic approach is unique, deriving from the naturopathic medical school experience, the principles of naturopathic medicine, and the ND professional community. Conventionally trained health care professionals may utilize nutritional, botanic, and homeopathic medicines from a holistic perspective, but experience has shown that there is a qualitative difference in the way such professionals treat their patients compared to NDs. "Green allopathy" is a term that has been used to describe conventionally trained professionals who merely substitute natural medicine for prescription drugs. On the other hand, there are certainly MDs, DOs, nurses, and other health care professionals who are just as holistic in their approach to patient care as NDs.

NDs have either founded many of the preeminent natural product companies in North America or serve as medical directors or consultants to this industry.

NDs understand the issue of natural product quality, and their expertise helps ensure accurate identification of raw materials, potency, purity, safety, and efficacy. With the aforementioned background of ND's expertise, let us consider the potential role of NDs in evaluating and managing dietary supplement use as well as coordinating that information with the rest of the patient care team, including conventional physicians, dieticians, nurses, and pharmacists.

EVALUATION

NDs are trained to function as primary care providers, and, as such, are able to diagnose disease with the same tools as conventionally trained health care professionals. This includes patient history, physical examination, laboratory testing, and diagnostic imaging. However, these tools are sometimes used slightly differently by NDs. For example, patient history will almost always include a dietary survey, and patients are always asked about which dietary supplements they are taking. It is a well-known phenomenon that, for various reasons, patients are often not asked by conventional providers about their diet or use of supplements. With the exception of dieticians, patients do not generally view these providers as knowledgeable about nutrition, and in the United States, 47% or more do not divulge the fact that they are taking dietary supplements (8). Furthermore, only 11.8% of adults in the United States seek care from a licensed or certified complementary and alternative medicine practitioner, suggesting that most individuals who use dietary supplements self-prescribe and/or self-medicate (9). Naturopathic physicians often ask patients to keep a diet and exercise diary for 1 week to review the quality and quantity of this vital sign. Although this instrument is not without its shortcomings (i.e., it depends on accurate recall and reporting), it also serves as an effective behavioral modification intervention to know that an expert will be looking at food choices and physical activity level.

Standard laboratory test results are viewed somewhat differently by NDs, especially in the case of borderline or slightly abnormal results. Some examples of this are as follows:

1. A slightly elevated mean corpuscular volume may indicate vitamin B_{12} deficiency.
2. Slightly elevated liver function tests are a cause to investigate the possibility of chronic hepatitis, fatty liver, or medication side effect.
3. A borderline low free thyroxine, and a high normal thyroid-stimulating hormone, may suggest subclinical hypothyroidism.

NDs may order tests to assess risk status as well as for ascertaining a diagnosis. Examples are 25(OH) vitamin D, homocysteine, highly sensitive C reactive protein, urine heavy metal screening, and functional intracellular nutritional assays. The latter test is a very sensitive indicator of nutrient deficiencies.

MANAGEMENT

As experts in natural medicine, it would be ideal if NDs could always be consulted and participate as part of a coordinated patient care team. Because of their small numbers this is impractical. In cases in which an ND is part of a care team, the ND's role can be as follows:

1. Actively participate in patient evaluation (history, physical examination, differential diagnosis, and diagnostic testing).
2. Offer an expanded perspective of clinical assessment and treatment, as appropriate to the individual patient, based on an in-depth understanding of the patient's underlying condition (including his or her experience) and to effectively communicate relevant information to other members of the care team.

One of the areas in which NDs are particularly knowledgeable is with various types of interactions between medications. Herb–herb interaction is a phenomenon well documented in traditional Chinese medicine and Western botanic medicine. Drug–herb/nutrient interactions often focus on potential risk that is frequently exaggerated in medical literature and popular media. Therapeutic drug–herb/nutrient interactions focus on benefits, such as reduction of drug dosage, side effects, costs, and the maintenance and enhancement of positive effects. An example is with metformin, the insulin-sensitizing drug used for diabetes and polycystic ovarian syndrome. Metformin interferes not only with glucose absorption in the gut but also with the calcium-dependent cell membranes that absorb vitamin B_{12}. Long-term B_{12} deficiency manifests as peripheral neuropathy, a common complication of diabetes. Calcium and vitamin B_{12} supplementation can prevent the development of peripheral neuropathy in patients with diabetes taking metformin.

Although some principles and tools of naturopathic practice are different from those of conventional health care, many of the goals of naturopathic medicine parallel those of other practitioners in providing for and maintaining the well-being of the patient. Collaboration is growing between conventional and naturopathic communities in evaluating and managing a broad range of conditions.

KEY WEB SITES/ORGANIZATIONS

American Association of Naturopathic Physicians—www.naturopathic.org
Association of Accredited Naturopathic Medical Colleges—www.aanmc.org
Bastyr University—www.bastyr.edu
Boucher Institute of Naturopathic Medicine—www.binm.org
Canadian College of Naturopathic Medicine—www.ccnm.edu
Canadian Association of Naturopathic Doctors—www.naturopathicassoc.ca
Council on Naturopathic Medical Education—www.cnme.org
National College of Natural Medicine—www.ncnm.edu
National University of Health Sciences—www.nuhs.edu
Southwest College of Naturopathic Medicine—www.scnm.edu
University of Bridgeport College of Naturopathic Medicine—www.bridgeport.edu/naturopathy
Homeopathic Academy of Naturopathic Physicians—www.hanp.net
American Association of Naturopathic Midwives—www.naturopathicmidwives.org
Oncology Association of Naturopathic Physicians—www.oncanp.org
Naturopathic Academy of Therapeutic Injection—www.nati.org

References

1. Elizabeth Goldblatt, et al. *Clinicians' and Educators' Desk Reference on the Licensed Complementary and Alternative Healthcare Professions*. 2009. http://accahc.org/index.php?option=com_content&view=article&id=42&Itemid=24
2. Hough H, Dower C, O'Neil E. *Profile of a Profession: Naturopathic Practice*. University of California, San Francisco: Center for the Health Professions; 2001.
3. Snider P, Zeff J. *Definition of Naturopathic Medicine: AANP Position Paper*. Rippling River, Oregon, 1989.
4. Health Professions Advisors Guide. National Association for Advisors of the Health Professions; 2007.
5. American Association of Naturopathic Physicians, 1998.
6. Dunne N, Benda W, Kim L, et al. Naturopathic medicine: what can patients expect? *J Fam Pract* 2005;54:12.
7. Bureau of Naturopathic Medicine. Findings and recommendations regarding the prescribing and furnishing authority of a naturopathic doctor. Presented to the California State Legislature by Bureau of Naturopathic Medicine January 2007. http://www.naturopathic.ca.gov/formspubs/formulary_report.pdf
8. Eisenberg DM, Kessler RC, Foster C, et al. Unconventional medicine in the United States. Prevalence, costs, and patterns of use. *N Engl J Med* 1993;328(4):246–252.
9. Eisenberg DM, Davis RB, Ettner SL, et al. Trends in alternative medicine use in the United States. 1990–1997: results of a follow-up national survey. *JAMA* 1998;280(18):1569–1575.

CHAPTER 40

The Role of the Traditional Chinese Medicine (TCM) Practitioner

Justine Greene

BRIEF HISTORY

Traditional Chinese medicine (TCM) herbal practices likely had their beginnings in medicinal substances and rituals described in texts dating back to approximately 2,000 to 3,000 years BCE. Herbal practitioners during that time were probably local shamans. In the later Han Dynasty (25 to 220 AD) texts were written such as the Yellow Emperor's Inner Classic that described some herbal remedies and purported the philosophy that health and illness were a result of natural forces of which humans were a part. Treatment of illness and maintenance of health would involve knowledge of our place within this natural order. The Classic of the Materia Medica was also written in this same time period and describes individual herbal medicinals. TCM herbal therapies developed from a combination of folk remedies and scholarly input and were influenced by multiple cultural forces over the years including various languages, politics, economics, geographic circumstances, religions, and philosophies regarding health and illness all culminating in how this medicine is used in modern times (1).

WHAT ARE TRADITIONAL CHINESE MEDICINE HERBALS?

The substances used in TCM herbology are mostly plant-based but can also be derived from animal and mineral sources. These medicinals can be used in many forms:

- whole raw herbs cooked into teas
- powdered and taken as a tea
- swallowed in a capsule or tablet
- poultices and patches
- extracted into tinctures of the whole herb
- standardized extracts of what is thought to be the active ingredient in the herb
- cooked into foods
- granulated
- eaten raw

Herbal substances can be used:

- Orally
- Topically

- As aromatherapy
- In a soak or bath
- As a sterile solution for injection

Herbal substances are categorized on the basis of multiple factors including their actions, taste, temperature, and which TCM energy meridians or organ systems they influence. A medicinal's properties can also be influenced by where and when it is produced and harvested and what processing it has undergone.

TCM herbals are not generally used individually. They are usually prescribed in combinations called formulas. Each formula has particular functions for restoring and maintaining health. Within the formulas, each herbal substance has one or more functions that contribute to the overall properties of the formula. Some herbs also mitigate any untoward effects of the other herbs in the formula. There are basic formulas used for TCM conditions with standard herb ingredients and dosages. For each formula, other herbals can be added and the dosages increased or decreased depending upon the patient's unique needs. This allows a high level of individualization of an herbal prescription. Brand new formulas can be created by the seasoned practitioner. Formulas can be combined and used together.

BRIEF OVERVIEW OF TRADITIONAL CHINESE MEDICINE DIAGNOSIS

TCM herbal formulas are prescribed on the basis of the TCM diagnostic system, so it would be helpful to have some understanding of how these diagnoses are made. Obviously, more than the briefest view of this diagnostic process is beyond the scope of this chapter.

As with other systems of medicine, there is a method for gathering information about the patient and his/her state of health. A TCM patient history would include the usual chief complaint and history of the present illness as expected. There is, however, more emphasis placed upon overall health and the relationship of the current issue to other health indicators, the environment, psychosocial/spiritual factors, nutrition, and other lifestyle elements. There are the traditional "Ten Questions" similar to a Western review of systems that ask the patient about:

1. Fevers/chills
2. Perspiration
3. Head and body
4. Defecation/urination
5. Lifestyle and bearing
6. Food/appetite/taste/thirst
7. Sleep
8. Eyes and ears
9. Chest/abdomen
10. Old illnesses (2, 3).

TCM physical examinations focus on elements that may be unfamiliar to Western practitioners. Much emphasis is placed upon visualization of the tongue because it gives information about the condition of TCM internal organ systems. The pulses at the wrists are ascribed to TCM organ systems and palpation by an experienced practitioner can lend important insights into the inner workings of the body. Visualization of the patient's body shape and size, skin color, facial characteristics, general demeanor, nail condition, and areas of TCM meridians is used to develop a diagnosis. More diagnostic clues may be found in other areas of examination such as listening to characteristics of a patient's voice, noting various odors, or palpating acupuncture points.

The totality of the information gained from the patient is then used to develop a working diagnosis based on TCM principles. One of these principles is that of qi or universal energy that is used by the body and may be normal or diminished in its presence and flow. Blood, which represents such concepts as fluidity, nourishment, and interconnection, may also be replete or deficient and show constraint in its normal motion within the body leading to disease. Bodily conditions may also be described in terms of hot or cold. Disease conditions can also be classified as interior (more to do with the visceral organs) or exterior (more involving skin, hair, and superficial musculoskeletal system; possibly stemming from external pathogens such as wind or dampness).

As mentioned above, there are organ systems in TCM: spleen, liver, large intestine, small intestine, heart, pericardium, gallbladder, lung, kidney, san jiao, stomach, urinary bladder. Some of these organs and their functions bear a resemblance to Western organs and some do not. Of course, there is the baseline concept of the duality of yin and yang and all organs, conditions, and so forth can be described in these terms and their relationship to the yin and yang of the world surrounding the patient.

So, it is possible for a patient to be given a very individualized TCM diagnosis such as spleen qi vacuity with liver qi depression and liver blood stagnation; or lung yin vacuity with acute external wind, and so forth.

Herbal formulas would then be chosen to address the patient's acute and chronic/underlying diagnoses.

CLINICAL CASE EXAMPLES

Case 1

A 52-year-old female presents for assistance with menopausal hot flushes. She has not had any menstruation for 15 months. She reports hot flushes each day in the afternoon, mostly over the face and upper chest; vaginal dryness; insomnia; low back and knee pain; and irritability. Her tongue is red with a peeled appearance. The pulse is rapid and thready.

TRADITIONAL CHINESE MEDICINE DIAGNOSIS

Kidney and liver yin vacuity with yang rising.

- The kidney and liver organs are often affected during menopause.
- The dryness associated with yin vacuity and the heat of rising yang energy are responsible for the symptoms of dryness and hot flashes.
- Heat and irritability often reported during menopause.

TRADITIONAL CHINESE MEDICINE HERBAL FORMULA

Six ingredient pill with Rehmannia (Liu Wei Di Huang Wan) (4).

TRADITIONAL CHINESE MEDICINE FORMULA FUNCTION

Nourishes kidney and liver yin.

FORMULA DESCRIPTION (5):

Herb Ingredient Name (pharmaceutical/pin yin)	**Herb Function in the Formula**
Radix Rehmanniae Glutinosae/Shu Di Huang	Enriches kidney yin and essence
Fructus Corniae Officinalis/Shan Zhu Yu	Nourishes liver
Radix Dioscoreae Oppositae/Shan Yao	Stabilizes essence by nourishing the spleen
Sclerotium Poriae Cocos/Fu Ling	Clears/drains liver heat; prevents side effects of shan zhu yu
Cortex Moutan Radicis/Mu Dan Pi	Aids spleen and digestion and prevents digestive side effects of other herbs
Rhizoma Alismatis Orientalis/Xe Xie	Clears/drains heat from kidney; prevents side effects of rich herb like shu di huang

Case 2

A 55-year-old male reports fatigue, lack of libido, and erectile dysfunction. He has been told by his physician that his testosterone levels are low and was given a diagnosis of hypogonadism (6, 7). He reports a previous history of frequent sexual activity with a multitude of sexual partners for many years. The patient also reports chronic prostatitis and nocturia, knee and low back pain for which he sees a chiropractor as needed, and getting cold easily.

Tongue: pale, swollen, wet, thin white coating

Pulse: deficient and weak especially kidney positions (2, 8)

TRADITIONAL CHINESE MEDICINE DIAGNOSES

Kidney qi and yang vacuity

- In TCM, the kidneys are associated with sexual/genital function, knees, lower back, and some forms of fatigue.

TRADITIONAL CHINESE MEDICINE HERBAL FORMULA

Restore the right kidney pill (you gui wan).

FORMULA FUNCTIONS

Warms and replenishes kidneys.

FORMULA DESCRIPTION (5):

Herb Ingredient Name (pharmaceutical/pin yin)	**Herb Function in the Formula**
Radix Lateralis Aconiti/fu zi	Warm and tonify kidney yang
Cortex Cinnamomi Cassiae/rou gui	Warm and tonify kidney yang

Colla Cornu Cervi/lu jiao jiao	Warm and tonify kidney yang
Radix Rehmanniae Glutinosae Conquitae/shu di huang	Nourish kidneys, spleen, liver
Fructus Corni Officinalis/shan zhu yu	Nourish kidneys, spleen, liver
Radix Dioscoreae Oppositae/shan yao	Nourish kidneys, spleen, liver
Fructus Lycii/gou qi zi	Nourish liver, spleen, and kidneys; help low back pain
Semen Cuscutae Chinensis/tu si zi	Nourish liver, spleen, and kidneys; help low back pain
Cortex Eucommiae Ulmoidis/du zhong	Nourish liver, spleen, and kidneys; help low back pain
Radix Angelicae Sinensis/dang gui	Tonify blood

WHO ARE TRADITIONAL CHINESE MEDICINE PRACTITIONERS?

Most of the US practitioners prescribing TCM herbal formulas are graduates of schools of Oriental Medicine and receive the degree of Masters of Traditional Oriental Medicine. Schools are accredited by the Accreditation Commission for Acupuncture and Oriental Medicine. At this writing there are just more than 50 accredited Masters Degree programs in the United States (9). Programs are now becoming available and accredited to bestow the degree of Doctor of Acupuncture and Oriental Medicine (9). Some practitioners have been educated at prestigious universities in other countries. Most, but not all, states require practitioners to pass licensing examinations (state-specific or nationally administered) in order to be licensed and practice in their state. This licensure will give the practitioner credentials such as LAc. (Licensed acupuncturist), A.P. (Acupuncture Physician), or RAc (registered acupuncturist). Some states accept a nationally recognized examination administered by the National Certification Commission for Acupuncture and Oriental Medicine (10). The accepted scope of practice for an acupuncturist may vary from one state to the next but generally includes the use of herbal medicines. There are more than 12,000 practicing acupuncturists in the United States today (11). Some other licensed clinicians such as naturopathic doctors (ND), medical doctors (MD), and doctors of osteopathy (DO) will practice herbal medicine. They usually must have special training to practice Oriental Medicine and may need to meet state-specific requirements. Naturopaths may receive training in TCM herbs as part of their basic schooling. MDs and DOs may attend schools of TCM or other courses of study to become educated in prescribing TCM herbs. In some states, other health care providers such as holistic health practitioners or herbologists recommend herbs as part of their treatments. Overall, TCM herbal medicine is considered to be complex and requires a clinician to invest years of study and practice in order to become truly proficient in its use. It is important that patients who are using TCM herbal formulas should be under the care of a well-trained and experienced clinician.

HOW TO LOCATE AN APPROPRIATE PRACTITIONER

Of course, you want to make sure that the practitioner you refer patients too is well-trained, experienced, and shares your interest in providing quality patient care. But how do you identify practitioners with whom you can work comfortably? Some questions you might investigate are as follows:

- Does the practitioner meet the requirements in the state in which he/she practices? Most states have a registry online that will list appropriately trained practitioners.
- Has the practitioner completed national testing?
  The National Certification Commission for Acupuncture and Oriental Medicine maintains listings of practitioners who have passed their national examinations (12).
- Has the practitioner been accepted into any professional organizations?
  The American Association of Acupuncture and Oriental Medicine (AAAOM) (13) lists its members who have completed requirements for admission to its professional organization.
- How long has the herbal professional been in practice?
- Does the practitioner have significant experience treating patients with the conditions you might often see in your practice and would like to refer?
- Does the practitioner accept the forms of payment your patients are used to using?
- Have colleagues had success with this TCM practitioner in the past?
- Do the practitioner's office, staff, and operating procedures including appointment scheduling, confidentiality, and availability meet you and your patient's expectations?
- What types of herbal preparations do they routinely use? How do they monitor the quality of the herbs that they recommend?
- Is the practitioner willing to communicate openly with you as you co-manage a patient?

TRADITIONAL CHINESE MEDICINE HERBAL SAFETY

One issue that is raised about herbal medicines in general is whether or not they are safe to use with Western pharmaceuticals. Many patients are using over-the-counter (OTC) and prescription drugs along with herbs and other dietary supplements. How do we know whether this is safe or not? In China, herbs and drugs are used simultaneously. There is not, however, abundant research available about drug–herb interactions in English describing this practice in China.

TCM practitioners might argue that, because Chinese herbs are used in formulas that are intricately fashioned to promote the positive effects and curb any side effects, they are safe and unlikely to cause adverse interactions. They purport that the use of herbal formulas may decrease dosages needed of Western medications, thereby decreasing side effects and cost. The combination of drugs and herbs is felt to provide overall better therapeutic effect than either herbs or pharmaceuticals alone.

Some interactions (inhibitions or potentiations) between herbs and drugs are known and some can be theorized on the basis of knowledge of the substances involved. Medications and herbs can affect each other's bioavailability by increasing or decreasing absorption in the GI tract. For instance, one medicinal can bind another or change the pH and thereby alter absorption of other substances. A drug that alters GI motility might change the absorption of herbs. Medicinals that affect the liver and kidney may alter the breakdown of herbs and drugs and necessitate changes in dosaging.

Western pharmaceuticals, like herbals, are thought to have effects on the physiology that can be described in terms of TCM. For example, pharmaceuticals like testosterone are considered to nourish yang such as in case #2 above. Chemotherapy agents are generally thought to cause significant heat and dryness in the body and therefore are considered to contribute to yin (fluid) vacuity in TCM. Western medications may alter the patient's presentation in terms of TCM diagnosis. It is important to diagnose the patient by how he/she presents taking into account Western medicines being used.

How might drugs and herbs be used more safely together? First, it would be important to document all substances ingested—prescription, OTC, all herbal preparations and any other dietary supplements, and so forth. Then a careful patient history reveals what each medicinal is being used for, how it is being used, and any benefits or side effects that have been noted. TCM practitioners are generally trained to not discuss Western pharmaceuticals with their patients, instead referring them back to their prescribing health care practitioners for assistance. TCM practitioners may start on a low dose of the formula if concerned about interactions with medications and then work up gradually as tolerated. Treating TCM practitioners or the patient's Western physician may measure any parameters such as blood pressure that might be of concern while starting treatment and then adjust treatment depending upon the results. Of course, patients must be cautioned appropriately and educated about what to expect from their treatments; when and how to call their practitioner for assistance. TCM practitioners are available to their patients who are taking herbs in case of questions or any adverse events. Beneficial use of pharmaceuticals and herbs together is an especially good example of how Western health care practitioners and TCM practitioners might work well together (7, 14–17).

The second main safety issue is the quality and purity of Chinese herbal medicines. There have been concerns about contamination with pesticides, heavy metals, bacteria, molds, prescription drugs, and other chemicals. These issues are discussed below.

Many Chinese herbs are harvested in the wild and are not exposed to pesticides. Whenever possible, natural pesticides are used. Some herbs are grown with pesticides, even those that are banned for some crops in the United States. American companies have tested for pesticides and generally find that there are no significant levels of these compounds found in Chinese herbs. Some American companies refuse to use herbs that have been exposed to pesticides, so pesticide-free herbs are available.

Concern arose over the use of sulfur in herb processing. This has not been shown to cause problems with sulfite-sensitive patients. There are companies in America that promise sulfur-free products.

Herbs may be irradiated for sterilization. This is thought not to be dangerous or lead to contamination by radioactivity. Raw herbs contain a certain amount of naturally occurring bacteria and mold that is not pathogenic. Levels higher than acceptable indicate improper storage and handling. Raw herbs and the manufacturer's finished products are tested in the United States for microbial contamination.

Heavy metals that may be detected in herbs such as mercury and arsenic are usually the result of intentional additions of herbals to the formulas to increase their effectiveness (i.e., cinnabar that contains mercury or realgar that contains arsenic.) Western manufacturers do not add these ingredients.

Some herbal products from China had been found to contain Western pharmaceuticals. The practice of adding pharmaceuticals to the herbs is common in China but banned in the United States. There are reports of drugs in Chinese herbal preparations sold in some Chinese herb stores in the United States. There have been incidences of severe illness and even death associated with the use of Chinese herbal medicines. One example is the renal toxicity associated with aristolochic acid. Patients who were using a specific herb mix for weight loss in the United Kingdom were exposed to aristocholic acid. The Food and Drug Administration stopped imports of aristolochia products after learning of several cases of kidney failure in Belgium and Great Britain. The illnesses in Europe were likely from using the incorrect forms of herbs that contained this toxic substance.

Chinese manufacturers who want to supply products to the West are improving their quality control, and regulations regarding manufacturing practices are being more stringently enforced. Some manufacturers in China would meet US GMP (Good Manufacturing Practices) and others would not. American herb companies and importers are now more savvy and aware of what to look for in herbal products. Reputable American companies test herbal products purchased from China. Some companies avoid Chinese-made products altogether and use herbs from more regulated countries or produce their own herbs in controlled circumstances within the United States.

Well-trained TCM practitioners are versed in choosing appropriate raw herbs and prepared products for their practices. This is another example of how partnering with a TCM practitioner would improve patient care and safety (18–20).

CONCLUSION

It is important to remember that, while TCM herbology is an exceptionally useful medicine in its own right, it is only one therapeutic modality available to the well-rounded practitioner of TCM. Acupuncture, Chinese nutritional principles, lifestyle modification, oriental movement and exercise practices, various forms of massage and other manual medicine, and moxibustion are just some of the other therapeutics in the TCM practitioner's tool kit. It is these diagnostic and therapeutic capabilities that can make the TCM practitioner a valued asset in patient care. A well-versed TCM practitioner can help alleviate illnesses, increase preventive care options, provide community education, and improve the safety of patients using herbal formulas and Western pharmaceuticals conjointly.

Regardless of the types of practitioner or the medicine they utilize, patients and their health and safety always remain the center of focus. Communication and collaboration among health care providers holds the promise of the ultimate in safe, effective patient care.

References

1. Bensky D, Gamble A. *Chinese Herbal Medicine Materia Medica*. Rev ed. Seattle: Eastland Press; 1993.
2. Maciocia G. *The Foundations of Chinese Medicine*. New York: Churchill Livingstone; 1989.
3. Beinfield H, Korngold E. *Between Heaven and Earth*. New York: Ballantine Books; 1991.
4. Dharmananda S. *The Treatment of Menopausal Syndrome with Chinese Herbs*. Institute for Traditional Medicine. www.itmonline.org. Accessed November 23, 2008.
5. Bensky D, Barolet R. *Chinese Herbal Medicine Formulas and Strategies*. Seattle: Eastland Press; 1990.
6. Maclean W. *Clinical Handbook of Internal Medicine—The Treatment of Disease with Traditional Chinese Medicine*. Macarthur, Australia: University of Western Sydney; 1998.

7. Sperber G, Flaws B. *Integrated Pharmacology*. Boulder, CO: Blue Poppy Press; 2007.
8. Ehling D. *The Chinese Herbalist's Handbook*. Santa Fe: InWord Press; 1996.
9. Accreditation Commission for Acupuncture and Oriental Medicine. www.acaom.org. Accessed November 16, 2008.
10. National Certification Commission for Acupuncture and Oriental Medicine. www.nccaom.org. Accessed November 16, 2008.
11. Acufinder. www.acufinder.com. Accessed December 6, 2008.
12. National Certification Commission for Acupuncture and Oriental Medicine. www.nccaom.org. Accessed December 15, 2008.
13. American Association of Oriental Medicine. www.aaaomonline.org. Accessed December 1, 2008.
14. Chen J, Chen T. *Chinese Medical Herbology and Pharmacology*. City of Industry Art of Medicine Press; 2004.
15. Chen J. Prevention of herb–drug interaction. www.medicalacupuncture.org/aama_marf/journal/vol10_2/herb-drug.html. Accessed December 18, 2008.
16. Hu Z. Herb–drug interactions: a literature review. *Drugs* 2005;65(9):1239–1282.
17. Fugh-Berman A. Herb–drug interactions. *Lancet* 2000;355(9198);134–138.
18. Chen J. Chinese herbs recalled due to possible contamination. *Acupunct Today* 2001;2(2) www.acupuncturetoday.com/mpacms/at/article.php?id=27762.
19. Dharmananda S. *How Clean and Pure are Chinese Herbs?* Institute for Traditional Medicine. www.itmonline.org. Accessed December 22, 2008.
20. Dobos GJ, Tan L, Cohen MH, et al. Are national quality standards for traditional Chinese herbal medicine sufficient? Current governmental regulations for traditional Chinese herbal medicine in certain Western countries and China as the Eastern origin country. *Complement Ther Med* 2005;13(3):183–190.

VII

Resources and Education

CHAPTER 41

Dietary Supplement Learning: Resources and Education

Robert Alan Bonakdar

As previous sections have pointed out, clinician and patient education are highly linked with the level of disclosure and discussion. With clinicians existing as dynamically evolving professionals who must adapt to changes in their field, educational resources are key for improving care. With that in mind, new paradigms of learning which are point-of-care, individualized, patient centered, and at the same time evidence-based are highly sought. The chapters in this section attempt to do that in different ways. Paula Gardiner, Rebecca Costello, and Julie Whelan summarize available resources to help clinicians find those that best address their needs and practice demands. Having seen Drs. Gardiner and Costello present this topic as an interactive workshop at the yearly conference: *Natural Supplements: An Evidence-Based Update* has provided examples of the real-world application of these resources for clinicians searching for point-of-care answers.

Dr. Sierpina then reviews strategies for clinician educators attempting to provide resources to those in training. As many clinicians are emerging, it is often noted that the education they receive is at times anything but emerging, but often based on outdated guidelines or consensus. Thus, to prepare the clinicians of tomorrow to address the areas of dietary supplement discussion, education, and management, it is pertinent to match their education to these evolving needs. Dr. Sierpina describes the innovative programs and case-based learning incorporated at his institution and others for meeting these important goals. The fundamental point of both chapters is that education should not be an obstacle but hopefully an accessible and fulfilling component of dietary supplement management.

CHAPTER 42

Resources on Dietary Supplements

Paula Gardiner, Julia Whelan, and Rebecca Costello

INTRODUCTION

There are many types of resources including textbooks, handbooks, pharmacopeias, monographs, Web sites, handheld computer databases, and online databases that provide information on dietary supplements. Every resource has its strength and weaknesses. It is up to the clinician to figure out what type of resource works for them. This chapter will focus on resources for the busy clinician.

TYPES OF RESOURCES: THEIR STRENGTHS AND WEAKNESSES

Although the quality of resources is improving, in the past dietary supplements resources were not always reliable. Many recommendations on safety and efficacy are based on traditional use, pharmacologic studies, in vitro and animal data, and case reports.

Much of the herbal literature comes from historical interpretation and poorly designed clinical trials which are difficult to interpret. This creates a challenge to the clinicians as they try to provide the best evidence-based information for their patients.

Evidence-based resources on dietary supplements should meet the following criteria: well referenced, written by authorities in the field, up-to-date, objective, evidence-based, noncommercial, and clinically relevant to the health care professional. In addition, information to be included in dietary supplement entries includes dietary supplement names, common names, basic pharmacology, dosage form, therapeutic uses, and information on special populations such as pregnancy, lactation, children, contraindications, adverse reactions, and interactions with pharmaceuticals or laboratory tests.

Throughout this chapter we will present several types of helpful resources available to quickly research dietary supplements. These include Web sites, handbooks, and monographs.

For our resources in this chapter, we used the following criteria.

- Are well referenced using evidence-based citations from primary literature based on high-quality data (such as clinical trials, systematic reviews, and meta-analyses)
- Evaluates the scientific accuracy of empirical data, how well the information is referenced, and whether the information is current

- Appropriate site text is intended for educational or clinical purposes and is clearly written and logically organized
- Organization is reputable and long-standing (government sites, professional organizations, educational institutions, nonprofit businesses)
- Nonbiased in text (balanced coverage in representing all the arguments)
- Includes information on adverse reactions, interactions with drugs, laboratory tests and diseases, safety in pregnancy, and lactation and adverse reactions
- "Clinically useful" in providing patient care
- Site is reviewed and updated on a regular basis and notice of last review date should be posted on the site
- Easy to use and navigate the Web site
- Web designer clearly states who they are and how to contact them.

WEB SITES BY SUBSCRIPTION SERVICES

These require an annual subscription or that the user purchases a license for the product.

AltMedDex

www.micromedex.com/products/altmeddex
More than 300 supplements are covered in excellent monographs, summaries, and consults, as well as entries on toxicological management. Patient information sheets on dietary supplements and medical conditions are included. The database is updated semiannually. This is a component of the larger Micromedex product, published by Thomson and cannot be purchased separately. (Handheld version and patient information sheets available.)

LexiComp

http://www.lexi.com/web/index.jsp
Lexi-Natural Products, published by LexiComp, is a palm-based, online, or desktop available software that covers 175 commonly used dietary supplements including herbs, vitamins, minerals, and other dietary supplements. Each monograph includes dosage and standardization, reported uses, active forms, pharmacology, general warnings, and other key information. (Individual subscriber $75.00 to $150.00.) (Handheld and handbook available.)

Natural Medicines Comprehensive Database

www.naturaldatabase.com
Created by the publishers of the *Pharmacist's Letter*. You can search by supplement or commercial product name. More than 1,000 monographs include extensive information about common uses, evidence of efficacy and safety, mechanisms, interactions, and dosage. Monographs are extensively referenced and updated daily. There is a drug/supplement interactions checker. Also CME, listserv, effectiveness checker, and personalized interaction profiles information are available. NMCD has consistently and independently been rated as a top resource for herb and supplement information (1, 2). (Individual subscriber full database $92/y, Handheld version $59. Available as a book (3) and patient information sheets available.)

Natural Standard

www.naturalstandard.com
Natural Standard is an independent collaboration of international clinicians and researchers who create evidence-based monographs on dietary supplements and other modalities available online. This extensive database can be searched by subject or by medical condition. There is a drug/supplement interactions checker, brand name database. The quality of evidence is graded for each supplement. (An abridged version is available for the desktop computer or hand held. Patient information sheets, handbook and desk reference (4) also available. PDA version is $79 for individual subscriber.)

HerbMed

www.herbmed.org
HerbMed is an herbal database that provides scientific data underlying the use of herbs. HerbMedPro, an enhanced version of HerbMed, is available for subscription, licensing, and data streaming. The public site has 40 herbs; HerbMedPro has an additional 128 herbs and continuous updating and also has a pay per day program for $5.99. (Free/subscription/other.)

WEB SITES FOR FREE

CAMline

http://www.camline.ca/about/about.html
Created in Canada, CAMline is an evidence-based nonprofit Web site on complementary and alternative medicine (CAM) for health care professionals and the public. It represents a successful collaboration of conventional and integrative medicine organizations, their interests, and expertise. It has 35 monographs on dietary supplements written for the consumer and health care professional. (Patient information sheets available.)

MD Anderson Cancer Center

http://www.mdanderson.org/departments/CIMER/dIndex.cfm
This Web site is sponsored by the University of Texas MD Anderson Cancer Center. It is a clearing house for patients with cancer on dietary supplements and CAM. The site includes approximately 60 dietary supplement monographs from Natural Standard, Cochrane Review Organization, National Cancer Institute—Office of Cancer Complementary and Alternative Medicine, and the National Center for Complementary and Alternative Medicine. (Patient information sheets available.)

Memorial Sloan-Kettering Cancer Center

www.mskcc.org/mskcc/html/11570.cfm
Approximately 340 monographs on dietary supplements are available on the Memorial Sloan-Kettering Cancer Center Web site. These dietary supplement monographs are comparatively brief with only the most salient references, but their summaries are generally accurate. The Web site provides easy access to clinically relevant information about botanics, vitamins, and related products for health care professionals and consumers. The Web site is updated daily as new findings or warnings

are released and a site-wide review of each monograph is performed twice a year. (Patient information sheets available.)

GOVERNMENT RESOURCES

National Library of Medicine

PubMed[1]

http://www.ncbi.nlm.nih.gov/entrez/query.fcgi?DB=pubmed
PubMed is a service of the United States National Library of Medicine that includes more than 17 million citations from MEDLINE and other life science journals for biomedical articles back to the 1950s. PubMed includes links to full text articles and other related resources and a number of very helpful online tutorials. For dietary supplement research we recommend you use the clinical queries search on PubMed located on the left-hand tool bar. PubMed can be helpful for looking up rare or unusual dietary supplements. (Free)

MEDLINE PLUS—ALTERNATIVE MEDICINE

http://www.nlm.nih.gov/medlineplus
This consumer health database from the National Library of Medicine offers extensive information on CAM treatments.

Links to CAM sites are organized using the same alternative medicine medical subject headings used by the National Library of Medicine. (Free) Some of the Natural Standard abridged monographs are available under the dietary supplements link. http://www.nlm.nih.gov/medlineplus/druginformation.html

Food and Drug Administration Dietary Supplements Page

http://vm.cfsan.fda.gov/~dms/supplmnt.html
The Food and Drug Administration (FDA) regulates foods including dietary supplements. Helpful information on its Web site includes updates on policy, regulation, and product warning notices as well as many consumer-oriented documents. (Free)

The National Center for Complementary and Alternative Medicine

http://www.nccam.nih.gov
The National Center for Complementary and Alternative Medicine (NCCAM) is the federal government's lead agency for scientific research on CAM. The mission of NCCAM is to explore complementary and alternative healing practices in the context of rigorous science, train CAM researchers, and disseminate authoritative information to the public and professionals. Look for the Alerts and Advisories, treatment information, resources, and links to other organizations (FDA, AHRQ, ODS etc.) *Herbs at a Glance*, a series of patient information sheets, is listed at http://nccam.nih.gov/health/herbsataglance.htm

[1] Primary literature: use these databases to search for original scientific studies and reviews of the medical literature. PubMed and IBIDS are examples listed in this chapter.

National Institutes of Health Office of Dietary Supplements

http://ods.od.nih.gov/

The mission of Office of Dietary Supplements is to strengthen knowledge and understanding of dietary supplements by evaluating scientific information, stimulating and supporting research, disseminating research results, and educating the public to foster an enhanced quality of life and health for the US population. This is a very helpful site; under Health Information you will find excellent dietary supplement fact sheets. http://ods.od.nih.gov/Health_Information/Information_About_Individual_Dietary_Supplements.aspx. (Free) (Patient information sheets available.)

International Bibliographic Information on Dietary Supplements[1]

http://ods.od.nih.gov/showpage.aspx?pageid=48

IBIDS is produced by the Office of Dietary Supplements, National Institutes of Health, along with the Food and Nutrition Information Center, National Agricultural Library, and United States Department of Agriculture. The IBIDS database provides access to bibliographic citations and abstracts from published, international, and scientific literature on dietary supplements. IBIDS contains more than 750,000 citations on the topic of dietary supplements from four major database sources: biomedical-related articles from MEDLINE, botanic and agricultural science from AGRICOLA, worldwide agricultural literature through AGRIS, and selected nutrition journals from CAB Abstracts and CAB Health. IBIDS is available free of charge.

HANDHELD RESOURCES

Handheld computers or PDAs have become extremely popular with medical professionals especially for drug information. Many of the drug information publishers also offer information on herbs and dietary supplements. Table 42.1 provides brief entries on general drug information applications which have some information on herbs and dietary supplements. A recent review rated LexiDrugs Platinum highest for drug information but noted, "this version contained virtually no information on dietary supplements, including information on herb-drug interactions . . ." (5). The inclusion of dietary supplement information is one of the principal differences between the free ePocrates version, which is available only for Palm, and ePocrates Rx Pro (5).

Table 42.2 lists PDA applications which focus on herb and supplement information. In a recent comparative review, National Medicines was selected as the most comprehensive whereas others were considered adequate for the occasional lookup (6). However, the PDA version of Natural Medicines does not have the mechanism-of-action field as well as the references which are included in the online and print versions. A major problem with mobileMICROMEDEX is that its dietary supplement content is not integrated with its drug interaction utility, so it cannot monitor for herb—drug interactions. The Guide to Natural Products was the only application that has pictures of dietary supplements and a section on their history, but this information is not typically useful to clinicians (5).

HANDBOOKS

The publishing of references on herbs and dietary supplements intended for clinicians continues to grow at a rapid pace making it difficult to choose from a crowded

TABLE 42.1 PDA Drug Information Resources with Information on Herbs and Dietary Supplements

Title	Web Site	Notes
ClinicalPharmacology OnHand	http://www.clinicalpharmacologyonhand.com/	Monographs, drug-natural product–nutritionals interactions, updated daily
DrDrugs	Davis's Drug Guide for Physicians http://www.skyscape.com/estore/ProductDetail.aspx?ProductId=220	Natural products monograph, drug-natural product and food interactions
ePocratesPro	http://www.epocrates.com	Inclusion of DS information is major difference between ePocrates and ePocratesPro (5). Alternative section >400 herbals, info comes from Natural Medicines Comprehensive Database. MultiCheck drug interactions program up to 30 drugs-natural products at once
Lexi-Drugs	http://www.lexi.com	Drug–herbal interactions can link to Lexi-Natural Products (see Table 2)
Natural Standard	www.naturalstandard.com	
mobileMICROMEDEX	http://www.micromedex.com	Alternative medicine monographs can not monitor for interactions
Physician's Drug Handbook	Physician's Drug Handbook, http:lww.com	Appendices on herbs
Pocket PDR	http://www.PDR.net	Has alternative medicine section
Tarascon Pocket Pharmacopoeia	http://www.tarascon.com	Herbal and alternative therapy section

field of similar references. With the time involved in writing, editing, and publishing these books, the information in handbooks quickly becomes out of date. Recent studies have evaluated handbooks by looking at how well they answer drug information questions, which ones are used in drug information centers, and by evaluating them against a set of objective criteria (11–13). Table 42.3 lists the three handbooks, *Natural Standard Herb and Supplement Handbook: The Clinical Bottom Line*; *Mosby's Handbook of Herbs and Supplements and Their Therapeutic Uses*; and *Mosby's Handbook of Herbs & Natural Supplements*, that have been rated highly.

The information presented in these three books was more balanced, well-referenced, and more complete than in the other handbooks. However, handbooks

TABLE 42.2 PDA Applications Focused on Herb and Supplement Information

Title	Source	Notes
5-Minute Herb and Dietary Supplement Consult	Online version of Fugh-Berman's book—Skyscape's technology allows herbal information to cross-index with other clinical and drug products (7).	Succinct, reliable information on herbs, minerals, vitamins, amino acids, probiotics, enzymes, over-the-counter hormones, and other dietary supplements. An A-to-Z list. Also claims, indications, scientific evidence, benefits, adverse effects, contraindications, drug interactions, and dosage, frequently asked questions.
Alticopeia	DDH Software Only available for PDA. Written by David I Rappaport, a medical student at Jefferson Medical College, Philadelphia. Inexpensive. http://www.ddhsoftware.com/description.html?II=rtalticope&UID=	Overview and uses for 400 herbs and dietary supplements. Includes names, scientific/Latin name, uses, scientific information, and findings of German Commission E, cautions, usual daily doses, references. Search by indications and sort by uses.
Guide to Popular Natural Products—also called GNP3	Facts and Comparisons. http://www.factsandcomparisons.com Skyscape. Abridged from Review of Natural Products (8)	Entries on 125 most popular herbs. Scientific/common names, patient information, references and abridged sections on botany/source, history, pharmacology, and toxicology. Lacks vitamins and minerals and standard dose. Has pictures and a full history of HDS—information may not be useful to clinicians (5).
Herballx	Facts and Comparisons http://www.factsandcomparisons.com Skyscape Print equivalent is Drug Interaction Facts: Herbal Supplements and Food, Facts and Comparisons (9)	Covers only possible drug/herb and drug/food interactions for >100 herbs. Organized by herbal product. Discusses significance, onset, severity, documentation, effects, mechanism, and management and reference sections.

(continued)

TABLE 42.2 *(Continued)*

Title	Source	Notes
Lexi-Natural Products	http://www.lexi.com Information from Natural Therapeutics Pocket Guide (10)	>175 natural products (neutraceuticals, vitamins, minerals, glandulars, herbs, amino acids). Each monograph includes dosage and standardization, reported uses, active forms, pharmacology, general warnings, and other key information.
Natural Medicines	Abridged from Natural Medicines Comprehensive Database http://naturaldatabase.com Palm and Pocket PC versions	Evidence-based info on herbs, vitamins, minerals. *Effectiveness Checker*, *Natural Product/Drug Interaction Checker*, updated daily, info on interactions, uses, and adverse effects; Brands, ingredients, and manufacturers; Ratings on efficacy and safety.
Natural Standard	Abridged version of full database http://naturalstandard.com Skyscape links to other applications.	Includes complementary and alternative therapies in addition to HDS. Evidence-based reviews. New release.

have their own strengths and weakness, some have more details on dosing or interactions whereas others emphasize indications or safety. In light of this, clinicians may want to consider their information priorities when making a selection or purchasing complementary references (14). Handbooks written for nurses generally offer more patient information such as the well-reviewed *Nursing 2006 Herbal Medicine Handbook* (15) and *Mosby's Handbook of Herbs & Natural Supplements* (16). The

TABLE 42.3 Handbooks for Clinicians

Basch EM, Ulbricht CE. *Natural Standard Herb and Supplement Handbook: The clinical bottom line.* St. Louis, MO: Elsevier Mosby; 2005. ISBN 0323029930 $37.95

Bratman S, Girman A. *Mosby's Handbook of Herbs and Supplements and Their Therapeutic Uses*. St. Louis, MO: Mosby/Healthgate; 2003. ISBN 0323020151 $37.95

Skidmore-Roth L. *Mosby's Handbook of Herbs & Natural Supplements.* 3rd ed. St. Louis: Mosby; 2006. ISBN 0323037062 $39.95

Natural Therapeutics Pocket Guide (10) also received favorable comments but an updated edition would be welcome (1, 2).

INFORMATION ON THIRD-PARTY TESTING FOR QUALITY SUPPLEMENTS

United States Pharmacopeia Dietary Supplement Verification Program

www.uspverified.org

The United States Pharmacopeia has recently initiated this volunteer program that manufacturers of dietary supplements can enter which is very rigorous. Manufacturers need to demonstrate Good Manufacturing Practices to earn the United States Pharmacopeia certification.

ConsumerLab

www.consumerlab.com

ConsumerLab evaluates commercially available dietary supplement products for composition, potency, purity, bioavailability, and consistency of products. The Natural Pharmacist database offers consumer-oriented information. Products that meet its criteria can receive a ConsumerLab seal of approval. (Annual subscription fee of $24)

National Health Products Directorate, from Health Canada

http://www.hc-sc.gc.ca/dhp-mps/prodnatur/index_e.html

This Web site is maintained by the national health products directorate from Health Canada. It contains a list of all the dietary supplements that have been licensed in Canada.

NSF International

http://www.nsf.org

NSF is a nonprofit company that provides rigorous third-party testing of dietary supplements. Its Web site provides a list of all the supplements companies that have passed its inspection.

MONOGRAPHS AND OTHER HELPFUL RESOURCES

There are a few more helpful resources that we wanted to mention that are not listed above. They are very helpful in the clinical setting.

ABC Clinical Guide to Herbs

Blumenthal M, Brinckmann J, and Wollschlaeger B. *The ABC Clinical Guide to Herbs*. Austin, TX: American Botanic Council; 2003. This book has very thorough monographs, patient information sheets, and excellent summary charts of clinical trials on specific herbs and brands (helpful for dosing). Very helpful resource from an independent science-based nonprofit organization: www.herbalgram.org.

American Herbal Pharmacopoeia and Therapeutic Compendium

www.herbal-ahp.org

American Herbal Pharmacopoeia is a nonprofit organization founded in 1995 that writes excellent scientifically based monographs that focus on the identity, purity, and quality of herbs. It has currently published 18 monographs that are available on the Web. Each monograph is $89.95.

World Health Organization

http://whqlibdoc.who.int/publications/1999/9241545178.pdf

Many of the World Health Organizations herbal monographs are available on the Internet for free. They are very comprehensive monographs compiled and reviewed by scientific experts.

References

1. Chambliss W, Hufford C, Flagg M, Glisson J. Assessment of the quality of reference books on botanical dietary supplements. *J Am Pharm Assoc* 2002;42(5):723–724.
2. Sweet B, Gay W, Leady M, Stumpf J. Usefulness of herbal and dietary supplement references[see comment]. *Ann Pharmacother* 2003;37(4):494–499.
3. Jellin J. *Natural Medicines Comprehensive Database*. 8 ed. Stockton, CA: 2005.
4. Ulbricht C, Basch E. *Natural Standard Herb & Supplement Reference: Evidence-Based Clinical Reviews*. St. Louis, MO: 2005.
5. Clauson KA, Seamon MJ, Clauson AS, Van TB. Evaluation of drug information databases for personal digital assistants. *Am J Health Syst Pharm* 2004;61(10):1015–1024.
6. Kupferberg N, Hartel L. Herbal databases for PDAs: advice from two librarians. *Journal Electronic Resour Med Libr* 2004;1(3):43–55.
7. Fugh-Berman A. *The 5-Minute Herb and Dietary Supplement Consult*. Philadelphia: 2003.
8. DerMarderosian A. *The Review of Natural Products: The Most Complete Source of Natural Product Information*. 4 ed. St. Louis, MO: Facts and Comparisons; 2005.
9. Tatro D. *Drug Interaction Facts: The Authority on Drug Interactions*. St. Louis, MO: Facts and Comparisons; 2006.
10. Krinsky D. *Natural Therapeutics Pocket Guide*. 2 ed. Hudson, OH: Lexi-Comp; 2003.
11. Shields KM, McQueen CE, Bryant PJ. Factors affecting dietary supplement resource selections in drug information centers. *J Am Pharm Assoc (Wash DC)* 2004;44(6):716–718.
12. Dvorkin L, Whelan J, Timarac S. Harvesting the best: evidence-based analysis of herbal handbooks for clinicians. *J Med Libr Assoc* 2006;94(4):208–213.
13. Walker J. Evaluation of the ability of seven herbal resources to answer questions about herbal products asked in drug information centers. *Pharmacotherapy* 2002;22(12): 1611–1615.
14. West P. Telephone service for providing consumers with information on herbal supplements. *Am J Health Syst Pharm* 2001;58(19):1842–1846.
15. Staff S. *Nursing 2006 Herbal Medicine Handbook*. Philadelphia: 2005.
16. Skidmore-Roth L. *Mosby's Handbook of Herbs & Natural Supplements*. 2 ed. St. Louis: 2004.

CHAPTER 43

Dietary Supplement Education in Health Care Training

Victor S. Sierpina

The doctor of the future will give no medicine, but will interest his patients in the care of the human frame, in diet, and in the cause and prevention of disease.—Thomas Alva Edison

Integrative Medicine is healing oriented medicine that takes account of the whole person (body, mind, and spirit), including all aspects of lifestyle. It emphasizes the therapeutic relationship and makes use of all appropriate therapies, both convention and alternative.—University of Arizona Center for Integrative Medicine (www.integrativemedicine.arizona.edu)

Integrative Medicine is the practice of medicine that reaffirms the importance of the relationship between practitioner and patient, focuses on the whole person, is informed by evidence, and makes use of all appropriate therapeutic approaches, healthcare professionals and disciplines to achieve optimal health and healing.—Consortium of Academic Health Centers for Integrative Medicine (www.imconsortium.org)

INTRODUCTORY WEB CASE FOR THIRD-YEAR FAMILY MEDICINE CLERKSHIP STUDENTS

"Flaxseed Case" (Synopsized)

A healthy, independent 84-year-old female comes to establish care with me because she has heard I am willing to discuss nutritional supplements. Her history includes atrial fibrillation, hypertension, and osteoporosis. She is on four prescription medications for these including warfarin and a calcium channel blocker. In addition, she brings a hand-written list of more than 20 supplements that she uses for nutritional support and disease prevention/management. While I am familiar with most of these, some are novel and I inquire to the patient as to why she is taking them.

{Web-Case presents a hand-written copy of patient supplements plus a somewhat more legible typed version for students to review.

Students are asked how they would approach this patient, how they would find information about her supplements, and are provided with links to both general information and potential drug–herb-supplement interactions. They need to submit their responses and answers to questions about interactions.}

As it turns out, there are at least five possible interactions, primarily with warfarin. These include ginkgo, Co-enzyme Q10, ginseng, vitamin E, and fish oil that are easily identified through the library-server hosted databases.

{Students are asked how to manage the issue of potential drug–supplement interactions and to post their responses Their responses are reviewed online by faculty.}

The patient is informed of interactions but has been on the combination of medications and supplements for years without difficulty and does not wish to change anything. She thanks us for our advice and leaves for one of her three seasonal homes in as many states.

At least three learning opportunities are presented here: (i) How to access information about unfamiliar herbs or supplements, (ii) How to determine potential or significant interactions with prescription medications and realistically assess risk, and (iii) How to communicate in a relationship-centered way with a patient using multiple supplements and medications.

This case was presented at a Society of Teachers of Family Medicine national conference as an example of "just in time learning." Adult learning is best done in the context of problem solving and this "Flaxseed case" presented several immediate issues. This approach is on one of "teaching by doing." Students learning from being presented with a real-life cases that require them to identify reliable, evidence-based databases regarding herbs and supplements. Furthermore, they observe a model or approach on how to communicate with an elderly but cognitively sharp year 84 old who has "done quite well, thank you" on this combination. Of note, this patient had a mild stroke this year at age 87. (To see complete case, go to http://www.designacase.org. Username: flaxseed. Password: guest)

Other online cases required for student's completion of the clerkship imbed learning issues about culturally based treatments, supplements, herbs, and other complementary therapies into disease-specific problems such as hypertension, headache, diabetes, and so on. A useful Design-a-Case software is available to utilize existing cases and to design new cases appropriate to local populations, culture, and student or resident usage. (For further information, contact http://www.designacase.org.)

BACKGROUND

The physician of the future must be trained today to practice medicine that does not yet exist. Competencies needed by health care practitioners of the future will to be defined by the kind of future in which they will practice (1, 2).

Integrative medicine is an ideal foundation onto which to base the future of health care. Combining the best evidence from both conventional and alternative practices, this holistic worldview that sees people as complete in mind, body, and spirit offers the most comprehensive and suitable method of providing health care. Lifestyle, culture, religious and health care beliefs, noninvasive and cost-effective treatments, and interdisciplinary, team-based care are all parts of this model.

Clearly, with the rapid pace of information dissemination, new knowledge, and techniques in both conventional and alternative medicine, **critical thinking skills** are essential to create an "informed intermediary" between the patient and glut of information and misinformation now available.

Lifelong learning skills are equally important as both the information presented in medical schools and other health care curricula as well as the context in which it is delivered becomes outdated or even obsolete. Flexibility of thinking and behavior and maintaining a robust self-directed learning program are essential behaviors for providers of the future. These must be taught and role-modeled in medical school and residency.

Finally, a **knowledge base in the domain of integrative medicine** is essential to provide a solid foundation on which to scaffold future learning and practice. Students and residents are highly challenged to learn the basic skills and information necessary to pass their required national step examinations and in-service and board examinations. Adding a requirement to learn information about dietary supplements is not necessarily good news as it requires additional time and effort.

However, by integrating such information into cases, clinical care, problem solving, and critical thinking exercises and by making it easily available through books, online databases, personal digital assistant hardware, and open discussion of supplement usage with patients and faculty, the context and content of such knowledge becomes part of everyday practice.

A new approach to the challenges of residency training in this area is the Integrative Medicine in Residency pilot project. Integrative Medicine in Residency is a 200-hour curriculum development project of the University of Arizona Center for Integrative Medicine that will create and deliver competency-based online integrative medical training to residents. Integrative Medicine in Residency is initially being piloted in eight family medicine residencies with the goal of expanding to primary care and subspecialty training programs throughout the United States and abroad.

This competency-based curriculum in Integrative Medicine is designed to be incorporated into the typical 3-year residency program, with a common Web-based curriculum, program-specific experiential exercises, and group process-oriented activities. Active online discussions will cross individual residencies and a larger community of learners will develop. The curriculum will have a comprehensive evaluation system.

Perhaps the best teachers in this realm are the patients themselves as they are often high users of supplements, vitamins, herbals, probiotics, and other over-the-counter products. Simply by asking patients during the medication history what "other OTC products such as nutritional supplements, herbs, or similar medications" they are taking, opens the learner (and experienced practitioner as well) to a universe of new learning opportunities.

CASE STUDY

Well, I take alpha lipoic acid, fish oil, CoQ10, nattokinase, ginseng, ginkgo, a multivitamin, Vitamins C, D, and E, as well as magnesium, calcium, and a probiotic, reported an 86-year-old retired veterinarian who is in vibrant health mentally and physically.

Again, this case presents the learner with an opportunity to (i) dismiss all of this information as irrelevant, (ii) warn the patient that none of these products are standardized, safe, or evidence-based, (iii) recommend stopping all since several may interact with current medications, or (iv) inquire as to why the patient has selected each product and then to research and learn current data on evidence of safety, efficacy, and product quality.

In the view of the patient, she has taken considerable time and expense to create this supplement plan to improve her cardiovascular risk, reduce neuropathic pain, improve her immunity and energy, manage her osteoporosis, and more. In the view of the busy but uninformed resident or medical student, this information is "noise" in the context of getting a disease-focused history and physical and coming up with an assessment and medical therapeutic plan.

A more productive learning experience is selecting option #iv above and taking time to listen to the patient's own knowledge and experience and then perhaps at a later time when clinic is over, to access books, journals, and databases that can further inform the clinical student or practitioner on these supplements.

PUTTING RESOURCES, LEARNING, AND PATIENT CARE TOGETHER

In truth, major issues in educating future health care practitioners are effective communication, building trust, and developing a style of practice that enhances patient-centered care (3). This also means looking for opportunities as in the cases above to understand the what, why, and how of the patient's choices of supplements.

This is hard work for the busy practitioner, resident, or student and cannot all be done at the point of care. Yet the point of care, the patient experience itself, and the trend of increased usage of supplements among patients all require increased attention to matters we would perhaps prefer to avoid.

A general introduction to the usage of supplements is often best done in the context of a classroom lecture, CME, grand rounds, or hospital staff conference. This orients attendees to the general issues, evidence, safety, efficacy, and interaction issues. It also presents an opportunity to address concerns, share resources, and provide validation for supplement use as part of medical practice. Such role modeling, be it before practicing physicians, nurses, or students at any level, has a major impact in changing culture and directing change toward more integrative approaches to care.

The most efficient method of addressing many learning issues at any point in the professional training process is to identify usable, reliable sources of information about natural products, supplements, botanics, and the like. We easily look at our PDA or the PDR for information about drugs and their dosages, interactions, and so forth. Now, we easily have similar access to information about herbs and supplements online, on a PDA, and free or subscription services. A detailed review of these resources is presented in chapter 42.

Some of the references we find particularly useful in teaching in the clinical setting are ePocrates, Natural Medicines Comprehensive Database, the PDR Herbal version, HealthNotes Online, AltMedex, Natural Standard, Consumer Lab, National Institutes of Health (NIH) Office of Dietary Supplements (ODS), International Bibliographic Information on Dietary Supplements (IBIDS) among others.

In addition to online resources, there are a number of reliable textbooks that provide excellent background in this area for students, residents, and graduate health care practitioners. Recommended textbooks are reviewed in Table 43.1. While I modestly recommend my own book, Integrative Healthcare: Complementary and Alternative Therapies for the Whole Person (now out of print but available through Amazon.com), a number of up-to-date sources are highly useful. Dr. David Rakel's Integrative Medicine is excellent for practicality, evidence-based, usable information. He has assembled a vast array of information on common problems and therapies that is both readable and immediately applicable. Each chapter has a Therapeutic Review in which the various supplements and other therapies useful

TABLE 43.1 Textbooks Available in the Area of Dietary Supplements and Integrative Medicine

Textbook	Author/Editors and Publishing Information
Integrative Healthcare: Complementary and Alternative Therapies for the Whole Person	Victor S. Sierpina, MD Publisher: Davis FA Pub. Date: December 2000 ISBN-13: 9780803607040
Integrative Medicine; 2nd Edition	David Rakel, MD Publisher: Elsevier Health Sciences Pub. Date: February 2007 ISBN-13: 9781416029540
Integrative Medicine: Principles for Practice	Benjamin Kligler, MD, Roberta A. Lee, MD Publisher: The McGraw-Hill Companies, Pub. Date: April 2004 ISBN-13: 9780071402392
The Desktop Guide to Complementary and Alternative Medicine: An Evidence-Based Approach; 2nd Edition	Edzard Ernst, M.D, PhD, FRCP, Max H Pittler, MD, PhD, Barbara Wider, MA (Editors) Publisher: Elsevier Health Sciences Pub. Date: August 2006 ISBN-13: 9780723433835
The ABC Clinical Guide to Herbs	Mark Blumenthal, Josef Brinckmann, Bernd Wollschlaeger, MD Publisher: Thieme Medical Publishers, Incorporated Pub. Date: April 2003 ISBN-13: 9781588901576

for say, diabetes, atopic dermatitis, heart disease, dysmenorrhea, and so forth, are neatly summarized along with icons for levels of evidence and safety. These reviews are also available through a PDA download enhancing portability and accessibility.

I recommend to my residents and students that once they have seen a particular problem, for example, hypertension, CHF, depression, they leaf through the pertinent chapter in Rakel's Integrative Medicine with special attention to the Therapeutic Review. A few times doing this helps promote an integrative approach that addresses prevention, exercise, mind–body approaches, pharmaceuticals, as well as botanics, nutrition, and supplements.

Another excellent text reference which includes a CME test component booklet is Drs. Benjamin Kligler and Roberta Lee's Integrative Medicine: Principles for Practice. It is organized by body system with numerous case reviews. Dr. Edzard Ernst has published a second edition of his highly useful evidence-based summaries, The Desktop Guide to Complementary and Alternative Medicine. The American Botanic Council's The ABC Clinical Guide to Herbs by Mark Blumenthal contains

TABLE 43.2 Continuing Medical Education (CME) Courses Available in the Area of Dietary Supplements and Integrative Medicine

CME Course (Sponsor)	Further Information
Natural Supplements: An Evidence-Based Update (Scripps Center for Integrative Medicine/Scripps Clinic)	www.ScrippsIntegrativeMedicine.org
Nutrition in Health (University of Arizona/Columbia University)	www.nutritionandhealthconf.org/
Food as Medicine (Center for Mind-Body Medicine)	www.cmbm.org
Applying Functional Medicine in Clinical Practice (The Institute for Functional Medicine)	www.functionalmedicine.org
American Board of Integrative and Holistic Medicine Annual Review and Board Preparation Course	www.holisticboard.org www.scripps.org
American Holistic Nursing Association Annual Conference	http://www.ahna.org/

thorough monographs, patient information sheets, and summaries of clinic trials on 28 common herbs.

In addition, many conferences are offered annually for physicians, nurses, and other health care practitioners who provide practical clinical information in the area of supplement use. These courses are summarized in Table 43.2.

ONLINE LEARNING

The University of Minnesota has several Web-based modules that we require of our students and residents. These provide a useful background to the rational prescribing of herbs and supplements and are freely available online (http://www.csh.umn.edu/modules/index.html). Other courses that learners may use include Drs. Kathy Kemper and Paula Gardiner's online course on Dietary Herbs and Supplements which was developed through an NIH grant through Wake Forest University (www1.wfubmc.edu/phim/About/Misc/Herbs+Supplements.htm). Their research documents the benefit of this mode of dietary supplement education for health care providers (4).

CREATING LEARNING OPPORTUNITIES

The key issues in the training context are (i) make learners aware of the broad use of supplements by the general public, (ii) teach them to inquire nonjudgmentally about patient use of supplements, and (iii) provide easily accessible, reliable, evidence-based resources (databases, Web sites, books, etc.) where they can research and learn about the wide array of products patients are taking.

Getting these resources into students' hands is relatively easy. I have purchased a number of the above-mentioned books for interns, students, hospital and clinic workrooms, the library, and so forth, through various educational funds. Although students and residents more and more rely on online and PDA references for their learning issues, an easily accessible handbook (like this one) or textbook is still a highly practical and efficient source of needed clinical information. Encouraging the library at your hospital or medical center to have at least one reliable online reference and a few key print resources related to supplements is not generally difficult nor inordinately expensive for its budget. Natural Medicines Comprehensive Database would be my choice if you can afford only one license (institutional license is around $1,800 for five users currently and about $125 for individuals). The Rakel Integrative Medicine textbook would be my choice if you only have room on the shelves or in the budget for one text (under $100).

Creating the opportunities for students to then actually *use* these materials in their study and practice is a matter of curriculum design whether through problem-based learning, team-based learning, bedside teaching, clinical cases, standardized patient examinations, written or oral examination, or other realistic incentives for study and application. Indeed, just having taken the American Board of Family Medicine recertification examination as well as their Maintenance of Certification examination, I noted an increasing number of questions related to supplements and other complementary therapies. This is true in other specialty board examination as well, for example, Internal Medicine, Obstetrics and Gynecology, Psychiatry, and Pediatrics. The Licensing Commission for Medical Education (LCME sets the standards for medical school accreditation) has incorporated complementary and integrative medicine into its educational standards. The American Board of Integrative and Holistic Medicine also offers an overview course and certification examination (see Table 43.1) that is a useful curriculum on supplements for the postgraduate physician (www.holisticboard.org). All of these are examples of how this area is gradually entering mainstream medical training.

CONCLUSION

There are many forces influencing changes in medical education including efforts by individual medical schools, the National Center for Complementary and Alternative Medicine at the NIH (http://nccam.nih.gov/), and groups such as the Consortium of Academic Health Centers for Integrative Medicine (www.imconsortium.org). Increasing sophistication of patients about supplement use, concerns by public policy-making bodies about such use, and the need for education of health care providers all will continue to be hydraulic forces in moving learners into becoming more sophisticated in their use and knowledge of supplements. Two important background documents which reinforce this trend include the White House Commission on Complementary and Alternative Medicine Policy Report and the Institute of Medicine Report on Complementary and Alternative Medicine in the United States (5, 6). Additionally, the Institute of Medicine held a national its most highly attended Summit on Integrative Medicine and the Health of the Public in February 2009 (http://iom.edu). The Summit explored the role of integrative health care within the

US and international health care systems. Topics included education, workforce, science, economics, policy, clinical models, and a vision of the future of health care (7). As educators, we need to ensure that in the area of herbs and supplements, students presented with relevant clinical problems, high-yield, time-efficient resources, and proper faculty mentoring and encouragement will be well prepared for the medicine of the future.

ACKNOWLEDGMENTS

The author thanks Wanetta Prelow for her work in manuscript preparation and many of the authors for their extensive work, Web site designers, and educators cited in the references for creating a broad body of information on supplements and their use. Dr. Sierpina's work is supported in part by the W.D. and Laura Nell Nicholson Family Professorship in Integrative Medicine and the University of Texas Medical Branch Academy of Master Teachers (http://www.utmb.edu/amt). The author also thanks National Center for Complementary and Alternative Medicine including their Educational Enhancement Grant (R25 AT000586-02) for their extensive support of education and information in this area. HRSA/BHPR Predoctoral Grant D56 HP 08345, Longitudinal Exposure to Complex Medical/Societal Problems in Family Medicine 2007–2010 (Principal Investigator, G. Shokar)
{This grant funded the Design a Case project cited at the beginning of the chapter}.

References

1. Sierpina VS. Teaching integratively: how the next generation of doctors will practice. *Integr Cancer Ther* 2004;3(3):201–207.
2. Sierpina VS, Schneeweiss R, Frenkel MA, et al. Barriers, strategies, and lessons learned from complementary and alternative medicine curricular initiatives. *Acad Med* 2007;82 (10):946–950.
3. Waters D, Sierpina VS. Goal-directed health care and the chronic pain patient: a new vision of the healing encounter. *Pain Physician* 2006;9(4):353–360.
4. Beal T, Kemper KJ, Gardiner P, Woods C. Long-term impact of four different strategies for delivering an on-line curriculum about herbs and other dietary supplements. *BMC Med Educ* 2006;6:39.
5. White House Commission on Complementary and Alternative Medicine Policy. http://www.whccamp.hhs.gov/fr4.html. Accessed July 22, 2008.
6. Institute of Medicine (IOM) Report: Complementary and Alternative Medicine in the United States. http://www.nap.edu/catalog.php?record_id=11182. Accessed July 22, 2008.
7. Institute of Medicine. *Integrative medicine and the health of the public: a summary of the February 2009 summit*. Washington, DC: The National Academies Press, 2009.

VIII

Case Studies

CHAPTER 44

HERBAL Mnemonic in Practice: Patient Case Studies

Robert Alan Bonakdar

The following section provides case studies in which clinicians provide guidance on the treatment of common conditions with a deliberate focus on dietary supplements. This section is provided to demonstrate how dietary supplement can be practically incorporated in sometimes complex patient scenarios. Moreover, it is provided as a real-world example on evidence-guided care. As the reader is introduced to the quick reference section with information from the Natural Medicines Comprehensive Database as well as other resources discussed in the book, there can be a plethora of choices. It is often important to put these choices and evidence into a patient-centered framework. Of note, with the exception of Dr. Low Dog's chapter on Pregnancy and Lactation, the chapters will attempt to take the reader through the clinical scenario using the stepwise approach of the H.E.R.B.A.L. Mnemonic. Hopefully, the chapters will provide some guidance into how other clinicians frame the discussion and supplement choices so that similar steps may be incorporated into your practice.

CHAPTER 45

Acne

Stephanie Bethune and Michael Traub

Case: *Shannon is 32-year-old with severe nodulocystic acne.*

BACKGROUND

- Acne vulgaris is a skin condition that affects 85% to 100% of people at some time during their lives.
- Twelve percent of women and five percent of men at age 25 years have acne. By age 45 years, 5% of both men and women still have acne (1).
- In general, acne is the #1 problem treated by dermatologists
  - Diet is generally disregarded as a major factor in the pathogenesis of acne, yet there is considerable evidence that foods that promote hyperinsulinemia and inflammation, and that contribute to an already imbalanced hormonal state, do in fact aggravate acne.

BACKGROUND TO CONDITION AND TREATMENTS

The clinical features of acne include open and closed comedones, erythematous papules, pustules, nodules, cysts, and scars. The severity of acne can be classified by the following index: Grade I—comedonal—open/closed, Grade II—papular, Grade III—pustular, Grade IV—nodular (not a cyst); number of lesions: mild 1 to 10, moderate 11 to 20, severe >20 lesions. **Comedonal acne** consists of comedones, which can be open (blackheads) or closed (whiteheads). These result from keratinized cells and sebum (oil). **Papular and cystic acne** most commonly affects the face but can involve the back and chest. Premenstrual flares are common. **Inflammatory acne** appears as erythematous papules (3 to 10 mm). These develop into **pustules** or resolve into fading erythematous macules. Inflammatory lesions may leave postinflammatory hyperpigmentation. Patients with **nodulocystic acne** experience firm, erythematous, tender nodules which become fluctuant or form cysts. Fluctuant sinuses result in postinflammatory pigmentary changes and scarring.

Propionibacterium acnes is an anaerobic bacterium in sebaceous follicles. It is not a pathogen, per se, but it does stimulate inflammation. In fact, the therapeutic effect of tetracycline antibiotics may relate more to their well-established anti-inflammatory effect than to their direct bactericidal effect against *P. acnes*. Subantimicrobial doses of doxycycline can improve acne without changing *P. acnes* counts at all.

Barriers and disadvantages of conventional acne therapy include increased incidence of bacterial resistance, increased incidence of methacillin-resistant *Staphylococcus* aureus, patient fears of antibiotics, negative media coverage of the side effects of isotretinoin, and regulatory pressures on the prescription of isotretinoin.

*H*EARING THE PATIENT OUT WITH RESPECT

Shannon is a 32-year-old female who experienced severe nodulocystic acne 4 months after discontinuing her oral contraceptive. She had a history of oral contraceptive use since age 12 due to menorrhagia and irregular menses.

Pertinent Medical History

She had a ruptured ovarian cyst at age 25 and has a history of hypoglycemia. Her father has had diabetes mellitus type 2 since age 20. Her paternal uncle may have molested her when she was aged 10 to 12. She has no memories of this.

She also has very pruritic patch on her right labia majora since age 12. This lesion itches and burns constantly. She uses topical steroid sparingly, which does not help. The itching keeps her awake at night. She wears cotton panties and avoids synthetic underwear. A dermatologist biopsied the labial lesion 3 years ago: "chronic eczematoid dermatitis with superimposed lichen simplex chronicus." The dermatologist referred her to an allergist for testing. She tested positive only to cockroach.

Lifestyle History

Shannon was raised on a diet of Sloppy Joes, yogurt, grapes, cheese and crackers, and candy bars. She desires sweets, sugar, and milk. She tends to skip meals and has had anorexic tendencies since age 6 when her parents separated. At that time, she began a habit of hiding food. She kept sugar under the bed and ate it with a spoon. She rarely had dinner, as her parents did not cook. Shannon has been celibate for 13 years because of religious beliefs. She sleeps only 3 hours a night since age 16 due to her labial itching. She usually naps 2 to 6:30 pm and gets a second wind of energy at 10 pm.

Treatment History

Shannon was on Depo progesterone for 11 years. During that time, she had no menses and no acne. After 9 years, a DEXA scan showed bone loss. After 2 more years, she discontinued Depo progesterone and started **Yasmin** (drospirenone and ethinyl estradiol. Then she had her menses every 3 months for 2 years with no acne. She discontinued Yasmin 4 months ago and severe cystic acne returned. She recently started getting peels (pumpkin, glycolic) from an aesthetician.

Physical Examination

Shannon had multiple red papules and tender nodules and cysts on her face, chest, and back. Examination of the right labia majora revealed a lichenified patch measuring 2 cm in diameter. She weighed 120 lb and was 5′7″ tall.

Assessment

Shannon was diagnosed with severe nodulocystic acne and lichen simplex chronicus (LSC). Polycystic Ovarian syndrome was also considered and the following blood work was ordered: CMP, lipids, TSH, insulin, prolactin, LH, FSH, DHEA-s, 17-OH progesterone, and testosterone. Atopiclair, a nonsteroidal topical anti-inflammatory cream, was prescribed tid for the LSC. Atopiclair contains extracts from licorice root, Aloe vera, chamomile, Grape seed, and Shea butter.

EDUCATING THE PATIENT

Naturopathic acne therapeutics are based on removing the "obstacles to cure," that is, identifying and removing the underlying causes of the disease, including androgen excess, *P. acnes,* oil-based cosmetics, dietary factors, chronic irritation, stress, and medications.

A study of 47,355 female nurses found a positive correlation between high school milk intake and acne prevalence. This may be due to the hormonal content of milk (estrogens, progesterone, androgens, glucocorticoids, and IGF-1). Soda, french fries, chocolate, and pizza were not associated with acne (2). Shannon had a high fasting blood glucose and a family history of diabetes. A high–glycemic-load diet increases sex hormone binding globulin, free androgen index, insulinlike growth factor-I, insulin insensitivity, and lesion counts, compared with a low–glycemic-load diet (3). She was informed that a diet that encourages a high insulin response chronically could promote acne by resulting in hyperinsulinemia and increased levels of IGF-1. Insulin and IGF-1 both stimulate the sebaceous gland and androgen production. IGF-1 promotes keratinocyte proliferation and sebum production, causing plugging of pores (4). Moreover, triglycerides in sebum offer "food" for bacteria. These triglycerides break down into free fatty acids, which promote inflammation.

Discussion with Shannon, regarding botanics and nutraceuticals, included safety during pregnancy and potential side effects as with any internal therapies. Shannon was informed that vitamin A should not be used at the prescribed dose during pregnancy, as it is teratogenic. Moreover, there are signs associated with vitamin A toxicity (discussed below). Other choices, including conventional therapy, were discussed and remain possibilities for future treatment.

OVERVIEW OF SUPPLEMENT CONSIDERATIONS

Vitamin A: high-dose vitamin A is a first-line therapy. It prevents comedones from forming, thus stopping acne at its inception. Vitamin A prevents keratinocytes from sticking so tightly together, thereby keeping the follicular canals patent. It also decreases sebum production (5, 6).

Zinc: involved in hormone activation, retinol-binding protein formation (enhances effect of retinoid therapy), wound healing, and enhanced immunity. Zinc sulfate has shown efficacy similar to tetracycline but with fewer side effects (7). Zinc gluconate, 30 mg daily, has also shown significant efficacy (8).

Pyridoxine: Women with premenstrual aggravation of acne often respond to B_6. This reflects its role in normal metabolism of steroid hormones (9).

Nicotinamide (Nicomide): A prescription oral preparation of nicotinamide, 750 mg, zinc oxide, 25 mg, cupric oxide, 1.5 mg, and folic acid, 500 mg. It inhibits leukocytic chemotaxis, leukocytic release of lysosomal enzymes, lymphocytic transformation, release of vasoactive amines, and the activity of *P. acnes* lipase. Nicomide T 4% cream and gel is available for topical anti-inflammatory acne treatment and causes virtually no dryness, burning, redness, and irritation commonly associated with use of prescription or over-the-counter acne medications, and with no risk of inducing bacterial resistance (10). In one study, Nicomide bested clindamycin gel in reducing lesion count and severity in moderate inflammatory acne (11).

Topical tea tree oil: 5% is comparable in efficacy to 5% benzoyl peroxide, with fewer side effects. A 15% concentration may be even more effective (12), but be aware that tea tree oil can produce contact dermatitis.

RECORD/RECOMMENDATIONS

After review of laboratory tests ordered (all were WNL except fasting glucose 100), the following recommendations were made:

Name	Brand	Dose	Notes
Vitamin A	Seroyal A-Mulsion 10,000 IU/drop	15 drops = 150,000 IU QD	Cinnamon flavored. Not water soluble, so taken by spoon.
Nicomide	Nicotinamide 750 mg, zinc oxide 25 mg, cupric oxide 1.5 mg, folic acid 500 mcg	1 BID	Combination formula for increased efficacy.
Homeopathic Staphysagria	Boiron	1M 1 dose	This remedy was prescribed at the 2-wk follow-up. See below for case analysis

Additional Recommendations

She should try to decrease the sweets, milk, and red meat in her diet. A rational alternative or adjunct to doxycycline is an anti-inflammatory diet which is low in saturated fat, trans fats, hydrogenated oils, and glycemic load but high in essential fatty acids from cold water fish, nuts and seeds and their butters, avocados and extra virgin olive oil, and flaxseed oil; and high in anti-inflammatory foods and spices such as garlic, ginger, turmeric, and onions.

Lastly, stress management is an essential aspect of managing acne, since the stress response increases cortisol, which may thicken sebum. The *stress of having acne* compounds the problem, so anything that can help reduce stress in a positive and healthy way will be a valuable adjunct to the medical treatment of acne. Shannon may want to try meditation, deep breathing, yoga, or journaling to help work through her thoughts.

BE AWARE OF REACTIONS AND INTERACTIONS

Make sure that female patients understand the teratogenic side effects of the therapeutic dose of vitamin A. Serum vitamin A levels correlate poorly with toxicity. Informed consent should be obtained when vitamin A is prescribed to females of childbearing age. Moreover, patients should be made aware that the early signs of vitamin A toxicity are dry, rough skin, cracked lips, sparse coarse hair, and eyebrow alopecia.

Late signs include irritability, headache, pseudotumor cerebri (benign intracranial hypertension), elevated liver function tests, hyperlipidemia, reversible noncirrhotic portal hypertension, hepatic fibrosis, and cirrhosis. Oral contraceptives may increase serum retinol and the use of topical retinoids may add to toxicity. Vitamin A therapy may decrease absorption of vitamin K. Close monitoring of lipids, transaminases, and psychological state is strongly recommended in high-dose vitamin A therapy.

AGREE TO DISCUSS AND FOLLOW UP

At her 2-week follow-up, Shannon's acne was significantly improving. She did not get the Nicomide because it was too expensive ($90!). It was decided to take her homeopathic case and prescribe a remedy.

Facts/rubrics pertinent to the homeopathic case were:

- Acne
- Genital LSC: vaginal itching, burning
- Irregular menses
- Sexually abused
- Secretive
- Passionate
- Religious
- "Night owl"
- Desires sweets, sugar, milk, ice
- Uncovers feet in bed

Staphysagria 1M was prescribed. Staphysagria covers the symptoms of suppressed anger and grief, especially in patients with a history of sexual abuse. In addition to anger, these patients often suppress their sexuality. A patient that needs staphysagria will tend to be passionate, sleepy all day and sleepless at night, crave sweets, and have itchy lesions on the genitalia.

At her 2-month follow-up, her face was much clearer and there were no new lesions. Her skin showed mild residual hyperpigmentation. At first, the LSC was worse, then got better, with no itching or burning. Her sweet craving got worse; it was deeper than ever before. She now felt no control and the cravings were overpowering. Insomnia persisted, but due to alertness, not itching. It was decided that the vitamin A was effective and the homeopathic remedy was acting. With homeopathic treatment, symptoms frequently worsen before improving, as the medicine stimulates a healing response. Daily sunscreen and skin lightener was recommended for residual hyperpigmentation. She was also encouraged to continue to journal at night to express her thoughts. At 6 month follow-up, her face remained clear with no outbreak of new acne lesions. Her sweet craving had disappeared. The patch of LSC had cleared since she it had stopped itching and she was no longer scratching the area. She was happy and no complaints.

LEARN

The patient is referred to the following resources for updated information on acne and dietary supplements:

- Traub M. Essentials of Dermatological Diagnosis and Integrative Therapeutics; 2008.

- Perricone N. The Acne Prescription: The Perricone Program for Clear and Healthy Skin at Every Age. 1st ed. Collins; 2003.
- Acne at MedicineNet.com. http://www.medicinenet.com/acne/index.htm. Accessed May 6, 2008.

SUMMARY

Acne is caused primarily by hormonal factors which contribute to excess sebum, follicular huyperproliferation and plugging, and inflammation. *P. acnes* plays a role in the inflammation. Although conventional medical and procedural treatments are effective for acne, they are often used without attention given to the underlying causes of the hormonal imbalance. A naturopathic approach to treatment focuses on addressing the obstacles to cure. Diet is generally disregarded as a major factor in the pathogenesis of acne, yet there is considerable evidence that foods that promote hyperinsulinemia and inflammation, and that contribute to an already imbalanced hormonal state, do in fact aggravate acne.

The sudden onset of severe acne suggests an underlying state of hyperandrogenism. Contraceptive medications block the ovarian production of androgens, and their abrupt discontinuation, as we saw in the above case, can result in an eruption of nodulocystic acne. Treatment with high-dose vitamin A, a low-glycemic anti-inflammatory diet, homeopathic medicine, and stress management can lead to rapid resolution.

References

1. Harper J. *Acne Vulgaris*. emedicine. http://www.emedicine.com/DERM/topic2.htm. Published January 23, 2007. Accessed May 6, 2008.
2. Adebamowo CA, Spiegelman D, Danby FW, Frazier AL, Willett WC, Holmes MD. High school dietary dairy intake and teenage acne. *J Am Acad Dermatol* 2005;52: 207–214.
3. Smith RN, Mann NJ, Braue A, et al. A low-glycemic-load diet improves symptoms in acne vulgaris. *Am J Clin Nutr* 2007;86(1):107–115.
4. Cordain L, Lindeberg S, Hurtado M, Hill K, Eaton SB, Brand-Miller J. Acne vulgaris: a disease of Western civilization. *Arch Dermatol* 2002;138:1584–1590.
5. Kligman AM. Acne–fact and folklore. *West J Med* 1979;131(6):547–548.
6. Kligman AM, Mills OH Jr, Leyden JJ, Gross PR, Allen HB, Rudolph RI. Oral vitamin A in acne vulgaris. *Int J Dermatol* 1981;20:278–285.
7. Michaelsson G, Juhlin L, Ljunghall K. A double-blind study of the effect of zinc and oxytetracycline in acne vulgaris. *Br J Dermatol* 1977;97:561–566.
8. Meynadier J. Efficacy and safety study of two zinc gluconate regimens in the treatment of inflammatory acne. *Eur J Dermatol* 2000;10:269–273.
9. Snider BL, Dieteman DF. Pyridoxine therapy for premenstrual acne flare. *Arch Dermatol* 1974;110:130–131.
10. Griffiths CEM. Nicotinamide 4% gel for the treatment of inflammatory acne vulgaris. *J Dermatol Treat* 1995;6:S8–S10.
11. Shalita AR, Smith JG, Parish LC, et al. Topical nicotinamide compared with clindamycin gel in the treatment of inflammatory acne vulgaris. *Int J Dermatol* 1995;34:434–437.
12. Bassett IB, Pannowitz DL, Barnetson RS. A comparative study of tea-tree oil versus benzoylperoxide in the treatment of acne. *Med J Aust* 1990;153:455–458.

CHAPTER 46

Benign Prostatic Hyperplasia

David Rakel

Case: *Robert is a 74-year-old male with difficulty urinating.*

BACKGROUND

- Prostate enlargement is present in half of men in their 60s and 90% of men in their 70s. One third of men more than 50 years of age develop symptoms of prostate enlargement (1).
- As the male passes the fifth decade, there is a decrease in serum testosterone and a rise in estrogen. Estrogen increases the number of receptors of dihydrotestosterone (DHT) which inhibits prostatic cell death and promotes cell proliferation that increases the size of the gland.
- As urinary outflow obstruction develops, the detrusor muscles of the bladder try to compensate by increasing pressure to expel urine, which leads to instability of the muscle and worsening symptoms.
- Factors that promote the accumulation of DHT and estrogens lead to lower urinary tract symptoms (LUTS).
- Lifestyle factors can play a major role in the severity of benign prostatic hyperplasia (BPH). Elevated cholesterol, obesity, and symptoms of the metabolic syndrome can all worsen symptoms by promoting inflammation through hormonal influences (2).

*H*EARING THE PATIENT OUT WITH RESPECT

Robert is a 74-year-old male who reports a decreased force of his urinary stream and dribbling after voiding. He wakes 2 to 3 times during the night to urinate. These symptoms have gradually worsened over the past 5 years and now are starting to interfere with his quality of life. He denies any hematuria or pain with voiding. He has no family history of prostate cancer and his prostatic-specific antigen (PSA) is 4.8. He scored 14 on the American Urological Association symptom questionnaire (>8 = moderate symptoms, >20 = severe symptoms).

Pertinent Medical History

Robert has dyslipidemia with a total cholesterol of 230, low-density lipoprotein of 145, high-density lipoprotein of 32, and a triglyceride level of 220. He has an elevated fasting blood sugar of 115 consistent with prediabetes.

Alleviating and Exacerbating Factors

Robert does not associate anything with improvement of his symptoms but he has noticed worsening of his symptoms as he gained weight.

Treatment History

For 2 weeks, Robert took an over-the-counter "herbal" product for prostate health. He stopped using it because he did not notice any change.

Lifestyle History

Robert eats a "meat and potatoes"–based diet. He includes one to two servings of fruits and vegetables each day and enjoys bread and bagels. He drinks one to two beers daily, more on special occasions. He also drinks one to two cups of milk and has a bowl of ice cream before bed. He has been trying to cut back on sweets since his physician told him that his blood sugar was elevated. He has no regular exercise routine and sits most of the day during work as a business executive. He does not smoke.

Physical Examination

Robert has trunkal obesity with a body mass index of 31. His prostate is diffusely enlarged on examination with no specific nodules. His blood pressure is 138/84.

EDUCATING THE PATIENT

Robert is educated regarding how lifestyle choices can influence the severity of his BPH symptoms and result in not only improvement of his LUTS but also reduction of his risk of stroke, heart disease, and cancer.

He is made aware of the importance of a regular exercise routine to help reduce his trunkal obesity, which worsens systemic inflammation.

A Mediterranean type diet was encouraged that includes seven to eight servings of fruits and vegetables daily, fiber, soy protein, and omega-3 fatty acids. This diet will help reduce cholesterol, which is a building block for the hormones (estrogen and testosterone) that can worsen BPH. Cholesterol's metabolites (epoxycholesterols) have been found to accumulate in the hyperplastic and cancerous prostate gland. This helps explain why hypocholesterolemic drugs (HMG-CoA reductase inhibitors or "statins") have been associated with a lower risk of BPH and prostate cancer (3).

Foods rich in omega-3 fatty acids such as cold-water fish (salmon, mackerel, and sardines), vegetables, and ground flaxseed or flaxseed oil were recommended. Lignan-rich flaxseed oil, 500 mg two to four capsules twice a day or grinding whole flaxseeds and consuming two tablespoons of flax daily. Ground flax can be sprinkled on salads, yogurt, or placed in a smoothie. Flaxseed has the added benefit of lignan fiber, which helps bind estrogen in the gut promoting its removal. A pilot study of 15 men with BPH showed that a low-fat diet with flaxseed supplementation of 30 g daily reduced PSA and cholesterol levels, while decreasing prostate epithelial proliferation at repeat biopsy after 6 months (4).

Eating more vegetables increases the intake of plant sterols and stanols that have also been found to reduce cholesterol and BPH. One of these phytosterols, beta-sitosterol has been found to be helpful in treating BPH (see below). Food sources with high concentrations can be found in dark greens, rice bran, wheat germ, peanuts, corn oils, and soybeans.

A case-control study comparing the dietary habits of 1,369 patients younger than 75 years of age who were surgically treated for BPH with 1,451 controls demonstrated that higher intake of cereals, bread, eggs, or poultry can increase the risk for BPH. Conversely, soups, cooked vegetables, legumes, and citrus fruit may be protective (5).

In summary, nutritional changes that would benefit Robert's LUTS include increasing fruit, vegetable, beans, and foods rich in omega-3 fatty acids. He should reduce meat, dairy, and bread consumption. He can continue his alcohol use in moderation. Light to medium alcohol consumption has been associated with a protective effect on BPH and LUTS. This is lost once consumption goes beyond two drinks a day (6).

OVERVIEW OF SUPPLEMENT CONSIDERATIONS

Saw Palmetto (*Serenoa repens*)

This product is the most researched botanic for BPH. It is thought to work through three different mechanisms to enhance prostate health. It is an inhibitor of 5-alpha reductase, it reduces the number of estrogen and androgen (DHT) receptors, and it has an anti-inflammatory effect. It is also very rich in beta-sitosterol, which has been found to improve BPH symptoms and lower cholesterol (7). Saw palmetto reduces the inner prostatic epithelium but does not appear to reduce the size of the whole gland.

Research has been supportive for its positive effect on symptom scores, nocturia, residual urine volume, and urinary flow for those with mild to moderate symptoms of BPH (8). A Cochrane review of the literature supports a mild to moderate effect of saw palmetto on BPH symptoms (9). It was found to be as effective as finasteride (Proscar) without the sexual side effects and unlike finasteride, does not artificially lower PSA levels (10). It is less likely to be of benefit for those with moderate to severe symptoms. A study of 225 men with moderate to severe BPH did not show benefit after 1 year of treatment (11).

Saw palmetto is safe and adverse reactions are rare but can include diarrhea, nausea, headache, and dizziness.

Beta-Sitosterol

This is a steroid that is found in plants (phytosterol). Sterols are similar in composition to cholesterol and inhibit cholesterol absorption. They are commonly used in margarines (Take Control, Benecol) used to lower cholesterol. Unlike human cholesterol, beta-sitosterol cannot be converted to testosterone. Many botanics (saw palmetto, pygeum, stinging nettles, rye grass pollen) that are used to treat BPH are rich in beta-sitosterol and may support a common mechanism of action. Like saw palmetto, it does not reduce the size of the gland.

Two randomized studies have shown benefit with little potential harm in treating BPH with beta-sitosterol (12, 13). A Cochrane review found beta-sitosterol to improve urinary symptoms and flow measures for BPH (14). The benefits of this therapy have been maintained after 18 months of use (15). Eating a diet rich in plants will also give the body ample amounts of bete-sitosterol and would likely reduce the need for supplementation.

Pygeum (*Prunus africana*)

Pygeum is obtained from the bark of the African plum tree. It likely works by having antiproliferative and anti-inflammatory effects on the prostate. There is evidence to support that pygeum suppresses epithelial growth factor, shrinking epithelial cells (16).

A meta-analysis has shown pygeum to have a 19% reduction in nocturia with a 24% reduction in residual urine volume. Peak urine flow was increased by 23% and side effects were mild and similar to placebo (17).

A Cochrane review of 18 randomized controlled trials involving 1,562 men showed that pygeum provided a moderately large improvement in the combined outcome of urologic symptoms and flow measures. Men using pygeum were more than twice as likely to report an improvement in overall symptoms (18).

Rye Grass Pollen (*Secale cereale*)

Compared to the other treatments discussed for BPH, rye grass pollen (also known as grass pollen) has more of an anti-inflammatory effect and has been found to be a beneficial therapy for prostatitis (19). It contains a substance that has been found to inhibit prostate cell growth (20) as well as reduce inflammation of the prostate by inhibiting prostaglandins and leukotrienes (21).

Rye grass pollen extract has been used in Europe to treat BPH for 35 years. Double-blind clinical studies have found it to be effective with an overall response rate near 70% (22). The most benefit has been seen in nocturia, urinary frequency, and residual urine volume (23).

Most of the research on rye grass pollen has been completed using a formulation called Cernilton (flower pollen). Although the majority of studies have been of limited power, of short duration, and often without an adequate control, a Cochrane review reports that Cernilton is well tolerated and modestly improves overall urologic symptoms including nocturia in those with BPH (24).

*R*ECORD SUPPLEMENT RECOMMENDATIONS

Supplement	Brand/ Formulation	Dose	Notes
Saw palmetto	• Nature's Way Saw Palmetto Standardized Extract, 160 mg/capsule • Walgreens Saw Palmetto Standardized Extract, 160 mg/capsule • Enzymatic Therapy Super Saw Palmetto, 160 mg/capsule	160 mg twice daily	The extract should be standardized to at least 85% fatty acids and 0.2% sterols. (A 160-mg capsule should have at least 136-mg fatty acids and 0.32-mg sterols)
Beta-sitosterol	• Source Naturals, Beta-Sitosterol, 113 mg/tablet • Natrol Beta-sitosterol, 120 mg/tablet • Pure • Encapsulations Beta-sitosterol, 68 mg/capsule	60 mg twice a day Can be lowered to 30 mg twice a day for maintenance once symptoms improve.	Doses used for dyslipidemia are much higher; 700–1,000 mg before meals three times a day. Can use sterol-rich margarines (Take control, Benecol). One tbsp of spread ~ 1 gm of sterols.

(*continued*)

Pygeum	• Nature's Herbs, Pygeum Power, 60 mg/capsule • Nature's Way standardized pygeum, 50 mg/capsule (combination product)	100–200 mg daily	Often found in combination with saw palmetto.
Rye grass pollen	Graminex, Pollen Aid, 126 mg/capsule	126 mg three times daily before meals	Graminex obtained the marketing rights for cernitin and sells it under the name of Pollen Aid.

Additional Recommendations

Robert was encouraged to avoid sympathomimetics such as over-the-counter cold medications (pseudoephedrine) and anticholingergics (antispasmotics and antihistamine). He should also avoid environmental xenobiotics that may have a negative hormonal influence. These include pesticides, herbicides, and food products rich in bovine growth hormone such as dairy and drugs including dehydroepiandrosterone, androstenedione, testosterone, and human growth hormone.

Other Helpful Treatments

Other common botanic products used for BPH but with less evidence to support efficacy include stinging nettles, pumpkin seed extract, and African wild potato. If symptoms are severe or there is no response to therapy, the patient should be given alpha-blocker pharmaceutical therapy or be referred for urological evaluation and treatment.

BE AWARE OF REACTIONS AND INTERACTIONS

The supplements discussed are relatively safe and do not have serious adverse effects. The most common side effects are mild, GI related (nausea, constipation, and diarrhea), and comparable to placebo in clinical trials.

AGREE TO DISCUSS AND FOLLOW-UP

After stressing the importance of lifestyle measures to help reduce systemic inflammation including weight loss, exercise, and improved nutrition, Robert was started on a combination of saw palmetto 160 mg twice daily and beta-sitosterol 360 mg twice daily before meals. The beta-sitosterol was prescribed at a higher dose to not only improve his symptoms of BPH but also help lower his cholesterol. Robert was educated that this treatment can take 6 to 8 weeks to show its full benefit. He will return in 2 to 3 months at which time we will have him come in fasting to recheck his cholesterol. At this visit we will have him retake the American Urological Association BPH symptom index to assess improvement in his symptoms (8 or > = moderate, 20 or > = severe).

LEARN

To evaluate BPH symptoms through the American Urological Association BPH Symptom Index questionnaire, go to: http://godot.urol.uic.edu/~web/ASIS.html.

A good resource for obtaining evidence-based information on neutraceuticals and botanics can be found by going to the Natural Database Web site at: http://www.naturaldatabase.com/. This site has a subscription fee. Another alternative is to consult the National Institutes of Health International Bibliographic Information on Dietary Supplements (IBIDS) Database at: http://dietary-supplements.info.nih.gov/Health_Information/IBIDS.aspx.

SUMMARY

Nutritional supplements and botanics are a good first-line strategy for treating mild to moderate BPH. Once symptoms become more severe (American Urological Association score of 18 or greater), more aggressive therapy with pharmaceutical or urological interventions should be considered.

Start with one or more antiproliferative agents such as saw palmetto, beta-sitosterol, or pygeum. If after 6 to 8 weeks, this does not result in benefit, consider adding an anti-inflammatory agent such as rye grass pollen. Remember the importance of lifestyle factors including weight management and nutrition on systemic inflammation that can influence BPH symptoms. If symptoms remain inadequately controlled, consider alpha-blockade with pharmaceutical therapy.

References

1. Thorpe A, Neal D. Benign prostatic hyperplasia. *Lancet* 2003;361:1359–1367.
2. Rohrmann S, Smit E, Giovannucci E, Platz EA. Association between markers of the metabolic syndrome and lower urinary tract symptoms in the Third National and Nutrition Examination Survey (NHANES III). *Int J Obes Relat Metab Disord* 2004;29:310–316.
3. Padayatty SJ, Marcelli M, Shao TC, Cunningham GR. Lovastatin-induced apoptosis in prostate stromal cells. *J Clin Endocrinol Metab* 1997;82(5):1434–1439.
4. Demark-Wahnefried W, Robertson CN, Walther PJ, Polascik TJ, Paulson DF, Vollmer RT. Pilot study to explore effects of low-fat, flaxseed-supplemented diet on proliferation of benign prostatic epithelium and prostate-specific antigen. *Urology* 2004;63(5):900–904.
5. Bravi F, Bosetti C, Dal Maso L, et al. Food groups and risk of benign prostatic hyperplasia. *Urology* 2006;67:73–79.
6. Ptatz EA, Rimm EB, Kawachi I, et al. Alcohol consumption, cigarette smoking, and risk of benign prostatic hyperplasia. *Am J Epidemiol* 1999;149:106–115.
7. Rakel DP. Benign prostatic hyperplasia. In: Rakel DP, ed. *Integrative Medicine*. Philadelphia, PA: WB Saunders; 2007: 639.
8. Wilt TJ, Ishani A, Stark G, MacDonald R, Lau J, Mulrow C. Saw palmetto extracts for treatment of benign prostatic hyperplasia: a systematic review. *JAMA* 1998;280(18):1604–1609.
9. Wilt T, Ishani A, Mac Donald R. Serenoa repens for benign prostatic hyperplasia. *Cochrane Database Syst Rev* 2002;3(3):CD001423.
10. Carraro JC, Raynaud JP, Koch G, et al. Comparison of phytotherapy with finasteride in the treatment of benign prostate hyperplasia: a randomized international study of 1,098 patients. *Prostate* 1996;29:231.

11. Bent S, Kane C, Shinohara K, et al. Saw palmetto for benign prostatic hyperplasia. *N Engl J Med* 2006;354(6):557–566.
12. Berges RR, Windeler J, Trampisch HJ, et al. Randomised, placebo-controlled, double-blind clinical trial of beta-sitosterol in patients with benign prostatic hyperplasia. *Lancet* 1995;345:1529–1532.
13. Klippel KF, Hiltl DM, Schipp B. A multicentric, placebo-controlled, double-blind clinical trial of β-sitosterol (phytosterol) for the treatment of benign prostatic hyperplasia. *Br J Urol* 1997;80:427–432.
14. Wilt T, Ishani A, Mac Donald R, Stark G, Mulrow C, Lau J. Beta-sitosterols for benign prostatic hyperplasia. *Cochrane Database Syst Rev* 1999(3):CD001043. DOI: 10.1002/14651858.CD001043.
15. Berges RR, Kassen A, Senge T. Treatment of symptomatic benign prostatic hyperplasia with beta-sitosterol: an 18-month follow-up. *BJU Int* 2000;85(7):842–846.
16. Santa Maria Margalef A, Paciucci Barzanti R, Reventos Puigjaner J, et al. Antimitogenic effect of Pygeum africanum extracts on human prostatic cancer cell lines and explants from benign prostatic hyperplasia. *Arch Esp Urol* 2003;56:369–378.
17. Ishani A, MacDonald R, Nelson D, et al. Pygeum africanum for the treatment of patients with benign prostatic hyperplasia: a systematic review and quantitative meta-analysis. *Am J Med* 2000;8(109):654–664.
18. Wilt T, Ishani A, Mac Donald R, Rutks I, Stark G. Pygeum africanum for benign prostatic hyperplasia. *Cochrane Database Syst Rev* 2002;(1):CD001044.
19. Rugendorff EW, Weidner W, Ebeling L, Buck AC. Results of treatment with pollen extract (Cernilton N) in chronic prostatitis and prostatodynia. *Br J Urol* 1993;71:433–438.
20. Habib FK, Ross M, Lewenstein A, Zhang X, Jaton JC. Identification of a prostate inhibitory substance in a pollen extract. *Prostate* 1995;26:133–139.
21. Loschen G, Ebeling L. Inhibition of arachidonic acid cascade by extract of rye pollen. (Article in German) *Arzneimittelforschung* 1991;41(2):162–167.
22. Buck AC, Cox R, Rees RW, Ebeling L, John A. Treatment of outflow tract obstruction due to benign prostatic hyperplasia with the pollen extract, cernilton: a double-blind, placebo-controlled study. *Br J Urol* 1990;66(4):398–404.
23. Becker H, Ebeling L. Conservative therapy for benign prostatic hyperplasia (BPH) with Cernilton. *Br J Urol* 1988;66:398–404.
24. Wilt T, Mac Donald R, Ishani A, Rutks I, Stark G. Cernilton for benign prostatic hyperplasia. *Cochrane Database Syst Rev* 2000;2(2):CD001042.

CHAPTER 47

Diabetes

Victor S. Sierpina and Ryan Bradley

Case: *Denise M. is a 56-year-old female with an 8-year history of type 2 diabetes.*

BACKGROUND

- According to NHANES data, only 37% of patients with diabetes are in good glycemic control (hemoglobin A_{1c} <7.0%) (1).
- Surveys suggest 48% to 72% of people with diabetes use some form of complementary and alternative medicine therapy, with complementary and alternative medicine use associated with increased use of preventive services (2–4).
- Evidence ranking and mechanistic reviews of nutritional and botanic supplements in diabetes are available in the literature (5, 6).

*H*EARING THE PATIENT OUT WITH RESPECT

Denise M. is a 56-year-old female living in Seattle with an 8-year history of type 2 diabetes. She presents to discuss dietary approaches in order to prevent taking additional medications for her diabetes. She subscribes to numerous natural health newsletters online and has questions about "natural cures" for diabetes. Her regular primary care physician dismissed her interest in supplements and was unable to offer her specific recommendations. Denise reports fatigue (energy 6/10), depression, blurry vision, and distal foot pain and tingling as her current symptoms. She denies polyuria, polydipsia, polyphagia, or cardiovascular symptoms. Denise brought laboratory reports dated 6 months ago reporting a HbA_{1c} of 8.3%, LDL cholesterol of 105 mg/dl, HDL cholesterol of 32 mg/dl, and triglycerides of 278 mg/dl. She states that she is afraid of the side effects of more prescription medications and would "rather die" than take insulin.

Pertinent Medical History

Denise reports a medical history of gestational diabetes with her second child, aspirin-induced gastritis, and depression starting 3 years ago. Her depression impacts her self-management; she reports stopping her blood sugar monitoring for over a year. She developed a macrocytic anemia while taking metformin. Her parents are still living, though she reports family history of both myocardial infarction (MI) (father, age 60) and diabetes (mother, onset at age 62).

Alleviating and Exacerbating Factors

Denise reports that her depression is better during the summer and with exercise, but she "really suffers" during the winter. She has noticed that high carbohydrate intake worsens her blurry vision and her foot tingling.

Treatment History

Upon diagnosis, Denise's PCP started her on glyburide. She had multiple hypoglycemic episodes and so was switched to metformin after 1 year. Metformin controlled her diabetes for 3 years; she developed a macrocytic anemia while on metformin. Her HbA_{1c} started to rise about a year ago despite a full dose of metformin. Her PCP recommended a thiazolidinedione, which she started. Denise stopped her thiazolidinedione 6 months ago because of weight gain and because she read the drug may increase heart attacks. She remains on metformin. She also takes sertraline for her depression, lisinopril for her blood pressure, and simvastatin for her cholesterol.

Lifestyle History

Denise was referred to a nutritionist upon diagnosis and learned how to count her carbohydrate and learned her body mass index (BMI). She states that she restricts carbohydrates and eats "whole grains," although a 24-hour diet recall includes rice crackers, potatoes, and ice cream. Denise eats three to four servings of fruit and vegetables per day, rarely drinks alcohol, and has a cup of black coffee every morning. She has no food restrictions but limits red meat to twice per week. Denise states that she feels "much better" when she exercises, and she walks 20 to 30 minutes daily. She is married and her husband walks with her.

Physical Examination

Fundoscopic examination was unremarkable. Neck was without carotid bruits, cardiac rate and rhythm were regular, and S1 S2 were normal, without murmur. Lungs were clear to auscultation and percussion. Abdomen was soft, obese, nontender without organomegaly, or bruits. Monofilament testing demonstrated an inability to detect monofilament at four of the nine sites on the right foot and five of nine sites on the left foot. Vibratory sense, deep tendon reflexes (DTRs), [and sensory discrimination were normal. There were no ulcerations or fungal infections and peripheral pulses were +2 bilateral. Mild (+1) peripheral edema was noted bilaterally. Her BP was 142/92 mm Hg and BMI 29. She was referred to an ophthalmologist for a dilated retinal examination.

EDUCATING THE PATIENT

Denise was educated that nutritional supplements complement lifestyle changes. Supplements combined with a structured exercise program and dietary modification would be most likely to be beneficial for her. Denise was also informed that unlike some prescription drugs for diabetes, we do not know whether supplements impact cardiovascular outcomes and risk of death; however, some supplements have been studied in well-designed clinical trials and have demonstrated improvements on clinical biomarkers in diabetes. She agreed to regular (every 3 months) follow-ups to evaluate the effects of supplements.

To direct supplementation, additional laboratory assessment was recommended. RBC magnesium concentration, vitamin D (25-hydroxycholecalciferol), a complete blood count (CBC), and methylmalonic acid (MMA[1]) were ordered as well as routine HbA_{1c}, lipids, hepatic functions, and urine microalbumin.

REVIEW OF NUTRITIONAL SUPPLEMENTATION

Omega-3 Fatty Acids/Eicosapentaenoic Acid and Docosahexaenoic Acid

Eicosapentaenoic acid (EPA) and docosahexaenoic acid (DHA) are essential fats for human nutrition and have antithrombotic, antiarrhythmic, and antiischemic effects as well as raising HDL cholesterol and reducing triglycerides. Regular intake of EPA and DHA (200 to 250 mg/d) has been clearly shown to reduce overall mortality and coronary death by 17% and 36% respectively, with higher doses (1,000 mg/d) recommended for patients with known cardiovascular disease (10). Furthermore, prescription EPA/DHA (Lovaza) is available and FDA-approved for the treatment of hypertriglyceridemia (see the "Record/Recommendations" section).

Chromium Picolinate

Chromium is an essential mineral in human nutrition and functions as a critical cofactor in the insulin-signaling pathway (11). Chromium picolinate appears to be the most absorbable form of those readily available (some amino acid chelates may be superior but are less available) (12).

Chromium picolinate has been studied in a number of randomized, double-blind, placebo-controlled trials (RDBPCTs). These studies have found that chromium improves glucose control with attenuation of weight gain, improved insulin sensitivity, reduced triglycerides, and reduction in HbA_{1c} of between 0.54% and 1.76% (9, 10).

Magnesium

Serum magnesium levels correlate well to both fasting blood glucose and glucose disposal during glucose tolerance testing in insulin-treated and noninsulin-treated patients with diabetes (13).

An RDBPCT of magnesium supplementation using magnesium chloride demonstrated improvement in measures of insulin sensitivity, reduced fasting blood glucose, and reduced HbA_{1c} 2.1% on average compared to placebo (14).

Vitamin D

Because Denise lives in the Pacific Northwest, assessment of vitamin D status is an essential part of her diabetes management.

Vitamin D is required in the pancreatic beta cell for normal insulin gene transcription and insulin secretion; hypovitaminosis D has been correlated to insulin resistance and carotid intima media thickness in diabetes (15–17). Hypovitaminosis D is common in the diabetic population, with prevalence from trials measured

[1]With Denise's history of macrocytic anemia, and because she remains on metformin, vitamin B_{12} status should be evaluated (7). Serum B_{12} alone is not a sensitive indicator of B_{12} status; multiple measures of B_{12} status have greater sensitivity, for example, MMA combined with a mean corpuscular volume (MCV), serum B_{12} combined with MCV, and so forth (8, 9).

between 36% and 57% (17, 18). 25-Hydroxycholecalciferol is the recommended laboratory test for assessment of vitamin D status (16).

Vitamin D replacement has been studied in controlled trials. Borissova et al (19) administered 1332 IU of vitamin D to 17 patients with type 2 diabetes, using nondiabetic, age- and BMI-matched women as controls. Significant improvements in fasting insulin sensitivity index (34.3% increase) in patients with diabetes were observed with the change highly correlated to changes in vitamin D concentration (P <.018) (19).

Coenzyme Q10 (CoQ10)

Consideration of supplemental coenzyme Q10 (CoQ10) is indicated because of Denise's diabetes, stage I hypertension, and her use of an HMG-CoA reductase inhibitor medication. CoQ10 is a coenzyme present in every ATP-producing cell in our bodies, serving as an electron carrier during oxidative phosphorylation in the mitochondria.

CoQ10 is transported in lipoproteins in the bloodstream and helps prevent LDL oxidation. CoQ10 concentrations are reduced by HMG-CoA reductase medications, that is, statins. Although the clinical significance of this reduction is not known fully due to a lack of RDBPCT addressing this specific question, concern has been voiced in the medical literature based on the known mechanisms of CoQ10 (20, 21).

RDBPCTs of CoQ10 have shown significant positive results in hypertension and diabetes including reductions in systolic blood pressure and HbA_{1c} (22, 23). Typical dosing is 200 mg per day. Absorption of CoQ10 varies depending on the form used; to date Q-Gel appears to be more bioavailable (24).

FOR NEUROPATHY

Denise's neuropathy symptoms deserve attention as neuropathy can be an obstacle to exercise and restful sleep but also increases her risk for ulceration and amputation. The presence of peripheral neuropathy suggests probable early autonomic neuropathy due to her suboptimal glycemic control. Vitamin B_{12} and alpha-lipoic acid (ALA) are useful supplements for neuropathy.

Vitamin B_{12}

Vitamin B_{12} is a critical nutrient to nerve conduction and has recently undergone systematic review for the treatment of diabetic neuropathy with positive conclusions (25). Seven controlled, clinical trials of varying quality suggest benefit in autonomic or peripheral neuropathic symptoms.

A common clinical protocol involves evaluating clinical response to a 1 cc IM injection of B_{12} when effective, positive responses are rapid with most patients reporting improvement within 48 hours. Duration of response is variable ranging between days and weeks. Some patients prefer periodic repeat injections, whereas others maintain on B_{12} oral supplementation.

Alpha-lipoic Acid

Recently, a large dose-finding RDBPCT in 181 patients with diabetes found statistically significant positive results in stabbing and burning pain scores, the neuropathy symptom and change score, and global assessment of efficacy (26). Three doses tested (600 mg/1200 mg/1800 mg/d vs. placebo) demonstrated positive results without differences between groups. Nausea, vomiting, and vertigo occurred at higher doses.

Based on this study, 600 mg per day of ALA orally appears to be an effective and tolerable dose for routine clinical recommendation.

RECORD/RECOMMENDATIONS

Diabetes is considered a cardiovascular disease equivalent and Denise is in moderately poor glycemic control with mixed dyslipidemia including hypertriglyceridemia. Denise's laboratory testing demonstrated mild vitamin B_{12} and vitamin D deficiencies. Denise's RBC magnesium status was adequate. After reviewing the available evidence, her glycemic control, cardiovascular risk, early neuropathy, and concurrent stage I hypertension, the following supplement recommendations were made:

Supplement Recommendations

Name	Brand	Dose	Notes
EPA/DHA	Nordic Naturals Arctic Cod Liver Oil (410 mg EPA/625 mg DHA/tsp) Pharmax Finest Fish Oil (1050 mg EPA/750 mg DHA/tsp) Omacor (465 mg EPA/375 mg DHA/capsule)	4 g combined DHA/EPA/d	• Liquid more affordable at high doses, but intolerance is more frequent due to burping and taste • Pharmax and Nordic Naturals have capsules available • Freezing fish oil capsules provides burp-free "slow release" • Insurance does not always cover Omacor
Vitamin D_3	Biotics Research BioDmulsion (400 IU/gtt) BioDmulsion Forte (2,000 IU/gtt) Multiple brands (1,000 IU/capsule)	2,000 IU/d (5 gtts) or 2,000 IU/d (1 gtt) or 2,000 IU/d (2 capsules)	• Serum 25-hydroxy (OH) cholecalciferol should be monitored every 1–3 mo • Serum calcium monitored more frequently if higher doses are used (>4,000 IU/d) or in high-risk patient
CoQ10	Multiple brands; (all Q-Gel manufactured by Tiscon Gel-Tec)	100–200 mg/d	• Typically well tolerated
Chromium picolinate	Diachrome, Nutrition 21, Inc.	600 mcg ChrPic/ 2 mg biotin/d (1 capsule)	• Typically well tolerated • Improves mood and reduces carbohydrate cravings

(*continued*)

Name	Brand	Dose	Notes
Vitamin B_{12}	Thorne Research Natural Factors Key Pharmacy, Kent, WA	1000 mcg/d or 1000 mcg/d SL or Preservative-free B_{12} 1 cc single-unit vials for IM injection	• IM injections result in rapid improvement when needed • Laboratory monitoring is recommended to confirm adequate absorption of oral supplementation
Alpha-lipoic acid	Multiple brands including Thorne Research, Pure Encapsulations, and Metagenics	600 mg/d	• R-ALA may be more effective in some patients per clinical observations

Additional Recommendations

DIET AND EXERCISE

Denise was encouraged to restrict "white foods," eliminate *trans* fats, and to "eat a rainbow of vegetables every day." "Functional foods" were recommended including broccoli; green, leafy vegetables; onions; garlic; green tea; pomegranate juice; dark chocolate/cocoa; maitake and shitake mushrooms; tree nuts; oily, cold-water fish (Alaskan salmon); minimally processed soy protein; and less salt and more spices (cinnamon, basil, fenugreek, turmeric, and ginger) to improve her blood pressure, lipids, and/or blood glucose (27–30).

Specific recommendations were given for:

- Green leafy vegetables will assist in providing fiber and will help maintain magnesium status
- Cinnamon (1 teaspoon per day as tea or 1/2 teaspoon on food) for reducing fasting blood glucose.
- Pomegranate juice (6 oz/d) for reducing oxidized LDL cholesterol, improving cardiac perfusion, increasing antioxidant status, and lowering LDL cholesterol and blood pressure.

Denise was also educated on the importance of exercise in diabetes and she set goals for herself for both aerobic and resistance exercise. She set a goal to work out at least 30 minutes a day daily with aerobics daily and resistance exercise every 2 to 3 days and has found an exercise class and exercise coach/trainer to work with her on establishing a regular program.

Future Recommendations

Clinical trial data exist for many botanic medicines in addition to the food-based herbs recommended above. American ginseng, fenugreek, cinnamon, Gymnema, Momordica, bilberry, nopal, and Coccinia have clinical research support for their use. Similar laboratory monitoring strategies are recommended.

BE AWARE OF REACTIONS AND INTERACTIONS

Of the recommended supplements, fish oil is the most poorly tolerated due to burping, frank reflux, and taste. Taking fish oils with food or using capsules improves tolerance.

Theoretical risk exists for high-dose omega-3 oils and/or coenzyme Q10 plus anticoagulants including warfarin and aspirin, although the available data do not support risk. Monitoring is recommended in high-risk patients and patients on warfarin.

Interactions between prescription and supplement "insulin sensitizers," for example, chromium and metformin, are poorly researched and therefore the patient should self-monitor blood glucose for changes in addition to laboratory monitoring.

Vitamin D supplementation/replacement should be monitored with periodic, q 1 to 3 months, laboratory testing to ensure response to therapy and to monitor for hypervitaminosis D. Patients on high-dose replacement therapy should be advised to notify physician immediately if palpitations occur.

High-dose magnesium can cause loose stools; slow titration can limit this response. In laboratory models, pomegranate juice reduces clearance of HMG-CoA reductase inhibitors, that is, statins; clinical monitoring for myalgias and liver function elevations is prudent.

AGREE TO DISCUSS AND FOLLOW-UP

Denise agrees to get laboratory monitoring on schedule and agrees to self-monitor her blood glucose daily in the interim.

Denise followed up 2 weeks after receiving her first B_{12} injection stating dramatic improvement in her foot pain and numbness. She stated that the effects lasted about 10 days and she requests another injection. She has not yet noticed changes in her blood glucose and has not experienced any major adverse effects, though she requests switching to omega-3 capsules. Her mood has improved slightly and she states that her carbohydrate cravings are improving. She is working on diet and exercise recommendations.

Denise returned for her 3-month follow-up and stated that her fasting blood glucose 30-day average is 155 mg/dl on her meter. She has lost 7# and is sleeping better due to "dramatic improvement" in her foot pain. She denies any new symptoms and reports that her energy is now 8/10. Denise wants to stop her sertraline and agrees to wait 3 more months for a titration plan. Her labs indicate her HbA_{1c} is now 7.5%, her HDL increased to 42 mg/dl, and her triglycerides are reduced to 180 mg/dl. 25-Hydroxyvitamin D is now normal and her vitamin D dose is reduced to 1,000 IU per day. Vitamin B_{12} injections are discontinued due to normalized MMA and MCV; 1,000 mcg orally qod is recommended for maintenance. On physical examination her blood pressure is 135/85; her monofilament test remains the same. She agreed to begin monitoring her 2-hour postprandial glucose in addition to her fasting readings. She is still incorporating dietary suggestions and exercise.

At 6-month follow-up, Denise's 30-day blood glucose average is 158 mg/dl, including postprandial readings. She reports no new symptoms and denies myalgias and muscle weakness. She is still taking all of her medications and supplements as recommended and enjoys the pomegranate juice throughout her day as her "treat." Her labs now indicate her HbA_{1c} is 6.9%, HDL is 45 mg/dl, LDL is 95 mg/dl, and her triglycerides reduced further to 160 mg/dl. Her blood pressure is 128/83. She remains interested in stopping her sertraline and is provided a dose-titration plan. She agrees to continue glucose monitoring and to follow up in 3 months. She is encouraged to remain on omega-3 oils, Diachrome, 600 mg qd ALA, 200 mg qd CoQ10, 1000 IU qd vitamin D, and 1000 mcg qid vitamin B_{12} and to continue her new diet.

LEARN

Denise is interested in learning more about supplements in diabetes and is provided the following resource:

- Natural Medicines Comprehensive Database consumer version
  www.NaturalDatabase.com
- Office of Dietary Supplements
  http://dietary-supplements.info.nih.gov
- Medline Plus
  http://medlineplus.gov
- USDA
  http://www.nutrition.gov
- National Center for Complementary and Alternative Medicine (NCCAM)
  http://nccam.nih.gov
- Linus Pauling Institute Micronutrient Information Center
  http://lpi.oregonstate.edu/infocenter/

SUMMARY

Diabetes is a complex, multifaceted chronic disease with multiple comorbidities. Patients are frequently interested in discussing complementary treatments in hopes of reducing or avoiding additional medications and/or transition to insulin. Many nutritional and botanic medicines have support of clinical research which is of varying quality Thus, clinicians are responsible for educating patients on the available data including the limitations in scientific knowledge. Supplements should be recommended with all cardiometabolic risk factors in mind including lipid profile and blood pressure and also their interaction with medications. Patient self-monitoring of blood glucose is recommended for all patients, but is especially important when new supplements are added and if the patient uses insulin. Laboratory assessment can be maintained on a standard schedule, that is, every 3 months; however, some supplements may require more frequent monitoring, for example, vitamin D replacement. Clinical benchmarks that include a timeline and expected change should be established with the patient on therapeutic trials of supplementation. Optimizing weight, fitness, dietary patterns, stress management, as well as laboratory values such as $HgbA_{1C}$ are all important in managing this chronic disease to improve quality and length of life of patients with diabetes. The use of botanic and nutritional supplements can play an important role in improving patient autonomy, responsibility, and adherence to a treatment plan in addition to their biological benefits.

References

1. Saydeh, S. Poor control of risk factors for vascular disease among adults with previously diagnosed diabetes. *JAMA* 2004;291(3):335–342.
2. Bell RA, Suerken CK, Grzywacz JG, Lang W, Quandt SA, Arcury TA. Complementary and alternative medicine use among adults with diabetes in the United States. *Altern Ther Health Med* 2006;12(5):16–22.
3. Garrow D, Egede LE. National patterns and correlates of complementary and alternative medicine use in adults with diabetes. *J Altern Complement Med* 2006;12(9):895–902.

4. Garrow D, Egede LE. Association between complementary and alternative medicine use, preventive care practices, and use of conventional medical services among adults with diabetes. *Diabetes Care* 2006;29(1):15–19.
5. Yeh G. Systematic review of herbs and dietary supplements for glycemic control in diabetes. *Diabetes Care* 2003;36(4):1277–1294.
6. Bradley R, Oberg EB, Calabrese C, Standish LJ. Algorithm for complementary and alternative medicine practice and research in type 2 diabetes. *J Altern Complement Med* 2007;13(1):159–175.
7. Liu KW, Dai LK, Jean W. Metformin-related vitamin B12 deficiency. *Age Ageing* 2006;35(2):200–2001.
8. Lindenbaum J, Savage DG, Stabler SP, Allen RH. Diagnosis of cobalamin deficiency: II. Relative sensitivities of serum cobalamin, methylmalonic acid, and total homocysteine concentrations. *Am J Hematol* 1990;34(2):99–107.
9. Oosterhuis WP, Niessen RW, Bossuyt PM, Sanders GT, Sturk A. Diagnostic value of the mean corpuscular volume in the detection of vitamin B12 deficiency. *Scand J Clin Lab Invest* 2000;60(1):9–18.
10. Mozaffarian D, Rimm EB. Fish intake, contaminants, and human health: evaluating the risks and the benefits. *JAMA* 2006;296(15): 1885–1899.
11. Anderson RA. Chromium as an essential nutrient for humans. *Regul Toxicol Pharmacol* 1997;26(1 pt 2):S35–S41.
12. Anderson RA, Polansky MM, Bryden NA. Stability and absorption of chromium and absorption of chromium histidinate complexes by humans. *Biol Trace Elem Res* 2004;101(3): 211–218.
13. Yajnik CS, Smith RF, Hockaday TD, Ward NI. Fasting plasma magnesium concentrations and glucose disposal in diabetes. *Br Med J (Clin Res Ed)* 1984;288(6423):1032–1034.
14. Rodriguez-Moran M and Guerrero-Romero F. Oral magnesium supplementation improves insulin sensitivity and metabolic control in type 2 diabetic subjects: a randomized double-blind controlled trial. *Diabetes Care* 2003;26(4):1147–1152.
15. Mathieu C, Gysemans C, Giuliett A, Bouillon R. et al. Vitamin D and diabetes. *Diabetologia* 2005;48(7):1247–1257.
16. Targher G, Bertolini L, Padovani R, et al. Serum 25-hydroxyvitamin D3 concentrations and carotid artery intima-media thickness among type 2 diabetic patients. *Clin Endocrinol (Oxf)* 2006;65(5):593–597.
17. Chiu KC, Chu A, Go VL, Saad MF. Hypovitaminosis D is associated with insulin resistance and beta cell dysfunction. *Am J Clin Nutr* 2004;79(5):820–825.
18. Vieth R. Vitamin D supplementation, 25-hydroxyvitamin D concentrations, and safety. *Am J Clin Nutr* 1999;69(5):842–856.
19. Borissova AM, Tankova T, Kirilov G, Dakovska L, Kovacheva R. The effect of vitamin D3 on insulin secretion and peripheral insulin sensitivity in type 2 diabetic patients. *Int J Clin Pract* 2003;57(4): 258–261.
20. Langsjoen PH, Langsjoen AM. The clinical use of HMG CoA-reductase inhibitors and the associated depletion of coenzyme Q10. A review of animal and human publications. *Biofactors* 2003;18(1–4):101–111.
21. Hargreaves IP, Duncan AJ, Heales SJ, Land JM. The effect of HMG-CoA reductase inhibitors on coenzyme Q10: possible biochemical/clinical implications. *Drug Saf* 2005;28 (8):659–676.
22. Hodgson JM, Watts GF, Playford DA, Burke V, Croft KD. Coenzyme Q10 improves blood pressure and glycaemic control: a controlled trial in subjects with type 2 diabetes. *Eur J Clin Nutr* 2002;56(11):1137–1142.
23. Langsjoen P, Langsjoen P, Willis R, Folkers K. Treatment of essential hypertension with coenzyme Q10. *Mol Aspects Med* 1994;15(suppl):S265–S72.
24. Chopra RK, Bhagavan HN. On the bioequivalence and bioavailability of three coenzyme Q10 products. *J Med Food* 2006;9(1):131–132; author reply 133–134.

25. Sun Y, Lai MS, Lu CJ. Effectiveness of vitamin B12 on diabetic neuropathy: systematic review of clinical controlled trials. *Acta Neurol Taiwan* 2005;14(2):48–54.
26. Ziegler D, Ametov A, Barinov A, et al. Oral treatment with alpha-lipoic acid improves symptomatic diabetic polyneuropathy: the SYDNEY 2 trial. *Diabetes Care* 2006;29(11): 2365–2370.
27. Srinivasan K. Plant foods in the management of diabetes mellitus: spices as beneficial antidiabetic food adjuncts. *Int J Food Sci Nutr* 2005;56(6):399–414.
28. Aviram M, Rosenblat M, Gaitini D, et al. Pomegranate juice consumption for 3 years by patients with carotid artery stenosis reduces common carotid intima-media thickness, blood pressure and LDL oxidation. *Clin Nutr* 2004;23(3):423–433.
29. Esmaillzadeh A, Tahbaz F, Gaieni I, et al. Concentrated pomegranate juice improves lipid profiles in diabetic patients with hyperlipidemia. *J Med Food* 2004;7(3):305–308.
30. Riccardi G, Capaldo B, Vaccaro O. Functional foods in the management of obesity and type 2 diabetes. *Curr Opin Clin Nutr Metab Care* 2005;8(6):630–635.

CHAPTER 48

Migraine Headache

Robert Alan Bonakdar

Case: *Beth is a 36-year-old female with menstrual migraines and intended pregnancy.*

BACKGROUND

- Migraines affect approximately 28 million Americans with typical onset in the teen years.
- Migraine patient are satisfied or very satisfied with current care options < 25% of the time (1, 2).
- Approximately one third of migraine sufferers attempt some type of complementary and alternative medicine (CAM) therapy including supplements with the most common rationale being: "potential improvement of headache" (47.7%) (3).
- In comparison to prescription options, certain dietary supplement may provide a relatively similar number needed to treat (NNT) for benefit and a lower side effects profile (number needed to harm [NNH]). Example: as preventative agents, riboflavin and valproic acid have a NNT of 2.3 vs. 1.6, respectively. However, their NNH are 33.3 and 2.4, respectively, representing a higher much higher likelihood of tolerability for riboflavin (4).

*H*EARING THE PATIENT OUT WITH RESPECT

Beth is a 36-year-old female who has a strong maternal family history of migraines who has personally suffered from headaches since she was 14 years old. She describes her headaches as typically one-sided, throbbing, and lasting several hours to several days with severe episodes requiring rare emergency room treatment 1 to 2 times a year. Her headaches are worst during her menstrual cycle and can vary from 4 to 10 headaches per month both during work and nonwork times. Associated headache symptoms include preheadache visual disturbances as well as nausea and rare vomiting. She denies any motor or sensory abnormalities (hemiplegia) or changes/progression of the symptoms recently. During an emergency room visit last year, she had a normal brain MRI and serum chemistry panel.

Pertinent Medical History

Beth has associated dysmenorrhea which she correlated with more severe migraines. Other workup for gynecological abnormalities has been negative. She denies other medical problems.

Alleviating and Exacerbating Factors

Beth describes her menstrual cycle and low noises as triggers she notices. She used a quiet dark room and ice in addition to medication for her migraines when available.

Treatment History

Beth has attempted a number of acute/abortive therapies initiating with over-the-counter analgesics and more recently requiring triptans, which provide adequate but at times variable or incomplete relief. Currently, she uses analgesics including nonsteroidal anti-inflammatory drugs and triptans a minimum of 1 to 2×/wk. She has also tried a number of preventative agents including beta-blockers, calcium channel blockers, tricyclics, and recently anticonvulsants including topiramate. She has discontinued these either due to lack of response or reactions including fatigue and sedation, stating that "I am very sensitive to medication."

She has not tried any CAM treatments but is interested in dietary supplements and acupuncture.

Lifestyle History

Beth drinks two to three cups of coffee a day—at times more when she has a headache. She exercises with moderate intensity walking 2 to 3×/wk for 30 minutes. She does not describe work stress as a potential trigger and has not attempted any lifestyle measures including food trigger avoidance or stress management. Beth is happily married without children and describes a good social and spiritual network.

She is hoping to attempt her first pregnancy in the next 1 to 2 years and is wishes to decrease medication and looking for possible replacement treatment options in this setting. Her friend has suggested the use of feverfew for her headaches.

Physical Examination

Beth's examination is within normal limits with no neurological abnormalities noted. Vitals and body mass index are within normal limits.

EDUCATING THE PATIENT

Beth is provided an overview of several dietary supplements in the setting of migraine headache. She is made aware that most dietary supplements, similar to prescription agents, do not have clear pregnancy safety data in humans. Because of the upcoming attempt at pregnancy, magnesium, omega-3s, and low-dose riboflavin appear to be the safest choices (5). Other choices are discussed and are reserved for times when she is not attempting pregnancy. She is asked to attempt the recommended supplement for 3 months before reevaluating potential benefit.

Several supplements (such as feverfew with potential uterine stimulatory effects), should be avoided in the setting of pregnancy. (See appendix for Dietary Supplement Safety Section.)

OVERVIEW OF SUPPLEMENT CONSIDERATIONS

Magnesium

Magnesium is essential for numerous functions related to migraines including maintaining vascular stability, energy production, and calcium channel antagonism (6). Human subjects with poor neurovascular tone demonstrate low cerebrospinal fluid magnesium levels and lower ionized/intracellular magnesium levels have been correlated in those most likely to suffer with migraines as well as predict those most likely to respond to magnesium supplementation (7–9).

Intravenous magnesium has been found in studies to be of benefit in acute migraine at a standard dose of 1 g magnesium sulfate (10, 11). In oral form for migraine prevention, the most appropriate formulation and dose of magnesium remains unclear and some trials have been difficult to interpret because of formulation variability and dropout rates due to magnesium's gastrointestinal side effects. Overall, magnesium's safety profile and potential benefit (especially in decreasing migraine frequency) makes it worth a theraputic trial in most cases.

In a 12-week randomized, double blind, placebo controlled trial (RDBPCT) ($N = 81$), subjects with migraine who utilized 24 mmol (600 mg/d) trimagnesium dicitrate decreased headache frequency by 42% versus 16% with placebo ($P < .05$). Migraine days and drug consumption also decreased significantly. A nonsignificant trend for decreased intensity of migraine was also noted. Adverse events included diarrhea (18.6%) and gastric irritation (4.7%) (12).

There is also preliminary data of benefit in the setting of pediatric and menstrual migraine.

- **Pediatric migraine**: In a 16-week RDBPCT, children 3 to 17 years of age with at least weekly, moderate-to-severe headaches received magnesium oxide (9 mg/kg/d divided TID with food ($n = 58$) or placebo ($n = 60$). Significant decreases in headache frequency ($P = .0037$) and headache severity ($P = .0029$) were noted relative to placebo treatment (13).
- **Menstrual migraine:** In a 16-week RDBPCT (with a 2-month run-in period) ($N = 20$), subjects with menstrual migraines utilizing 360 mg of magnesium pyrrolidone carboxylic acid daily demonstrated a significant decrease in number of headache, total pain index, and premenstrual complaints versus placebo (7).

Patients should be started at a low dose (100 mg/d) and titrated on the basis of GI tolerability to 300 mg to 400 mg/d as appropriate based on the formulation attempted. In certain cases, chelated/reacted and long-acting forms of magnesium may possess better tolerability.

Riboflavin (Vitamin B-2)

Riboflavin is a coenzyme vital to energy metabolism through its role in the flavin adenine dinucleotide system. Disruption in this system has been linked to vascular instability and inflammation. Riboflavin has been tested in a number of open and comparative trials versus other preventative agents (beta-blockers). These initial trials, typically utilizing 400 mg/d, lead to the controlled trial noted below:

In an RDBPCT ($N = 55$), riboflavin at 400 mg/d demonstrating a responder rate (a 50% reduction in symptoms) of 59% versus 15% with placebo ($P = .002$). In this trial response took 3 months to become evidence with the most benefit noted with reduction in the frequency of headache. Side effects were minimal and included diarrhea. The NNT was 2.3 (4).

Butterbur (*Petasites hybridus*)

Butterbur is a traditional European herb used for conditions including allergy and more recently receiving attention in the prevention of migraine headache. The mechanism is unclear but may be due to reduction in vascular inflammation. A number of trials have been carried out including a recent well-controlled trial.

In a three-arm, placebo controlled trial, 150 mg/d of butterbur (Petadolex) over 4 month demonstrated a significant reduction in frequency of headache versus placebo (48% vs. 26%, [$P = .0012$]). Doses less than 150 mg/d did not appear significantly helpful. Side effects included mild gastrointestinal events, predominantly burping (14).

Unprocessed butterbur has been linked with hepatic dysfunction secondary to hepatotoxic alkaloids. This potential does not appear to be a problem with research-tested formulations including Petadolex which is processed to remove these potential alkaloids. Patients are cautioned to use only recommended brands and periodic chemistry panel is recommended to evaluate hepatic function in long-term use.

Coenzyme Q-10 (CoQ10)

Similar to riboflavin, CoQ10 is essential in energy metabolism, specifically efficient functioning of the electron transport chain. Suboptimal CoQ10 status has been linked to a number of neurological disorders including Parkinson disease, Huntington disease, and migraine.

In a 4-month RDBPCT ($N = 42$), subjects with migraine who utilized 300 mg of coenzyme Q10 daily had a significant decrease in attack-frequency as well as days with headache and nausea. Responder - rate for attack frequency was 47.6% for CoQ10 and 14.4% for placebo. CoQ10 was well tolerated and had an NNT of 3 (14).

Feverfew (*Tanacetum parthenium*)

Feverfew is a daisylike plant recognized by first century Greek physicians for its analgesic and antipyretic qualities. Its active ingredients include sesquiterpene lactones, particularly parthenolide, which demonstrate in vitro modulation of prostaglandins, serotonin, and platelet phospholipase, all of which may play a role in migraine (16).

In several RDBPCT, feverfew has demonstrated inconsistent results which may be due to the formulation utilized and product inconsistency (17). Most positive trials have used a freeze-dried formulation with 100 mg or more feverfew, typically standardized to 0.2% or higher parthenolide content. These trials have demonstrated a modest reduction in migraine frequency and severity (18). In some countries, parthenolide consistency is required for feverfew products with US studies demonstrating a significant variation in reported versus actual parthenolide content (19).

If attempted, feverfew may take 4 to 6 weeks before benefits are noted with side effects being minimal and including GI upset. Feverfew should be avoided in pregnancy. Withdrawal headache has been noted, so use should be tapered if appropriate (i.e., prior to surgery) to minimize this potential. Newer formulations with more consistent and stable dosing are anticipated.

Omega-3 Fatty Acids

Beth has coexisting dysmenorrhea with her migraines, which is not an uncommon scenario. Migraine is associated with decreased concentrations of omega-3 fatty acids in platelet and red blood cell membranes and dysmenorrhea has been associated with low omega-3 polyunsaturated fatty acid intake (20).

Both conditions have small trials demonstrating improvement with omega-3 supplementation (21, 22). Because of her history, an attempt at improving Beth's omega-3 intake with supplementation while improving her background diet appears a prudent approach that can be continued into pregnancy. She is instructed on an anti-inflammatory diet to increase omega-3 and decrease omega-6 intake. In addition, she is instructed on omega-3 supplementation with emphasis on finding well-regulated supplements high in the eicosapentaenoic acid (EPA) and docosahexaenoic acid (DHA) components.

RECORD/RECOMMENDATIONS

After review of appropriate supplements and testing which demonstrated a low RBC magnesium level and low normal coenzyme Q10 levels the following recommendation were made:

Supplements Recommendations

Supplement	Brand/Formulation	Dose	Notes
Magnesium	• Metagenics Mag glycinate (100 mg/ tablet) • Ortho Molecular Products: Reacted Magnesium (235 mg/ 2 tablets)	Start 100 mg/d advance as tolerated to 300–400 mg/d	• All supplements to be reevaluated in 8–12 wk • Titrate slowly to improve GI tolerability • Chelated/reacted formulation preferred • Effect on frequency > severity migraine
Riboflavin	Various	400 mg/d in trials	• Effect on migraine frequency > severity • Rare possibility of diarrhea
Omega-3	• Nordic Naturals Pro Omega (325 mg EPA/ 225 mg DHA/tablet) • Pro-EPA (425 mg EPA/ 100 mg DHA) • Ortho Molecular Products: Orthomega (420 mg EPA/300 mg DHA/tablet) • Lovaza[a] (465 mg EPA / 375 mg DHA/tab)	1 g/d (EPA/DHA) increase to 2–4 g/d as tolerated	May need to change formulation to decrease stomach upset, burping; Also available in liquid formulation when patients reach high doses

[a]Lovaza is currently FDA approved for hypertriglyceridemia.

Additional Recommendation

Beth is asked to keep a journal of headaches to monitor frequency, severity, and triggers. She is asked to avoid potential trigger foods (ripe cheese, wine, excess caffeine during the trial period) and to minimize use of analgesics, especially more than 2×/wk. She is also asked to contact your office if she is considered any other dietary supplements so you can review the safety and efficacy.

Other Helpful Treatments

Various mind body therapies including biofeedback and stress management as well as acupuncture can be considered in addition to dietary supplement suggestions.

BE AWARE OF REACTIONS AND INTERACTIONS

- Make the patient aware of potential GI side effects from magnesium and riboflavin (diarrhea), omega-3 (burping, bloating), and to call you office to discuss alternate dosing or brands. Other side effects are rare.
- Patient handouts provided for supplements above through Natural Medicines Comprehensive Database.
- Because of the upcoming pregnancy, advise patient to be especially diligent in discussing any planned supplements, prescription, and over-the-counter medications with her health care providers. Laboratory follow-up/monitoring: retest intracellular/ionized magnesium to ensure that she has reached therapeutic levels.

AGREE TO DISCUSS AND FOLLOW-UP

Patient follows up in 12 weeks stating that she was able to reach 400 mg of riboflavin, 200 mg of magnesium, and 1.5 g of omega-3 fatty acids with slow titration over the first 3 weeks. She states that she did not notice significant benefit until 6 weeks after use. Subsequently she has noticed a greater reduction in the frequency than severity of both her headaches and dysmenorrhea. She has been able to decrease her use of analgesics and triptans by approximately 30% over the last month. She describes less functional interference from her headaches including no days of work missed or visits to the emergency room for severe headaches. Beth's most recent magnesium level has reached a normal level and a recent chemistry panel is normal.

Beth is overall satisfied with the progress she is making although it has been slow in onset. She is asked to follow up in 3 months and to increase her omega-3 dose by 1 g, if possible.

At 6-month follow-up the patient has continued to find relief from the supplements recommended and is now at 400 mg of riboflavin, 300 mg of chelated magnesium, and 2 g of omega-3s a day. She is currently experiencing 1 to 2 migraines per month which she grades at 60% the severity of those she experienced before her initiating supplements. She continues to see parallel benefit in reduced symptoms of dysmenorrhea. She plans to begin biofeedback and acupuncture in the next month to help with remaining symptoms.

The patient will be followed every 3 months or sooner if there is any change in her status. She is asked to call if she has questions before her follow-up.

LEARN

The patient is referred to the following resources for updated information on migraine headache and dietary supplements.

- National Headache Foundation
  www.headaches.org
- Natural Medicines Comprehensive Database consumer version
  www.NaturalDatabase.com
- Office of Dietary Supplements
  http://dietary-supplements.info.nih.gov
- Medline Plus
  http://medlineplus.gov
- USDA
  http://www.nutrition.gov

SUMMARY

Migraines are complex, multifactorial disorders which continue to leave a significant number of patients under medical care with less than satisfactory improvement. This has prompted a greater interest in the use of dietary supplements which demonstrate preliminary benefit in the setting of migraine. Several of the supplements reviewed have the additional benefit of increased tolerability and medication sparing. The most common scenario of supplement use for migraines is unfortunately a less than optimal dietary supplement taken for too short an evaluation period. Clinicians are key in helping patients choose wisely and safely, continue treatment for an adequate period of time (typically 3 to 4 months), and schedule regular follow-ups to discuss benefits, side effects, monitoring, and modifications in the treatment plan.

The future of dietary supplements for migraine appears to point to additional attempts at standardized and combination products. This includes feverfew and other phyto anti-inflammatories (willow bark, ginger, etc.) (23). More dietary supplement choices for acute treatment of migraine are also expected. Finally, the use of supplements with hormonal capability, such as melatonin, is being investigated (24, 25).

References

1. Lake AE. Psychological impact: the personal burden of migraine. *Am J Man Care* 1999;5:S111–S121.
2. Lipton RB, Stewart WF. Acute migraine therapy: do doctors understand what patients want from therapy? *Headache* 1999;39:S20–S26.
3. Rossi P, Di Lorenzo G, Malpezzi MG, et al. Prevalence, pattern and predictors of use of (CAM) in migraine patients attending a headache clinic in Italy. *Cephalalgia* 2005;25(7): 493–506.
4. Schoenen J, Jacquy J, Lenaerts M. Effectiveness of high-dose riboflavin in migraine prophylaxis. *Neurology* 1998;50:466–470.
5. Welch KM. Migraine and pregnancy. *Adv Neurol* 1994;64:77–81.
6. Weaver K. Magnesium and migraine. *Headache* 1990;30:168.
7. Faccinetti F, Sances G, Borella P, et al. Magnesium prophylaxis of menstrual migraine: effects on intra-cellular magnesium. *Headache* 1991;31:298–304.

8. Ramadan NM, Halvorson H, Vande-Linde A, et al. Low brain magnesium in migraine. *Headache* 1989;29:590–593.
9. Mauskop A, Altura BT, Altura BM. Serum ionized magnesium levels and serum ionized calcium/ionized magnesium ratios in women with menstrual migraine. *Headache* 2002; 42(4):242–248.
10. Corbo J, Esses D, Bijur PE, et al. Randomized clinical trial of intravenous magnesium sulfate as an adjunctive medication for emergency department treatment of migraine headache. *Ann Emerg Med* 2001;38(6):621–627.
11. Bigal ME, Bordini CA, Tepper SJ, et al. Intravenous magnesium sulphate in the acute treatment of migraine without aura and migraine with aura. A randomized, double-blind, placebo-controlled study. *Cephalalgia* 2002;22(5):345–353.
12. Peikert A, Wilimzig C, Kohne-Volland R. Prophylaxis of migraine with oral magnesium: results from a prospective, multi-center, placebo-controlled and double-blind randomized study. *Cephalalgia* 1996;16:257–263.
13. Wang F, Van Den Eeden SK, Ackerson LM, et al. Oral magnesium oxide prophylaxis of frequent migrainous headache in children: a randomized, double-blind, placebo-controlled trial. *Headache* 2003;43(6):601–610.
14. Lipton RB, Gobel H, Einhaupl KM, et al. Petasites hybridus root (butterbur) is an effective preventive treatment for migraine. *Neurology* 2004;63(12):2240–2244.
15. Watanabe H, Kuwabara T, Ohkubo M, Tsuji S, Yuasa T. Elevation of cerebral lactate detected by localized 1H-magnetic resonance spectroscopy in migraine during the interictal period. *Neurology* 1996;47:1093–1095.
16. Sumner H, Salan U, Knight DW, Hoult JRS. Inhibition of 5-Lipoxygenase and Cyclo-oxygenase in Leukocytes by Feverfew. *Biochem Pharmacol* 1992;43:2313–2320.
17. Pittler MH, Ernst E. Feverfew for preventing migraine. *Cochrane Database Syst Rev* 2004;(1):CD002286.
18. Palevitch D, Earon G, Carasso R. Feverfew(Tanacetum parthenium) as a prophylactic treatment for migraine: a double-blind placebo-controlled study. *Phytother Res* 1997;11: 508–511.
19. Heptinstall S, Awang DVC, Dawson BA, et al. Parthenolide content and bioactivity of feverfew (Tanacetum parthenium). Estimation of commercial and authenticated feverfew products. *J Pharm Pharmacol* 1992;44:391–395.
20. Deutch B. Menstrual pain in Danish women correlated with low n-3 polyunsaturated fatty acid intake. *Eur J Clin Nutr* 1995;49(7):508–516.
21. Harel Z, Biro FM, Kottenhahn RK, Rosenthal SL. Supplementation with omega-3 polyunsaturated fatty acids in the management of dysmenorrhea in adolescents. *Am J Obstet Gynecol* 1996;174(4):1335–1338.
22. McCarren T, Hitzemann R, Smith R, et al. Amelioration of severe migraine by fish oil (omega-3) fatty acids. *Am J Clin Nutr* 1985;41:874.
23. Shrivastava R, Pechadre JC, John GW. Tanacetum parthenium and Salix alba (Mig-RL) combination in migraine prophylaxis: a prospective, open-label study. *Clin Drug Investig* 2006;26(5):287–296.
24. Peres MF, Zukerman E, da Cunha Tanuri F, Moreira FR, Cipolla-Neto J. Melatonin, 3 mg, is effective for migraine prevention. *Neurology* 2004;63(4):757.
25. Vogler B, Rapoport AM, Tepper SJ, et al. Role of melatonin in the pathophysiology of migraine: implications for treatment. *CNS Drugs* 2006;20(5):343–350.

CHAPTER 49

Hypercholesterolemia and Hypertension

Robert Alan Bonakdar

Case: *Claire, 38-year-old with hypercholesterolemia and prehypertension.*

BACKGROUND

- Prevalence of hypercholesterolemia in American adults from the National Health and Nutrition Examination Survey (NHANES) is approximately 50% with less than 40% of those affected being aware of it, less than 20% being treated, and less than 10% meeting treatment guidelines (1, 2).
- Although improved from the 10% rate of blood pressure control (<140/90 mm Hg) in the first NHANES data 1976 to 1980, the most recent rate of meeting treatment goals is still only 40% of those diagnosed with hypertension (HTN).
- NHANES data from 1999 to 2000 and US Census Bureau information demonstrated that 29% to 31% of the adult US population has hypertension which translates into 58 to 65 million Americans, an increase from 43.2 million estimated in the 1988 to 1991 NHANES III survey (3, 4).
- Currently, dietary supplements in the form of plant stanols/sterols and soluble dietary fiber are components of the National Cholesterol Education Program Adult Treatment Panel III (NCEP ATP III) Guidelines for therapeutic lifestyle changes for reaching goals in patients with elevated cholesterol (5).

HEARING THE PATIENT OUT WITH RESPECT

Claire is a 38-year-old woman whose recent preinsurance physical and laboratory evaluation revealed elevated cholesterol (as noted below) and prehypertension. She is currently asymptomatic but comes in for a checkup to discuss the results and treatment strategies, especially because of her positive family history. She is interested in pursuing lifestyle modification and also has questions about the possible use of CoQ10.

Her most recent basic lipid panel revealed:

- TC (total cholesterol) = 226
- LDL (low-density lipoprotein) = 166
- HDL (high-density lipoprotein) = 43
- TG (triglycerides) = 158 new 189

Pertinent Medical History

No other significant medical history is noted including obesity, diabetes, hyperglycemia, or cigarette use.

Treatment History

Patient has not previously been aware of her elevated cholesterol and not initiated any formal treatment.

Lifestyle History

Claire drinks one cup of coffee a day, one glass of wine three to four times per week and denies any current or previous use of cigarettes. She exercises aerobically three to four times a week for 30 to 40 minutes. Because of her family history she has attempted a low-cholesterol, low-fat diet but does describe having a "sweet-tooth." With this regimen she has achieved a 5-lb weight loss over the last 4 months. She does not describe significant situation stress at home or at her job where she works as an administrative assistant. Claire is married with 2 children and enjoys her home life.

Family History

Claire states that several family members have high cholesterol as well as two male members of her family, including her father, who have suffered heart attack in their 60s.

Physical Examination and Laboratory

Vitals: BP: 138/86 mm Hg (prehypertension); HR = 72; RR = 12; Weight = 180, height = 5′6″ (body mass index (BMI) at 29)

Claire's examination is within normal limits and does not demonstrate any. Her laboratory test values including her electrolytes, fasting blood glucose, and urinalysis are within normal limits. High sensitive C-reactive protein (hsCRP) is borderline. Vitamin D (25OH) is low at 16 ng/ml. Other labs are unremarkable.

EDUCATING THE PATIENT

Claire is educated that her total and LDL cholesterol as well as TG fall into the category of "borderline high" per the NCEP ATP III primary guidelines. Because of her prehypertension status (systolic pressure from 120 to 139 millimeters of mercury [mm Hg] or a diastolic pressure from 80 to 89 mm Hg) she has an additional risk factor and is at twice the risk to develop hypertension compared to normotensive individuals (6). For both scenarios she can pursue lifestyle modification to improve her status and which, such as the dietary approaches to stop hypertension (DASH), can have effects similar to single drug therapy (7, 8).

She has a discussion regarding the use of coenzyme q10 and told that although it may have some evidence in the setting of isolated systolic hypertension, the best evidence for this supplement appears to be when combined with prescription antihypertensives to provide additive effects. Claire is provided an overview of several diet and dietary supplement interventions she can pursue in the setting of dyslipidemia and hypertension.

TABLE 49.1 DASH Diet

- In a 2,000-calorie DASH diet, the following are recommended:
  - 7–8 servings of grains
  - 4–5 servings of fruits
  - 4–5 servings of vegetables
  - 2–3 servings of low-fat dairy products
  - 2 or less servings of lean meats
  - Snacks and sweets ≤5/wk

OVERVIEW OF CONSIDERATIONS

Dietary Overview

DASH DIET

Dietary changes can have a moderate to significant impact on dyslipidemia and hypertension and in some cases help decrease or avoid need for medications. In the setting of hypertension, two dietary approaches which appear helpful are the DASH diet and the Mediterranean diet. Claire has a dietary consultation and provided with techniques to incorporate the DASH diet (see Table 49.1), which focuses on increasing fruits and vegetables and reducing fat and cholesterol intake. This approach has been shown to provide an average systolic blood pressure reduction of 8 to 14 mm Hg.

MEDITERRANEAN DIET/LINOLENIC ACID

In addition, Claire has a discussion regarding the importance of incorporating foods high in alpha-linolenic acid which are typical in a Mediterranean diet. These foods are typically vegetable oils (flaxseed, canola, soybean oil) but also include nuts and green leafy vegetables. Consuming a diet high in alpha-linolenic acid appears to reduce the risk of hypertension by about one third (9). Handouts regarding these approaches are listed in the appendix.

BLOND PSYLLIUM

Blond psyllium is a water-soluble fiber that is used as a specific powder preparation (Metamucil) or found in cereals, breads, or snack bars. Soluble fibers appear to have beneficial cardiovascular effects and can be recommended for both dyslipidemia and (pre)hypertension. The Food and Drug Administration (FDA) has ruled that foods containing at least 1.7 g of psyllium per serving can be labeled with the claim that it may reduce the risk of heart disease when consumed as part of a diet low in fat and cholesterol.

In an randomized controlled trial (RCT) ($N = 41$), blond psyllium at 12 g/d added to a control amount of 15 g/d demonstrating a 5.9 mm Hg reduction in systolic blood pressure as compared to controls ($P = .002$). There also appeared to be additive benefit when protein (soy) intake was doubled from 12.5% to 25% of energy intake (10).

Blonde psyllium has also been found beneficial in the setting of mild to moderate hypercholesterolemia. This benefit seems to be found at doses of >10 g/d when consumed at mealtime (11).

In a meta-analysis of eight RCT adding 10 g psyllium per day to a low-fat diet for ≥8 wk in subjects with mild-to-moderate hypercholesterolemia was compared to a control diet control. Results demonstrated that psyllium intake lowered serum total cholesterol by 4% ($P < .0001$), LDL cholesterol by 7% ($P < .0001$), and the ratio of apolipoprotein (apo) B to apo A-I by 6% ($P < .05$). No significant effect on serum HDL or triglycerides were noted. Intake appeared well tolerated without severe adverse effects (12).

POTASSIUM

Low potassium intake, especially in the setting of higher than recommended salt intake, appears to be related to hypertension with supplementation associated with a mild reduction. Approved FDA health claims note that at least 350 mg of potassium per serving in foods that are low in sodium, saturated fat, and cholesterol might help reduce the risk of developing high blood pressure (13).

In a review of 33 RCTs (N = 2,609 participants), potassium supplementation was associated with a significant reduction in mean systolic (3.11 mm Hg) and diastolic (1.97 mm Hg) blood pressure. Effects were most pronounced in trials in which subjects had higher sodium intake (14).

In meeting with your clinic staff, Claire is educated on an optimal diet for her which uses elements of the DASH and Mediterranean diet while focusing on high potassium foods as well as use of fiber at mealtime.

PLANT STEROLS/STANOL

Plant sterols structurally resemble cholesterol and competitively inhibit both dietary and biliary cholesterol absorption. They are currently part of the NCEP ATPIII Guidelines for therapeutic lifestyle changes for reaching goals in patients with elevated cholesterol levels and available in various formulations including capsules, spreads, and additives to various foods such as juice. They have been shown to reduce LDL cholesterol by about 10% in normal circumstances and up to 20% when combined with a low-fat/cholesterol diet. The optimal dosing for plant sterols appears to be 2 g/d.

In a meta-analysis of 41 trials using 2 g/d of stanols or sterols, LDL was reduced by 10% without benefit noted at higher doses. No difference was noted with use of sterols and stanols. Effects appeared additive with diet with optimal combinations demonstrating LDL reduction of 20%. Of note, plasma levels of vitamins A and D are not affected by use of plant sterols (15).

FISH OIL

Fish oils have been used for both reduction of blood pressure and lipids/triglycerides. In the setting of blood pressure reduction, 4 g/d has typically been used with a high concentration of eicosapentaenoic acid (EPA) + docosahexaenoic acid (DHA), component.

In an RCT ($N = 32$) of mild essential hypertensive (diastolic BP: 95 to 104 mm Hg), subjects received either fish oil (total 4 g with EPA and DHA ethyl esters [2.04 g EPA and 1.4 g DHA] or a control of olive oil (4 g/d) for 4 months. Both systolic BP (−6 mm Hg, $P < .05$) and diastolic BP (−5 mm Hg, $P < .05$) decreased significantly during fish oil supplementation. The maximum effect was observed after 2 months with return to baseline after discontinuation (16).

For dyslipidemia, various dosages and formulations of fish oil have been utilized. The most robust benefit of fish oils appears to be in reduction of triglycerides which can be 20% or more. Other areas of change on the basic lipid profile may be modest or insignificant (slight increase in total LDL and HDL) with the most significant change likely being improvement in particle size, including LDL, which may decrease atherogenic potential (17). Four grams of prescription fish oil Lovaza is FDA approved in the setting of hypertriglyceridemia.

VITAMIN D

Population studies have demonstrated from a cardiovascular standpoint that low or deficient levels of vitamin D (25OH) (typically defined as level <20 ng/mL for deficiency and <30 ng/mL for insufficiency) are associated with higher likelihood of hypertension, hyperlipidemia, diabetes mellitus, and cardiovascular mortality. From a general health standpoint, *vitamin 25 (OH) D levels in the lowest quartile (<17.8 ng/ml) are independently associated with all-cause mortality in the general population* (18, 19). Vitamin D as an intervention does not have extensive research, but combining 400 IU of vitamin D with calcium may have additive effects on dyslipidemia in the setting of weight loss.

In a 15-week RCT (n = 63), vitamin D (400 IU) + calcium (1,200 mg/d) were examined versus placebo as part of a weight-loss intervention. At the end of the trial those on vitamin D plus calcium had significantly greater reductions in total:LDL and LDL:HDL ($P < .01$ for both) and of LDL cholesterol ($P < .05$) which were independent of weight loss. Also, a trend for beneficial changes in HDL cholesterol, triglycerides, and total cholesterol was noted in the calcium + Vitamin D group ($P = .08$).

For Claire whose level was quite low, a high-dose intervention as noted in the chart below is initiated to bring her to an adequate level. Subsequently, a maintenance dose will be determined to keep her within the normal range.

COCOA

Claire notes a "sweet-tooth" which usually takes the form of hard candy and other simple sugar choices. She is aware that these choices can be detrimental in her attempt to manage her medical state both by increasing caloric intake and by decreasing intake of health-promoting foods. She is given counseling on the incorporation of small amounts of dark and semidark chocolate into her diet both to satisfy her "sweet-tooth" and serve as a potential adjunctive agent for reaching her health goals. Certain types of dark chocolate have demonstrated mild benefit in the setting of hypertension. Overall, consuming 46 to 105 g/d (213 to 500 mg of cocoa polyphenols) lowers systolic blood pressure by 4.7 mm Hg and diastolic blood pressure by 2.8 mm Hg (20).

In an RCT with crossover ($N = 20$) consuming 100 g/d dark chocolate (containing 88 mg flavanols) was compared with 90 g/d flavanol-free white chocolate (control) for 15 days. Those consuming dark chocolate had improvement in 24-hour systolic BP of −11.9 mm Hg, $P < .0001$ and diastolic BP of −8.5 mm Hg, $P < .0001$. Dark chocolate also demonstrated benefit in flow-mediated dilation and LDL cholesterol ($P < .05$) (21).

In a trial ($N = 44$), consuming 6.3 g of dark chocolate per day (30 kcal and 30 mg of polyphenols) decreases systolic blood pressure by 2.9 mm Hg and diastolic blood pressure by 1.9 mm Hg when consumed for 18 weeks by patients with prehypertension or mild hypertension as compared with white chocolate. Subjects consuming dark chocolate also had an increase in active nitric oxide levels (22).

RECORD/RECOMMENDATIONS

After review of appropriate supplements and laboratory testing, the following supplement recommendations were made and are summarized for the patient and chart:

Supplements Recommendations

Supplement	Brand/Formulation	Dose	Notes
Plant sterols (Sitostanol)	• Cholest-off 2 tablets (900 mg plant sterols/stanols)/d • Spreads: Take Control Smart Balance	Goal = 2 g/d	• All supplements to be reevaluated in 8–12 wk
Blond psyllium (soluble fiber)	Various including Metamucil	10–25 g/d	Advance slowly and maximum dose may be limited by GI tolerability
Vitamin D	High dose: Various OTC formulation at 5,000 IU Vitamin D_3/capsule Prescription: 50,000 IU Vitamin D_2/capsule Low dose: Various formulations available in 1, 2, 5,000 IU/per serving. In liquid formulations: Bio-D-Mulsion liquid 400 IU Vitamin D_3/drop	D_3 or D_2 formulation (50,000 IU once/wk × 8–12 wk and then continue at appropriate doses to maintain optimal level.	
Omega-3	• Nordic Naturals Pro Omega (325 mg EPA/225 mg DHA/tablet) • Pro-EPA (425 mg EPA/100 mg DHA) • Ortho Molecular Products: Orthomega (420 mg EPA/300 mg DHA/tablet) • Lovaza[a] (465 mg EPA/375 mg DHA/tablet)	4 g/d (total fish oil with approximately 3 g EPA/DHA)	May need to change formulation to decrease stomach upset, burping; Also available in liquid formulation when patients reach high doses
Dark chocolate	Ritter Sport Halbbitter (Alfred Ritter GmbH & Co.)	6–30 g/d	Lower doses are recommended to decrease high caloric intake

[a]Lovaza is currently FDA approved for hypertriglyceridemia.

Additional Recommendation

Claire is asked to keep a journal of her dietary changes to monitor compliance and tolerability of the DASH/Mediterranean selections as well as finding foods with appropriate potassium to meet the suggested intake. She is also asked to monitor her blood pressure periodically prior to her follow-up.

BE AWARE OF REACTIONS AND INTERACTIONS

- Make the patient aware of potential GI side effects from fiber (loose stools, diarrhea) and omega-3 (burping, bloating) and to call you office to discuss alternate dosing or brands. Other side effects are rare.
- Patient handouts provided for supplements above through Natural Medicines Comprehensive Database.
- Laboratory follow-up/monitoring: repeat lipid testing (Vertical Auto Profile (VAP) panel), hsCRP, vitamin D, and electrolytes.

AGREE TO DISCUSS AND FOLLOW-UP

At the 16 week follow up, Claire states has been able stating that she was able to advance slowly and tolerate 4 g of fish oils and 15 g of psyllium per day with minimal GI disturbance. She finds that the dietary changes do not leave her hungry as she feared and is enjoying her daily amounts of dark chocolate and healthy nuts when she needs to snack. Her blood pressure readings have been consistently below 120/80, her BMI is now 28 based on a 5-lb weight loss since her last visit. Her newest laboratories reveal the following:

- TC = 189 (↓16%)
- LDL = 128 (↓ 22%)
- HDL = 47 (↑ 4%)
- TG = 123 (↓ 35%)
- Vitamin D 25(OH) = 39 ng/ml
  hsCRP is in the normal range,
  All other labs unremarkable.

Claire is pleased with the progress she is making and is asked to follow up in 3 months for repeat evaluation. She will continue on her diet and dietary supplement recommendations as previous with dosing of her vitamin D_3 done to keep her in the normal range.

LEARN

The patient and provider can utilize the following resources for updated information on cholesterol and blood pressure management.

- National Heart Lung and Blood Institute (Patient and clinician resources for high blood pressure and dyslipidemia including the DASH diet)
  - Health professionals site
    http://www.nhlbi.nih.gov/health/indexpro.htm
  - Consumer site
    http://www.nhlbi.nih.gov/health/index.htm
- Your Guide to Lowering Cholesterol with Therapeutic Lifestyle Changes (TLC)
  http://www.nhlbi.nih.gov/health/public/heart/chol/chol_tlc.htm
- Natural Medicines Comprehensive Database consumer version
  www.NaturalDatabase.com
- Office of Dietary Supplements
  http://dietary-supplements.info.nih.gov
- Medline Plus
  http://medlineplus.gov

- USDA
  http://www.nutrition.gov

SUMMARY

Dyslipidemia and (pre)hypertension are increasing in prevalence and represent modifiable risk factors for cardiovascular disease, the most common cause of death in the United States. Both conditions, when presenting in the borderline state, can be approached with the use of lifestyle and dietary/dietary supplement modification. The above case example represents the use of multiple interventions in a motivated patient with multiple risk factors. In other cases, the clinician may desire to start with a more focused plan with regular follow-up to observe changes, especially when first initiating use of dietary supplements.

Over time, the clinician will become more comfortable in knowing the correct setting for incorporation of various interventions based on factors including severity of disease, patient desire, compliance, and cost. In many cases, the dietary supplement, when incorporated in the borderline states allows the patient additional options to prevent the progression of a borderline state. In addition, the use of diet and dietary interventions can be empowering to patients in gaining control of their borderline state and ensuring better long-term adherence to lifestyle approaches.

References

1. Centers for Disease Control, and Prevention. NHANES 1999–2000 public data release file documentation. Available at: http://www.cdc.gov/nchs/about/major/nhanes/currentnhanes.htm.
2. Ford ES, Mokdad AH, Giles WH, Mensah GA. Serum total cholesterol concentrations and awareness, treatment, and control of hypercholesterolemia among US adults: findings from the National Health and Nutrition Examination Survey, 1999 to 2000. *Circulation* 2003;107(17):2185–2189.
3. Hajjar I, Kotchen TA. Trends in prevalence, awareness, treatment, and control of hypertension in the United States, 1988–2000. *JAMA* 2003;290(2):199–206.
4. Fields LE, Burt VL, Cutler JA. The burden of adult hypertension in the United States 1999 to 2000: a rising tide. *Hypertension* 2004;44(4):398–404.
5. Grundy SM, Cleeman JI, Merz CN. Implications of recent clinical trials for the National Cholesterol Education Program Adult Treatment Panel III Guidelines. *J Am Coll Cardiol* 2004;44(3):720–732.
6. Vasan RS, Larson MG, Leip EP, Kannel WB, Levy D. Assessment of frequency of progression to hypertension in non-hypertensive participants in the Framingham Heart Study: a cohort study. *Lancet* 2001;358(9294):1682–1686.
7. Sacks FM, Svetkey LP, Vollmer WM, et al. Effects on blood pressure of reduced dietary sodium and the Dietary Approaches to Stop Hypertension (DASH) diet. DASH-Sodium Collaborative Research Group. *N Engl J Med* 2001;344:3–10.
8. Vollmer WM, Sacks FM, Ard J, et al. Effects of diet and sodium intake on blood pressure: subgroup analysis of the DASH-sodium trial. *Ann Intern Med* 2001;135:1019–1028.
9. Djoussé L, Arnett DK, Pankow JS, Hopkins PN, Province MA, Ellison RC. Dietary linolenic acid is associated with a lower prevalence of hypertension in the NHLBI Family Heart Study. *Hypertension* 2005;45(3):368–373.
10. Burke V, Hodgson JM, Beilin LJ, et al. Dietary protein and soluble fiber reduce ambulatory blood pressure in treated hypertensives. *Hypertension* 2001;38(4):821–826.

11. Wolever TM, Jenkins DJ, Mueller S, et al. Method of administration influences the serum cholesterol-lowering effect of psyllium. *Am J Clin Nutr* 1994;59:1055–1059.
12. Anderson JW, Allgood LD, Lawrence A, et al. Cholesterol-lowering effects of psyllium intake adjunctive to diet therapy in men and women with hypercholesterolemia: meta-analysis of 8 controlled trials. *Am J Clin Nutr* 2000;71(2):472–479.
13. FDA, CFSAN. FDA-approved potassium health claim notification for potassium containing foods. www.cfsan.fda.gov/~dms/hclm-k.html. Published 2000.
14. Whelton PK, He J, Cutler JA, et al. Effects of oral potassium on blood pressure. Meta-analysis of randomized controlled clinical trials. *JAMA* 1997;277(20):1624–1632.
15. Katan MB, Grundy SM, Jones P et al. Efficacy and safety of plant stanols and sterols in the management of blood cholesterol levels. *Mayo Clin Proc* 2003;78(8):965–978.
16. Prisco D, Paniccia R, Bandinelli B, et al. Effect of medium-term supplementation with a moderate dose of n-3 polyunsaturated fatty acids on blood pressure in mild hypertensive patients. *Thromb Res* 1998;91(3):105–112.
17. Sanchez-Muniz FJ, Bastida S, Viejo JM, Terpstra AH. Small supplements of N-3 fatty acids change serum low density lipoprotein composition by decreasing phospholid and apolipoprotein B concentrations in young adult women. *Eur J Nutr* 1999;38(1):20–27.
18. *Arch Intern Med* 2007;167(11):1159–1165.
19. *Arch Intern Med* 2008;168(15):1629–1637.
20. Taubert D, Roesen R, Schomig E. Effect of cocoa and tea intake on blood pressure: a meta-analysis. *Arch Intern Med* 2007;167:626–634.
21. Grassi D, Necozione S, Lippi C, et al. Cocoa reduces blood pressure and insulin resistance and improves endothelium-dependent vasodilation in hypertensives. *Hypertension* 2005; 46(2):398–405.
22. Taubert D, Roesen R, Lehmann C, et al. Effects of low habitual cocoa intake on blood pressure and bioactive nitric oxide: a randomized controlled trial. *JAMA* 2007;298:49–60.

CHAPTER 50

Low Back Pain

Robert Alan Bonakdar

Case: *Richard, 42-year-old with recurrent low back pain.*

BACKGROUND

- Low back pain is the most common cause of activity limitation in those younger than 45 years of age and one of the top five reasons for visiting a physician (1, 2).
- Approximately 80% of adults will experience low back pain sometime in their lives.
- Americans spend more than $75 billion looking for relief from back pain with more than 10% of US adults reporting back problems (3).

*H*EARING THE PATIENT OUT WITH RESPECT

Richard is a 42-year-old office worker who has had recurrent episode of back pain since his late 30s with an episode starting yesterday. He describes these episodes as intermittent with episodes 2 to 3×/year, not typically based on activity or injury lasting up to 3–4 weeks. He describes the location of the pain as low in the back occurring in a beltlike fashion. He has rarely had any symptoms below the back and denies any lower extremity weakness or numbness. His episodes are typically characterized by moderate to severe spasm of the low back (feeling that it is "locked-up") associated with aching and at times sharp pain (maximum 8/10) which typically causes missed work and interference with daily activities. His pain is increased with extension of his back and relieved with rest, flexion, and certain seated positions.

Richard has received previous evaluation and imaging including x-ray and MRI that have been unremarkable. He denies any significant previous injury or trauma to the area. He has tried various short-term applications of physical therapy, massage, and acupuncture as well as over-the-counter anti-inflammatories, muscle relaxants, and on rare occasion, narcotic medication, when he has had to go to the emergency room for treatment. He has found these treatments variably helpful, but is interested in trying other options, including dietary supplements, which he can incorporate on his own to control these episodes.

Pertinent Medical History

No significant medical history is noted.

Treatment History

As above

Lifestyle History

Richard drinks two to three cup of coffee a day, one beer two to three times per week, and denies any current or previous use of cigarettes. He describes stress "all the time" as part of his sales job but cannot describe a direct relationship to his back pain. He does not describe any significant stress-coping strategies. He exercises less frequently when his pain is flaring, but typically exercises aerobically one to two times a week for 30 minutes. He denies any significant stretching or strengthening program.

Family History

Richard denies any significant family history of low back pain, arthritis, or other rheumatologic disorders in his first-degree relatives.

Physical Examination and Laboratory

VITALS: WITHIN NORMAL LIMITS; PAIN CURRENTLY 5/10 BODY MASS INDEX AT 28

His physical examination demonstrates hypertonicity of the lumbar paraspinal musculature and the infrailiac soft tissue region with associated point sensitivity. He does not have a positive straight leg test or abnormal deep tendon reflexes. No referred or radicular pain is appreciated and normal motor/sensory testing is noted. Extension of the low back causes discomfort and other movements are tolerated but demonstrate generalized reduction in range of movement. All labs, including vitamin D (25OH), are unremarkable.

EDUCATING THE PATIENT

Richard is educated on his condition and receives discussion of several dietary supplements that may be of benefit as listed below. In addition, he is provided discussion and resources on the importance of core strengthening and flexibility exercises which have been shown helpful in the setting of chronic back pain. Lastly, he has an overview of simple breathing exercise he can perform which may be of benefit in the setting of situation stress muscle tension (4).

OVERVIEW OF SUPPLEMENTS

White willow bark, devil's claw, and capsicum (topical) have been shown in a recent Cochrance Review to have moderate to strong evidence in the setting of herbal medicines for low back pain (5). These are reviewed below:

White Willow Bark

The bark of the willow bark tree contains a number of active compounds that may be anti-inflammatory. Most notably is the salicin component that is acetylated to provide aspirin products. In addition, willow bark contains flavonoids and tannins that may contribute antioxidant and antinociceptive properties and possibly decreased gastrointestinal irritation. Experiments of willow bark demonstrate inhibition of cyclooxygenase (COX)-2—mediated prostaglandin release but no significant direct COX-1 or COX-2 activity. Willow bark appears to be slower in onset of action than other anti-inflammatories and its onset of action is important to discuss with patients before initiating therapy.

In an randomized controlled trial (RCT) ($N = 210$) of exacerbation of chronic low back pain (VAS $\geq$ 5/10), subjects were assigned to willow bark 120 mg, 240 mg (salicin component), or placebo with tramadol as rescue medication. Pain-free subjects in the last week of treatment were 39% with high-dose, 21% with low-dose, and 6% with placebo ($P < .001$). The response to treatment became evident in the high-dose group after 1 week of treatment. Moreover, rescue medication use was significantly higher in the placebo group ($P < .001$) (6).

Devil's Claw (*Harpagophytum procumbens*)

Devil's claw is a "hooklike" (Greek "Harpagophytum") appearing plant containing iridoid glycosides including harpagoside, harpagide, and procumbide as well as other active constituents including acteoside, isoaceteoside, and stachyose. These compounds are believed to provide an anti-inflammatory effect through inhibition of predominantly cyclooxygenase (COX)-2, nitric oxide synthetase and tumor necrosis factor (TNF)-alpha. The most common side effect appears to be GI upset and diarrhea in <10% of subjects.

In a systematic review of 4 RCTs of devil's claw, there was moderate to strong evidence of effectiveness for the use at a daily dose of 50 to 100 mg harpagoside in the treatment of acute exacerbations of chronic nonspecific low back pain (7).

Capsicum (*Capsicum frutescens*)

Capsaicin is the active compound found in the fruit of the capsicum or hot pepper plant. When applied to skin repeatedly it appears to provide an anti-nociceptive effect through various mechanisms including substance P depletion. It is available in various topical and transdermal applications including gels, creams, as well as pads/plasters. The timing of application can be up to four times per day based on application. It is common for initial skin discomfort/irritation with gradual reduction in most cases.

An Randomized double-blind, placebo-controlled trial (RDBPCT) ($N = 320$) of capsicum plaster in nonspecific low back pain found that after 3 weeks of use there was a pain reduction of 42% (capsicum) and 31% (placebo) with a responder rate of 67% versus 49% ($P = .002$). The subject's efficacy rating "symptom free" or "improved" reached 82% versus 50%. Local skin reactions were noted in 7.5% of capsicum versus 3.1% of placebo subjects (8).

RECORD/RECOMMENDATIONS

After review of appropriate supplements and laboratory testing the following supplement recommendations were made and are summarized for the patient and chart:

Supplements Recommendations

Supplement	Brand/ Formulation	Dose	Notes
• Willow bark extract (WBE) (Salix spp)	Flexipert/ Assalix (Bionorica)	• Typically standardized to 120–240 mg of the salicin component daily	• All supplements to be reevaluated in 8–12 wk • Effect may seen within 1 wk • Possibility of allergic reaction
• Devil's claw (*Harpagophytum procumbens*)	Doloteffin (Ardeypharm) Harpadol (Arkopharma)	Typically standardized to 50–100 mg harpagoside component per day	Possible GI upset, diarrhea • maximum pain relief occurs after 3-4 month
Capsicum (*Capsicum frutescens*)	Various	Plaster or cream at 0.025%–0.075% applied up to 4×/d	Warn patient of initial reaction and skin irritation

Additional Recommendation

Richard is asked to increase activity as tolerated and to initiate a program focusing on core stabilization exercises, yoga and breath retraining.

BE AWARE OF REACTIONS AND INTERACTIONS

- Ask the patient about allergies to aspirin and aspirin-related products and make the patient aware of rate potential for allergic reaction to willow bark. Discuss the possibility of local irritation and discomfort with the use of capsicum.
- Patient handouts provided for supplements above through Natural Medicines Comprehensive Database.

AGREE TO DISCUSS AND FOLLOW-UP

Richard follows up in 8 weeks stating that he has had significant reduction in his pain that took approximately 10 days to become consistent (pain < 0–2/10). Since that point he notes less discomfort and increased range of motion that has improved his overall functional ability. He also notes less hesitancy with activity over the last 2 to 3 weeks as the pain relief has been more consistent. He noted some local discomfort with his topical capsicum for the first 4 to 5 days and since then he has tolerated application without a problem and does not report any other symptoms. He has noted steady increase in his physical activity including walking and stretching and core strengthening exercises, which has reached 30 minutes 3 times a week.

Richard is asked to reduce his white willow bark to 120 mg from 240 mg/d, decrease the frequency of his Capsicum continue with his other treatments including exercise, and to follow up in 3 months for repeat evaluation and reduction in his supplement regimine as appropriate.

LEARN

The patient and provider can utilize the following resources for updated information on dietary supplement and low back pain.

- Natural Medicines Comprehensive Database consumer version
  www.NaturalDatabase.com
- Office of Dietary Supplements
  http://dietary-supplements.info.nih.gov
- Medline Plus
  http://medlineplus.gov
- USDA
  http://www.nutrition.gov

SUMMARY

Low back pain is a common condition affecting the vast majority of Americans at some point in their life. Unfortunately, in many, the condition becomes a chronic and difficult to treat condition with functional and psychosocial sequelae. In the setting of chronic nonspecific low back pain with acute exacerbation there is often a need to find additional options in an attempt to obtain treatments that may provide meaningful reduction in pain and dysfunction. Dietary supplements as discussed above, with the appropriate addition of physical activity, can often be overlooked as helpful options. Patients attempting such a regimen are often motivated to incorporate such treatments in conjunction with other self-mangement approaches, in hopes of decreasing the frequency and severity of their back pain.

References

1. Hart LG, Deyo RA, Cherkin DC. Physician office visits for low back pain. Frequency, clinical evaluation, and treatment patterns from a U.S. national survey. *Spine* 1995;20:11–19.
2. Deyo RA, Mirza SK, Martin BI. Back pain prevalence and visit rates: estimates from U.S. national surveys, 2002. *Spine* 2006;31:2724–2727.
3. Martin BI, Deyo RA, Mirza S, et al. Expenditures and health status among adults with back and neck problems. *JAMA* 2008;299(6):656–664.
4. Mehling WE, Hamel KA, Acree M, Byl N, Hecht FM. Randomized, controlled trial of breath therapy for patients with chronic low-back pain. *Altern Ther Health Med* 2005;11(4):44–52.
5. Gagnier JJ, van Tulder M, Berman B, Bombardier C. Herbal medicine for low back pain. *Cochrane Database Syst Rev* 2006;(2):CD00450.
6. Chrubasik S, Eisenberg E, Balan E, et al. Treatment of low back pain exacerbations with willow bark extract: a randomized double-blind study. *Am J Med* 2000;109:9–14.
7. Gagnier JJ, Chrubasik S, Manheimer E. Harpgophytum procumbens for osteoarthritis and low back pain: a systematic review. *BMC Complement Altern Med*. 2004;4:13.
8. Frerick H, Keitel W, Kuhn U, et al. Topical treatment of chronic low back pain with a capsicum plaster. *Pain* 2003;106:59–64.

CHAPTER 51

The Use of Botanics During Pregnancy and Lactation

Tieraona Low Dog

BACKGROUND

Women are the largest consumers of health care and this extends to their utilization of complementary and alternative medicine. Researchers have attempted to uncover the reasons why women turn to complementary and alternative medicine in general and to botanic medicine in particular. Desire to have personal control over their health has been cited as the strongest motive for women to use herbal medicine. Second was dissatisfaction with conventional treatment and its disregard for a holistic approach as well as concerns about the side effects of medications (1). These concerns may explain, in part, the fact that many women use herbal remedies during pregnancy. A survey of 578 pregnant women in the eastern United States reported that 45% of respondents had used herbal medicines (2), whereas a survey of 588 women in Australia revealed that 36% had used at least one herbal product during pregnancy (2). Women probably feel comfortable using herbal remedies because of their perceived safety, easy access, and the widespread availability of information (i.e., Internet, magazines, books).

While it is true that many botanics are mild in both treatment effects and side effects, the data regarding safety during pregnancy are very limited. Given the small sample sizes in clinical trials studying botanics in pregnant women, only large differences in measures of pregnancy outcomes would likely be detected. For example, if an herb were thought to increase the rate of spontaneous abortion from 6% to 7%, a sample size of more than 19,000 women would be needed. It is highly unlikely that there will be any studies of a botanic (or drug) with this large sample size. So, when addressing the safety of an herb during pregnancy, we must look at the totality of the evidence, which includes traditional and contemporary use, animal studies, pharmacological studies, and clinical trial data, when available.

Survey data tell us that women often do not share their use of herbal remedies with their health care provider due to fear of offending the provider, or the belief that the clinician will be ignorant about their use. Practitioners should maintain an open and respectful demeanor when counseling pregnant and nursing women about the use of botanic medicines and they should know how to access unbiased and authoritative information sources so that they may reliably answer questions on inadvertent exposures and provide guidance on herbal products that might be beneficial. (Please refer to section 1 on the Herbal Mnemonic and chapter 42 on Resources on Dietary Supplements for further guidance).

The topic of herb use while pregnant or breastfeeding is very large and clearly cannot be extensively covered in this chapter. What follows is a review of several botanics that are either commonly used or have documented evidence of benefit for some of the common problems women encounter during these times.

NAUSEA AND VOMITING OF PREGNANCY

Nausea and vomiting of pregnancy (NVP) is a common experience for many women (33% to 50%), usually beginning by 4 to 8 weeks gestation and disappearing by the 16th. The etiology is not known. Mild cases of morning sickness generally pose no significant risk to mother or baby and can be safely treated at home with self-care measures. The diagnosis of *hyperemesis gravidarum* is made when NVP is serious enough to cause a weight loss of at least 5% of the prepregnancy weight, dehydration, electrolyte imbalance, and ketosis. This condition necessitates hospitalization (3).

Case: *Kathy is in the first trimester of her second pregnancy. She had a terrible time with nausea and vomiting during her first pregnancy and was hospitalized for dehydration. She is experiencing nausea, occasional vomiting, and is routinely late for work, as she feels too sick to drive. Kathy says that her employer and husband are sympathetic and supportive. She has no health problems and does not take any prescription or over-the-counter medications except for her prenatal vitamin. She recently read that ginger was helpful for morning sickness. Kathy mentioned it to her obstetrician who told her that ginger was not safe during pregnancy and that the FDA does not regulate dietary supplements, making them risky to use. He told her to try soda crackers and small frequent meals, which have not helped. Kathy knows that you practice integrative medicine and would like your opinion.*

In addition to its long history of use as a spice, ginger (*Zingiber officinale*) is also highly regarded as an antiemetic, anti-inflammatory, digestive aid, diaphoretic and warming agent. It is also the most extensively studied botanic for NVP. A systematic review of six published clinical trials found that ginger, at doses of 1.0 to 1.5 g, is effective for reducing NVP (4). Four of the six randomized controlled trials (RCT) (n = 246) showed superiority of ginger over placebo; the other two RCT (n = 429) found ginger as effective as vitamin B_6 in relieving the severity of nausea and vomiting episodes.

There has been some concern about the use of ginger during pregnancy, largely due to the publication of the German Commission E monographs in English, which states that ginger is contraindicated during pregnancy (5). However, in a controlled experimental rat study, ginger failed to demonstrate maternal or developmental toxicity at doses up to 1,000 mg/kg/d of body weight (6). When pregnant Sprague-Dawley rats were administered 20 g/l or 50 g/l ginger tea via their drinking water from gestation day 6 to 15 and then sacrificed at day 20, no maternal toxicity was observed; however embryonic loss in the treatment groups was double that of the controls ($P < .05$) (7).

Researchers at the Hospital for Sick Children in Toronto, Canada, conducted a prospective observational study in which they followed 187 pregnant women who used some form of ginger in the first trimester. The risk of these mothers having a baby with a congenital malformation was no higher than a control group (8). The follow-up of RCT consistently shows that there are no significant side effects or adverse effects on pregnancy outcomes (5).

In summary, based upon traditional use, modern use in the population as a spice, animal data, as well as clinical trials, we can assume with some degree of assurance that ginger at doses of 1.0 to 1.5 g per day is a safe and effective remedy for NVP.

Vitamin B_6, or vitamin B_6 plus doxylamine, is safe and effective and should be considered first-line pharmacotherapy. A single 25-mg of the antihistamine doxylamine (Unisom) tablet taken at night can be used in combination with vitamin B_6 (10 to 25 mg three times daily) (9). Acupressure was found in six of seven randomized trials to be effective for relieving morning sickness (10). Acupressure wristbands are readily available over-the-counter and many women find them a less expensive alternative to acupuncture.

Ginger can be considered a first-line approach for morning sickness. If ginger causes gastric upset, or is ineffective, consider switching to vitamin B_6, with or without doxylamine. I almost always recommend acupressure with either approach.

THREATENED ABORTION/MISCARRIAGE

A miscarriage, or spontaneous abortion, can be devastating for a woman desiring her pregnancy. Unfortunately, it is estimated that one in five pregnancies will end in this manner. An evaluation for threatened miscarriage, ectopic pregnancy, vaginal or cervical lesions, infection, or molar pregnancy should be performed if a woman experiences uterine irritability or vaginal bleeding during the first trimester. Women with recurrent miscarriages should be evaluated for antiphospholipid antibody syndrome (11). Women who experience threatened AB during the first trimester are more likely to deliver prematurely and so should be monitored closely during the third trimester (12).

Case: *Sarah is a 39-year-old healthy G1P0 who presents to the Indian Health Service urgent care clinic. She is 13 weeks pregnant by last menstrual period. She reports 2 days of uterine cramping and denies having any fever, dysuria, or trauma. Ultrasound confirms an intrauterine pregnancy. The pelvic examination reveals no cervical change and a small amount of blood in the vaginal vault. Sarah is very distraught. She and her husband have tried to conceive for almost a year and were elated when she found out she was pregnant. After some counseling, the physician sends Sarah home on bed rest and instructions to abstain from intercourse. She was told that there was nothing else to do but let nature takes it course. The following afternoon, Sarah calls the clinic and asks to speak to the midwife on staff. After a brief consultation, the midwife recommends that she take a tincture of black haw for 3 to 4 days and follow up with her in clinic. Sarah took 5 ml of the tincture in hot water 3 to 4 times per day for 4 days. She reported that the cramping and bleeding began to lessen almost immediately after using the herb. Over the course of her pregnancy, she used the black haw on 3 to 4 occasions and delivered a healthy baby boy at 38 weeks.*

A number of herbs have been traditionally used to prevent early pregnancy loss. In western herbal practice, the most common are black haw (*Viburnum prunifolium*) and cramp bark (*Viburnum opulus*). Indigenous women used black haw to prevent miscarriage and early American physicians praised it for "preventing abortion and miscarriage: whether threatened from accidental cause or criminal drugging" (13). King's American Dispensatory states "The condition for which black haw is most valued is threatened abortion" (14). Black haw was officially entered into the United States Pharmacopoeia in 1882 and remained in the National Formulary until 1960.

Contemporary herbalists commonly recommend black haw and/or cramp bark for painful menstrual cramps, threatened miscarriage, afterbirth pains, and muscle spasm. An in vitro study with an active glycoside from *V. prunifolium* noted relaxation in both animal and human uteri. Viopudial in *V. opulus* (15) and scopoletin in both *V. prunifolium* and *V. opulus* act as smooth muscle antispasmodics (16). Animal studies demonstrate complete relaxation of uterine muscle when administered extracts of black haw and cramp bark (17). Despite the praise of practitioners both past and present and the preliminary in vitro and animal data—there are no human studies evaluating the antispasmodic effects of either herb.

No adverse events in pregnancy are found in the literature and there are no known constituents that sound an alarm; however, given the widespread use of this botanic by herbalists and midwives for menstrual cramping and threatened miscarriage, some basic science, animal studies, and modern research would be welcome. The dose is typically 1 g of crude herb, or equivalent in tincture or extract, taken 3 to 4 times per day as needed.

> Women who experience a threatened miscarriage often feel that they have "done something wrong." Reassurance, active listening, and compassionate counsel are so important—no matter the outcome. Black haw and cramp bark are very effective for reducing uterine irritability and cramping, though, they would not likely prevent pregnancy loss in cases of significant fetal abnormalities.

URINARY TRACT INFECTION

Urinary tract infections (UTI) are common in pregnancy; up to 90% are due to the gram-negative bacteria *Escherichia coli*. Pregnancy increases the risk of UTI because increased bladder volume and decreased bladder and ureteral tone increase urinary stasis and ureterovesical reflux (18). Up to 70% of pregnant women develop glycosuria, which encourages bacterial growth in the urine (19). Untreated asymptomatic bacteriuria can lead to the development of pyelonephritis in up to 50% of cases and is associated with an increased risk of intrauterine growth retardation and low–birth-weight infants. Thus, routine screening is advocated. The US Preventative Services Task Force recommends a urine culture be obtained between 12 and 16 weeks of gestation (20).

Case: *Shelly is a G3P2 and is been seen for her first prenatal visit at 9 weeks. She has had two healthy children, born vaginally at term, and is excited about her current pregnancy. Her examination is normal, except for the presence of bacteria in her urine. She denies any dysuria, frequency, or urgency. Shelly is frustrated at the prospect of taking antibiotics, as she ended up on suppressive therapy during her last pregnancy because of recurrent asymptomatic bacteriuria. She wants to know whether there is anything else she can try.*

Cranberry (*Vaccinium macrocarpon*) reduces the frequency of UTI by preventing the adherence of pathogenic *E. coli,* and other fimbriated bacteria, to the urinary epithelium. A Cochrane review reported that cranberry significantly reduces the incidence of UTIs at 12 months (RR 0.65, 95% confidence interval, 0.46 to 0.90) as compared to placebo/control (21). Cranberry extracts in tablet form also reduce the risk of UTI and is often more convenient and better tolerated. There are no significant safety concerns for cranberry products during pregnancy and given the significant morbidity that can occur, it seems common sense to recommend it for prevention. While not studied to the same degree as cranberry, blueberries and blueberry juice appear to exhibit similar activity (22). The typical dose is 4 oz cranberry juice two times per day, or 400 mg cranberry extract twice daily.

Uva-ursi (*Arctostaphylos uva-ursi*), also known as bearberry, is endorsed by the European Scientific Cooperative on Phytotherapy and the German Commission E for minor infection/inflammatory disorders of the lower urinary tract. Arbutin, an active compound in uva-ursi leaf has antibacterial activity against *E. coli*, *Pseudomonas aeruginosa*, *Proteus mirabilis* and *Staphylococcus aureus* (23). Uva-ursi reduced the risk of recurrent UTI in a 12-month study of 57 women who had at least three documented UTI in previous year when compared to placebo (24). Unfortunately for Shelly, both the German Commission E and the American Herbal Products Association (25) contraindicate the use of uva-ursi during pregnancy, likely due to the potential for hydroquinone toxicity in the fetus. Exposure of human lymphocytes and cell lines to hydroquinone has been shown to cause various forms of genetic damage (26). Uva-ursi is also contraindicated during lactation (27).

The use of cornsilk (*Zea mays*) for afflictions of the kidney and bladder can be traced back to the Incas. Parke-Davis introduced a cornsilk product in the 1880s for the treatment of urinary pain and spasm. The *British Herbal Compendium* lists cornsilk as a mild diuretic and urinary demulcent. Cornsilk is quite safe and often included in herbal formulas designed to ease the pain of cystitis. No contraindications are found in the literature.

> It is common sense to recommend pregnant women drink cranberry juice, or take the extract, to reduce the risk of UTI, especially those at high risk. Women with asymptomatic bacteriuria can undergo a trial of cranberry extract 400 to 500 mg two times daily for 5 to 7 days and then recheck the urine.

PARTUS PREPARATORS AND LABOR AIDS

Case: *Kathy responded to the combination of an acupressure bracelet and ginger capsules for the nausea and vomiting she experienced during her first trimester. She has had an easy pregnancy and is now in her 34th week. She returns to your office with an herbal product her friend used during her last pregnancy. The label says it contains blue cohosh (Caulophyllum thalictroides), black cohosh (Actaea racemosa), and raspberry (Rubus spp). Kathy's friend said that it was "simply amazing" and that if a woman takes the product 6 weeks before her due date, it will "essentially guarantee a timely and painless birth." Kathy's first pregnancy ended in an induction when she went 2 weeks past her due date, and though she had prepared for natural childbirth, she had an epidural for the pain. She is feeling a little anxious and wants to know whether these herbs are safe and whether they can really help ensure a timely and less painful birth.*

Since ancient times, pregnant women have used, and midwives have recommended, herbs to facilitate labor. These preparations are often referred to as *partus preparators*. Depending upon the herb, these labor aids were taken anywhere from a few days to a month before the suspected due date. Indigenous North American women used blue cohosh to induce labor or stimulate sluggish, ineffective contractions. It was official in the United States Pharmacopoeia as a labor-inducing agent from 1882 to 1905 and then the National Formulary from 1916 to 1950. There has been little contemporary data to explore its effectiveness as a labor aid.

Blue cohosh is found in many formulations marketed to women as *partus preparators*. Many obstetricians are unfamiliar with its use but a survey of nurse midwives in 1999 found that 64% used blue cohosh, often in combination with black cohosh, to augment labor during delivery (28). While many used blue cohosh, they also reported having the least comfort with its use during pregnancy as compared to other herbs. A significant number reported observing an increased rate of meconium, tachycardia, and need for resuscitation in association with its use.

There have been a small number of case reports implicating blue cohosh, often in combination with black cohosh and/or other herbs, with myocardial infarction (29), multiorgan failure, congestive heart failure (30), and perinatal stroke (31) in infants born to mothers taking the herb several weeks before birth. While the published case reports are not conclusive, blue cohosh contains some potentially dangerous compounds that should give clinicians pause. Blue cohosh contains caulosaponin, a glycoside that has been shown to constrict coronary vessels and likely accounts for its oxytocic effects (32). It also contains N-methylcytisine, an alkaloid with action similar to nicotine, known to cause coronary vasoconstriction, tachycardia, hypotension, and respiratory depression (33). *In vitro* studies show that extracts of blue cohosh rhizome or pure N-methylcytisine (at 20 ppm) induce major malformations in cultured rat embryos (34). The concentration of N-methylcytisine in dietary supplements containing blue cohosh ranges from 5 to 850 ppm (35).

The question immediately before the health care professional is what to say to a woman regarding the safety and use of blue cohosh during pregnancy? Despite the shortcomings of published case reports, the chemistry and pharmacology of the plant are reasonably well known. The human case reports, as incomplete as they are, paint a picture that is consistent with the evidence provided by *in vitro* and animal studies. At this time, it is wise to err on the side of caution and counsel against its use during pregnancy.

Black cohosh (*A. racemosa; Cimicifuga racemosa*) is probably best known for its use in menopause, though it was traditionally used for rheumatic pain, uterine cramping, and ease melancholy. The German health authorities also recognize its use for dysmenorrhea. It is unrelated to blue cohosh but the two herbs are often used in combination to induce labor or as a partus preparator. Studies on other Cimicifuga species failed to show teratogenicity in female rats at doses up to 2,000 mg/kg per day (36); however, similar studies in *A. racemosa* have not been published. Both the British Herbal Pharmacopoeia (37) and American Herbal Products Association contraindicate the use of black cohosh during pregnancy (38). Reproductive toxicology studies are definitely needed for this herb.

Raspberry leaf (*Rubus idaeus, R. occidentalis*) can be found in many popular "pregnancy teas." It is often promoted to prevent miscarriage, ease morning sickness, and ensure a quick birth. A survey of 172 certified nurse midwives found that 63% of midwives using herbal preparations recommended red raspberry leaf (39).

A retrospective study of women taking raspberry leaf from 30 to 35 weeks onward failed to find any significant adverse outcomes in mother or infant compared to controls (40). A double-blind, placebo-controlled study randomized 192 low-risk, nulliparous women to receive raspberry leaf tablets (two tablets of 1.2 g/d) or placebo, from 32 weeks' gestation until delivery (41). Raspberry leaf was not associated with any adverse effects in mother or baby, but contrary to popular belief did not shorten the first stage of labor. Clinically significant findings were a shortening of the second stage of labor (mean difference, 9.59 minutes) and a lower rate of forceps deliveries between the treatment group and the control group (19.3% versus 30.4%). Contraindications for use in pregnancy or lactation are found in the literature.

The notion that women need to take an herb or drug during the last 4 to 6 weeks of pregnancy to ensure a healthy, timely birth is disconcerting, especially when the substances may be harmful. I prefer to give an expectant mother a jar of raspberry leaf tea with the suggestion to prepare a cup each evening or early morning, when it is quiet, and slowly sip it as she writes letters to her unborn child in a journal or notebook during the last month of pregnancy. The tea is gentle and tasty, the ritual connects her with her child, and along with childbirth classes, helps to prepare her for the journey.

LACTATION

Although the benefits of breastfeeding may be self-evident, they are also increasingly demonstrated by science. Benefits include the superior nutritional composition of breast milk (42), reduced incidence of feeding intolerance and necrotizing enterocolitis in preterm infants (43), and enhanced resistance to infectious disease (44). There is also a significant psychological benefit for both mother and infant. It is beyond the scope of this brief chapter to explore the myriad of ways botanic medicine could be safely used by breastfeeding women for conditions such as sore nipples, engorgement, early mastitis, nipple thrush, postpartum depression, and so forth. Instead, this chapter will be limited to a discussion of lactagogues.

LACTAGOGUES

Lactagogues, or galactagogues, are substances that aid in the initiation, maintenance, or augmentation of milk production. Common indications include increasing milk production after maternal or infant illness or separation, reestablishment of milk supply after weaning, or induction of lactation in a woman who did not give birth to the infant (e.g., adoption). Maternal milk production is a complex process. Dopamine agonists inhibit, whereas dopamine antagonists increase prolactin and milk production. Although some lactagogues act as dopamine antagonists, the mechanism of action for most is simply not known.

Case: *Anna is a 27-year-old single mother of a 9-week healthy son born at term. Anna has recently started back to work part-time and is concerned that her milk supply is faltering. She is trying to pump but "it isn't going very well." Anna had been successfully* *breastfeeding before returning to her job. The baby appears healthy and hydrated. You observe Anna using the breast pump and make appropriate recommendations. Anna returns 6 weeks later for the baby's immunizations and you ask how the breastfeeding is going. Anna tells you that her mother gave her a tea of fenugreek and shatavari and laughingly reports that she is making enough milk to feed the neighborhood.*

Around the world and throughout history, women have used herbs and foods to enhance their milk supply. In spite of formal scientific evaluation, many are widely recommended. Herbs commonly mentioned in the literature include fenugreek, goat's rue, milk thistle, blessed thistle, shatavari, aniseed, caraway seed, dill, borage, and comfrey.

Fenugreek (*Trigonella foenum-graecum*) has been valued as a spice and medicine throughout India and the Middle East for millennia. The seeds are used to relieve intestinal gas, respiratory congestion, and in larger doses it can reduce serum cholesterol and glucose levels. Fenugreek has a substantial reputation for increasing breast milk production in nursing mothers. A case report summarized the anecdotal use of fenugreek in at least 1,200 women who reported an increase in milk supply within 24 to 72 hours (45). Two small preliminary reports also suggest effectiveness (46, 47), yet, in spite of its widespread use, there are no rigorous trials for review. Well-tolerated, ingestion of fenugreek can impart a maplelike odor to sweat, milk, and urine, which could mistakenly lead a practitioner to consider the diagnosis of maple syrup–urine disease (branched-chain hyperaminoaciduria), a rare inherited metabolic disorder, in a breastfed infant whose mother is taking the herb. There is cross-reactivity in those with chickpea allergy. There are numerous cautionary statements in the literature regarding hypoglycemia with fenugreek use, though blood sugar lowering activity is mild and seen only at doses exceeding 25 g per day. The usual dose for lactagogue effect is 1 to 2 g of the dried powdered seeds taken three times per day. Fenugreek can also be prepared as tea, steeping ¼ teaspoon of seeds in 8 oz of water for 10 minutes.

The roots of wild asparagus (*Asparagus racemosus*), also known as shatavari, have been widely recommended in the Ayurvedic tradition to increase milk production in lactating women. The herb is considered to be a nourishing herb and is also recommended for those who are debilitated or convalescing. Nursing mothers often consume a combination of wild asparagus root and cardamom called Shatavari Kalpa. There are a handful of animal and human studies that support the lactogenic effect of wild asparagus, given either alone or in combination with other herbs (48); however a randomized controlled study of *A. racemosus* in women with lactational inadequacy failed to find any effect on milk production or prolactin levels (49). The dose is 1 g powdered root per day taken in milk or juice.

The lactagogue effect of goat's rue (*Galega officinalis*) leaf was first scientifically reported to the French Academy in 1873 after observing that it increased milk production in cows by 35% to 50%. These findings were later independently confirmed in 1913 (50). There are no modern studies for review. Goat's rue is found in numerous products, typically in combination with other herbs. The tea is generally prepared by steeping 1 teaspoon of dried leaves in 8 oz of water for 10 minutes, with one cup taken two or three times a day. One adverse event in the literature links the maternal ingestion of a lactation tea containing extracts of licorice (*Glycyrrhiza glabra*), fennel (*Foeniculum vulgare*), anise (*Pimpinella anisum*), and goat's rue with drowsiness, hypotonia, lethargy, emesis, and poor suckling in two breastfed neonates. An evaluation for infection yielded negative results, and symptoms and signs resolved after discontinuation of the tea and a 2-day break from breastfeeding (51). The tea was not tested for contaminants or adulterants, and there are no other published adverse events.

Milk thistle (*Silybum marianum*), best known for its liver-protecting effects, has been used as a lactagogue for centuries. Early Christian lore holds that the white leaf veins are a symbolic representation of the Virgin Mary's breast milk, hence the common names of milk thistle and St. Mary's thistle. There are no human studies evaluating its purported lactagogue effect. There are no known safety concerns with the seed. The tea is prepared by simmering one teaspoon crushed seeds in 8 oz of water for 10 minutes. The dose is one to three cups daily or 1 to 3 g of the ground seeds in capsule form. Note that this is not the standardized extract typically used for liver disorders but rather crude preparations of the seeds.

Aniseed, caraway seed, cinnamon, dill, and fennel seed are all aromatic spices that can be easily and safely added to the diet: dill to a tuna salad, cinnamon in applesauce, a cup of anise tea, or candied fennel after a meal. Raspberry and nettle can be easily consumed in tea. Of the herbs commonly recommended in lay literature, only comfrey and borage should be avoided as they contain pyrrolizidine alkaloids, which pass readily into breast milk and have the potential to cause severe liver damage (52).

> Most women are able to successfully breastfeed if given the proper support and guidance. I have found both fenugreek and milk thistle to be very effective lactagogues, especially when women are expressing milk because they are returning to work or when they are separated from their baby (i.e., premature infant). I often refer to lactation consultants, as they are well prepared to answer questions regarding positioning, sore nipples, and so forth.

CONCLUSION

Women have been the recipients, as well as the primary keepers, of botanic medicines for millennia. Women herbalists and midwives observed the effects that particular plants had on female reproduction, pregnancy, and breastfeeding, handing down their knowledge across the generations. While their expertise and wisdom can still be felt in various folk traditions, much of the wise woman knowledge was shared through oral, not written, traditions, thus some of the finer nuances of herbal ministrations have been lost. The lack of formal herbal training programs in Western countries over the past century has contributed to our gap in knowledge. While scientific research has exploded in the field of natural products, there has been shamefully little research aimed at assessing the safety and effectiveness of botanic remedies during pregnancy or lactation. When coupled with a marketplace filled with hundreds of products targeting women, including a considerable number with dubious efficacy and questionable quality, it becomes clear that there is strong need for a rigorous approach for assessing which herbs are of benefit and under what circumstances. Hopefully clinicians, researchers, and herbal manufacturers can work together to conduct rigorous scientific studies, both at the basic science level and in clinical trials; create reasonable practice guidelines for the use of botanic remedies during pregnancy and lactation; and design high-quality products that are based on sound formulation, scientific principles, and clinical need.

References

1. Vickers K, Jolly KB, Greenfield SM. Herbal medicine: women's views, knowledge and interaction with doctors: a qualitative study. *BMC Complement Altern Med* 2006;6:40.
2. Glover DG, Amonkar M, Rybeck BF, Tracy TS. Prescription, over-the-counter, and herbal medicine use in a rural, obstetric population. *Am J Obstet Gynecol* 2003;188(4): 1039–1045.
3. Cashion C. Endocrine and metabolic disorders. In: Lowdermilk DL, Perry SE, Bobak IM, eds. *Maternity and Women's Health Care*. 7th ed. St. Louis, MO: Mosby, 2000:861–886.
4. Borrelli F, Capasso R, Aviello G, Pittler MH, Izzo AA. Effectiveness and safety of ginger in the treatment of pregnancy induced nausea and vomiting. *Obstet Gynecol* 2005;105 (4):849–856.
5. Blumenthal M, Busse W, Goldberg A, et al. eds. *The Complete German Commission E Monographs Therapeutic Guide to Herbal Medicines*. Boston: Integrative Medicine Communications; 1998.
6. Weidner MS, Sigwart K. The safety of ginger extract in the rat. *J Ethnopharmacol* 2000; 73(3):513–520.
7. Wilkinson JM. Effect of ginger tea on the fetal development of sprague-dawley rats. *Reprod Toxicol (United States)* 2000;14(6):507–512.
8. Portnoi G, Chng LA, Karimi-Tabesh L, Koren G, Tan MP, Einarson A. Prospective comparative study of the safety and effectiveness of ginger for the treatment of nausea and vomiting in pregnancy. *Am J Obstet Gynecol* 2003;189(5):1374–1377.
9. Atanackovic G, Navioz Y, Moretti ME, Koren G. The safety of higher than standard dose of doxylamine-pyridoxine (Diclectin) for nausea and vomiting of pregnancy. *J Clin Pharmacol* 2001;41(8):842–845.
10. Fugh-Berman A. Acupressure for nausea and vomiting of pregnancy. *Alt Ther Women's Health* 1999;1(2):9–16.
11. Mezzesimi A, Florio P, Reis FM, et al. The detection of anti-beta2-glycoprotein I antibodies is associated with increased risk of pregnancy loss in women with threatened abortion in the first trimester. *Eur J Obstet Gynecol Reprod Biol*. 2007;133(2):164–168.
12. Johns J, Jauniaux E. Threatened miscarriage as a predictor of obstetric outcome. *Obstet Gynecol*. 2006;107(4):845–850.
13. Felter HW, Lloyd JU. *King's American Dispensatory* 18th Ed. 3rd Revision 1898; Cincinnatti: Ohio Valley Co.; 1898.
14. Felter HW, Lloyd JU. *King's American Dispensatory*. 18th ed. 3rd rev. Vol. 2. Portland: Eclectic Medical Publications; 1983:2059–2062.
15. Nicholson JA, Darby TD, Jarboe CH. Viopudial, a hypotensive and smooth muscle antispasmodic from Viburnum opulus. *Proc Soc Exp Biol Med* 1972;140(2):457–461.
16. Jarboe CH, Schmidt CM, Nicholson JA, Zirvi KA. Scopoletin, an antispasmodic component of *Viburnum opulus* and *V. prunifolium*. *J Med Chem* 1967;10:488–491.
17. Jarboe CH, Schmidt CM, Nicholson JA, Zirvi KA. Uterine relaxant properties of Viburnum. *Nature* 1966;212(5064):837.
18. Patterson TF, Andriole VT. Bacteriuria in pregnancy. *Infect Dis Clin North Am* 1987; 1:807–822.
19. Lucas MJ, Cunningham FG. Urinary infection in pregnancy. *Clin Obstet Gynecol* 1993; 36:855–868.
20. U.S. Preventive Services Task Force. *Guide to Clinical Preventive Services: Report of the U.S. Preventive Services Task Force*. 2nd ed. Baltimore: Williams & Wilkins; 1996.
21. Jepson RG, Craig JC. Cranberries for preventing urinary tract infections. *Cochrane Database Syst Rev* 2008;23(1):CD001321.
22. Jepson RG, Craig JC. A systematic review of the evidence for cranberries and blueberries in UTI prevention. *Mol Nutr Food Res*. 2007;51(6):738–745.

23. *European Scientific Cooperative on Phytotherapy Monographs on the Medicinal Uses of Plant Drugs*. United Kingdom: ESCOP, Exeter; 1997; Fascicule 5.
24. Larsson B, Jonasson A, Pianu S. Prophylactic effect of UVA E in women with recurrent cystitis: a preliminary report. *Curr Ther Res Clin Exp* 1993;53(4):441–443.
25. McGuffin M, Hobbs C, Upton R, Goldberg A. *American Herbal Products Association's Botanical Safety Handbook*. Boca Raton: CRC Press; 1997.
26. Smith MT, Zhang L, Jeng M, et al. Hydroquinone, a benzene metabolite, increases the level of aneusomy of chromosomes 7 and 8 in human CD34-positive blood progenitor cells. *Carcinogenesis (England)* 2000;21(8):485–490.
27. Blumenthal M, Goldberg A, Brinckmann J, et al., eds. *Herbal Medicine: Expanded Commission E Monographs*. Newton, MA: Integrative Medicine Communications; 2000: 389–393.
28. McFarlin BL, Gibson MH, O'Rear J, Harman P. A national survey of herbal preparation use by nurse-midwives for labor stimulation. Review of the literature and recommendations for practice. *J Nurse Midwifery* 1999;44(3):205–216.
29. Gunn TR, Wright IM. The use of black and blue cohosh in labour. *N Z Med J* 1996; 109(1032):410–411.
30. Jones TK, Lawson BM. Profound neonatal congestive heart failure caused by maternal consumption of blue cohosh herbal medication. *J Pediatr* 1998;132:550–552.
31. Finkel RS, Zarlengo KM. Blue cohosh and perinatal stroke. *N Engl J Med* 2004;351(3): 302–303.
32. de Smet PAGM. *Adverse Effects of Herbal Drugs*. Vol. 2. Berlin: Heidelberg; 1993:348
33. Scott C, Chin K. The pharmacologic action of N-methylcytisine. *Therapeutics* 1943;79:334.
34. Kennelly EJ, Flynn TJ, Mazzola EP, et al. Detecting potential teratogenic alkaloids from blue cohosh rhizomes using an in vitro rat embryo culture. *J Nat Prod* 1999;62(10): 1385–1389.
35. Betz JM, Andrzejewski D, Troy A, et al. Gas chromatographic determination of toxic quinolizidine alkaloids in blue cohosh (*Caulophyllum thalictroides* (L.) Michx.) *Phytochem Anal* 1998;9:232–236.
36. Liske E. Gerhard I, Wustenberg P. Menopause: herbal combination product for psychovegetative complaints. *TW Gynakol* 1997;10:172–175.
37. Bradley PR. *British Herbal Compendium*. Vol. 1. Dorset: British Herbal Medicine Association; 1992.
38. McGuffin M, Hobbs C, Upton R, Goldberg A (Eds). *American Herbal Products Association's Botanical Safety Handbook*. Boca Raton, FL: CRC Press; 1997.
39. McFarlin BL, Gibson MH, O'Rear J, Harman P. A national survey of herbal preparation use by nurse-midwives for labor stimulation. Review of the literature and recommendations for practice. *J Nurse Midwifery* 1999;44:205–216.
40. Parsons M, Simpson M, Ponton T. Raspberry leaf and its effect on labour: safety and efficacy. *J Aust Coll Midwives* 1999;12:20–25.
41. Simpson M, Parsons M, Greenwood J, Wade K. Raspberry leaf in pregnancy: its safety and efficacy in labor. *J Midwifery Womens Health* 2001;46(2):51–59.
42. Wagner CL, Anderson DM, Pittard WB. Special properties of human milk. *Clin Pediatr* 1996;35:283–293.
43. Lucas A, Cole TJ. Breast milk and neonatal necrotizing enterocolitis. *Lancet* 1990;336: 1519–1523.
44. Wright AL, Bauer M, Naylor A, et al. Increasing breastfeeding rates to reduce infant illness at the community level. *Pediatrics* 1998;101:837–844.
45. Huggins KE. Fenugreek: one remedy for low milk production. Retrieved from http://www.breastfeedingonline.com/fenuhugg.shtml. Accessed November 24, 2009.
46. Swafford S, Berens P. Effect of fenugreek on breast milk volume. Abstract, 5th International Meeting of the Academy of Breastfeeding Medicine; September 2000;11–13; Tucson, AZ.

47. Co MM, Hernandez EA, Co BG. A comparative study on the efficacy of the different galactogogues among mothers with lactational insufficiency. Abstract, AAP Section on Breastfeeding, 2002 NCE, October 21, 2002.
48. Goyal RK, Singh J, Lai H. *Asparagus racemosus:* an update. *Indian J Med Sci* 2003; 57(9):408–414.
49. Sharma S, Ramji S, Kumari S, Bapna JS. Randomized controlled trial of *Asparagus racemosus* (Shatavari) as a lactogogue in lactational inadequacy. *Indian Pediatr* 1996;33: 675–677.
50. Remington JP, ed: *The Dispensatory of the United States of America*. 20th ed. Philadelphia: Lippincott-Raven; 1918.
51. Rosti L, Nardini A, Bettinelli ME, et al. Toxic effects of a herbal tea mixture in two newborns. *Acta Paediatr* 1994;83:683.
52. Panter KE, James LF. Natural plant toxicants in milk: a review. *J Anim Sci* 1990;68(3): 892–904.

CHAPTER 52

Urinary Tract Infection

Wadie Najm

Case: *Ms. Stella Taylor is a 25-year-old female presenting with dysuria and frequency for 1 day.*

BACKGROUND

- Sixty percent of healthy adult females may experience a urinary tract infection (UTI).
- *Escherichia coli*, gram-negative bacilli, is the most common causative agent.
- Women, who have a first UTI caused by *E. coli*, appear to be more likely to develop a second UTI within 6 months.
- Dietary supplements could be used as first-line therapy in the prevention of UTI and as an adjunct to antibiotics to minimize the length of treatment and decrease the risk of resistance in uncomplicated UTI.

*H*EARING THE PATIENT OUT WITH RESPECT

Ms. Stella Taylor is a 25-year-old female. She presents today with a 1-day history of dysuria and increased urinary frequency. She reports some pressure sensation in the hypogastric area which started yesterday. She does not report any fever, chills, or blood in the urine. Ms. Taylor denies any back pain or discomfort.

Pertinent Medical History

She is Gravida 0, Para 0, her last menstrual period was 2 weeks ago and her menses are regular. She is married and sexually active with her husband. She has been on an oral contraceptive for birth control for the last 5 years. Her last UTI was approximately 5 months ago, she experienced similar symptoms, and was treated with a 3-day course of antibiotics by at an urgent care clinic. She has had a total of four episodes of UTI which occur mostly after intercourse. In all three previous episodes she was treated successfully with antibiotics. She is otherwise healthy. She denies any family history of renal lithiasis or urinary problems.

Ms. Taylor does not care very much for "medications/drugs" and would like to be proactive in the management of her symptoms. She is interested in dietary supplements and or complementary and alternative medicine approaches.

Lifestyle History

Ms. Taylor is married for 4 years. She has no children. She has never smoked and drinks socially (one to two drinks a week). Ms. Taylor drinks two to four cups of coffee a day but denies any soda. She works as an accountant. She is physically active and does Pilates three to four times a week. On the weekends she and her husband are avid bike riders.

She is hoping to attempt her first pregnancy in the next 2 years and is hoping to avoid any "medications/drugs" and she is looking for possible "natural" options in this setting. Her friend has suggested the use of cranberry for her symptoms.

Physical Examination

Ms. Taylor appears of stated age; she is in no acute distress. She is afebrile and her other vital signs are normal. Her examination reveals no costovertebral angle tenderness to percussion. She had a mild discomfort on deep palpation of the hypogastric area, otherwise the remaining examination was unremarkable.

The urine dipstick was noted as showing moderate leukocytes esterase and nitrites, negative blood, protein, or glucose.

EDUCATING THE PATIENT

Ms. Taylor is provided an overview of several dietary supplements in the setting of UTI. She is made aware that these dietary supplements are utilized in the prevention and early (1 to 2 days) management of symptoms, but that antibiotics are required for an established UTI. Ms. Taylor is advised that no clear evidence exists for the safety or harm of the dietary supplements during pregnancy.

OVERVIEW OF SUPPLEMENT CONSIDERATIONS

Cranberry

Cranberry is commonly used by the lay public for prevention and treatment of UTI. Several mechanisms of action have been advanced; however the most consistent evidence suggests that cranberry constituents (fructose and proanthocyanidins) inhibit bacterial adhesion to the uroepithelium, hence preventing colonization and infection (1–3).

A systematic review of available trials found a lack of good quality trials and no good evidence to suggest that cranberry juice or cranberry product (e.g., cranberry capsules) is effective for the treatment of UTIs (4).

Two systematic reviews looking at UTI prevention report that evidence from good quality studies show that cranberry juice may decrease the incidence of symptomatic UTIs over a 12-month period, particularly in women with recurrent UTIs (5, 6).

As much as 0.25 to 0.5 liters, once to three times per day of cranberry juice has been shown to be effective. Cranberry tablets are available for people with diabetes or those who want to avoid high sugar intake; however the evidence for tablets is not as strong as juice.

Uva-Ursi

Uva-Ursi is a shrub native to North America. The leaves contain hydroquinone derivative, the glycoside arbutin. When hydrolyzed by gastric fluid and if the pH of the urine is sufficiently alkaline (>7) then it will act as a direct antimicrobial agent (7).

In a randomized double-blind placebo controlled trial, 57 women with recurrent cystitis were randomized to 1 month of Uva-Ursi versus placebo. Those on Uva-Ursi had no recurrence of cystitis in the following year compared with 23% recurrence in women on placebo (8).

Uva-Ursi is commonly used in a dose of 400 to 800 mg arbutin/d. Long-term use is not recommended due to safety concerns (carcinogenesis). For best results, avoid using with animal products (acidifies the urine) or combine with 1 tablespoon of sodium bicarbonate to alkalinize the urine.

Uva-Ursi should be avoided during pregnancy and lactation due to its possible carcinogenic effect.

D-Mannose

D-Mannose is a naturally occurring sugar found in fruits such as apples, oranges, and some berries (e.g., cranberries and blueberries) that is excreted mainly intact in the urine. D-Mannose will adhere to lectins on *E. coli* bacteria hence inhibiting their adherence to the uroepithelial cell wall and minimizing the colonization (9, 10).

Laboratory studies demonstrated significantly lower bacteriuria in rats inoculated with bacteria and 10% D-Mannose than in controls on days 5 and 7 and the percentage of rats with less than 100 bacteria/ml was higher on day 7 in D-Mannose–treated rats (11).

The majority of the evidence for D-Mannose is anecdotal. Well-designed studies are not available to verify the effectiveness.

Common dosing of D-Mannose is 500 mg taken four times daily. Since this product is specific for the treatment of *E. coli*, it is important to consider other treatment options if symptoms do not improve within 24 hours.

RECORD/RECOMMENDATIONS

After review of appropriate supplements and testing which demonstrated positive nitrites and leukocyte esterase, the following recommendation were made:

Supplement Recommendations

Name	Brand	Dose	Notes
Cranberry	(1) Cranberry juice cocktail (sweetened) (2) 100% cranberry juice (unsweetened) (3) Capsules (of cranberry juice powder)	(1) A dose of 300 ml (10 oz) per day (2) A dose of 15 to 30 milliliters per day. (3) Between one and six 300- to 400-mg capsules twice daily by mouth have been taken with water 1 hr before or 2 hr after meals.	In very large doses (3–4 l/d of juice) cranberry can cause gastrointestinal upset and diarrhea.
D-Mannose	Pure encapsulations—D-Mannose 100 g powder	500 mg 2–4 times daily	Reevaluate effectiveness in 24–48 hr.

Additional Recommendation

Ms. Taylor is advised to drink plenty of fluids, avoid delays in emptying her bladder, and to wear cotton underwear. She was also instructed to empty her bladder prior to and after sexual intercourse to reduce the likelihood of infection.

BE AWARE OF REACTIONS AND INTERACTIONS

Make the patient aware of potential gastrointestinal side effects and risk of urinary stones from prolonged high doses of cranberry.

Drug Interactions

Advise the patient that initial reports suggest possible interaction with warfarin, but that additional studies are needed to validate this result (12). When counseling patients on dietary changes necessary during warfarin treatment, it does not seem necessary to eliminate daily cranberry juice consumption, but the International Normalized Ratio (INR) should be followed up closely (13, 14).

Advise the patient that cranberry could theoretically affect medications eliminated primarily through the kidney or dependent on the acidity of the stomach.

Also make Ms. Taylor aware that Uva-Ursi can cause nausea, vomiting, gastrointestinal discomfort, and a greenish-brown discoloration of the urine. Large amounts can be oxytocic, increasing the rapidity of labor. Other adverse effects due to uva-ursi include hepatotoxicity and irritation and inflammation of the urinary tract mucous membranes (15–17).

Patient handouts provided for supplements above through Natural Medicines Comprehensive Database and Natural Standard.

AGREE TO DISCUSS AND FOLLOW-UP

Ms. Taylor returns to the clinic in 2 weeks. Her urine analysis did show *E. Coli* at less than 50,000 colonies. She reports that she followed your recommendations and took the dietary supplements. Her symptoms improved within 24 hours and resolved within 3 days. She has not had any recurrence since the last visit.

Ms. Taylor comes back to see you after 1 year. She is 8 weeks pregnant. She reports having had some occasional symptoms of dysuria that she has self-treated with increased fluid intake, cranberry juice, and D-Mannose with good results. You remind her again that Uva-Ursi should not be used during pregnancy.

LEARN

The patient is referred to the following resources for updated information on UTIs and use of dietary supplements.

- Natural Medicines Comprehensive Database consumer version
  http://www.NaturalDatabase.com
- Natural Standard
  http://www.naturalstandard.com/

- Office of Dietary Supplements
  http://dietary-supplements.info.nih.gov
- Medline Plus
  http://medlineplus.gov
- United States Dietary Administration (USDA)
  http://www.nutrition.gov

SUMMARY

UTI covers a wide array of conditions and circumstances. When patients present with symptoms suggestive of an acute infection or possible renal involvement (fever, back pain, or chills), aggressive treatment with antibiotics is needed. Patients with diabetes or underlying immunosuppression should also be managed aggressively with antibiotics to minimize complications.

If patients are able to recognize/suspect early UTI symptoms, then a trial of natural approaches is warranted. Start with encouraging water intake (six 8-oz glasses a day), cranberry juice, or D-Mannose to limit adhesion of bacteria to the uroepithelium. If patients are not pregnant or breastfeeding, a trail of Uva-Ursi as antimicrobial can be helpful. If symptoms persist or progress within the next 24 to 48 hours obtain a urine culture and sensitivity.

Several common measures can help in preventing UTIs. These include avoiding holding urine for prolonged periods, increasing water intake, urinating before and after sexual activity, wearing loose cotton underwear, and considering cranberry juice or tablets.

The future of dietary supplements for UTI points toward the use of combination products. These include cranberry, D-Mannose, goldenseal, juniper, and Uva Ursi. Other natural supplements including probiotics and those with nitric oxide inhibitory action are also being considered.

References

1. Ofek I, Goldhar J, Sharon N. Anti-Escherichia coli adhesin activity of cranberry and blueberry juices. *Adv Exp Med Biol* 1996;408:179–183.
2. Howell AB, Reed JD, Krueger CG, Winterbottom R, Cunningham DG, Leahy M. A-type cranberry proanthocyanidins and uropathogenic bacterial anti-adhesion activity. *Phytochemistry* 2005;66(18):2281–2291.
3. Howell AB. Bioactive compounds in cranberries and their role in prevention of urinary tract infections. *Mol Nutr Food Res* 2007;51(6):732–737.
4. Jepson RG, Mihaljevic L, Craig J. Cranberries for treating urinary tract infections. *Cochrane Database Syst Rev* 2008;(2):CD001322.
5. Jepson RG, Craig JC. Cranberries for preventing urinary tract infections. *Cochrane Database Syst Rev* 2008;(1):CD001321.
6. Jepson RG, Craig JC. A systematic review of the evidence for cranberries and blueberries in UTI prevention. *Mol Nutr Food Res* 2007;51(6):738–745.
7. Frohne D. [The urinary disinfectant effect of extract from leaves uva ursi]. *Planta Med* 1970;18(1):1–25.
8. Larsson B, Jonasson A, Fianu S. Prophylactic effect of UVA-E in women with recurrent cystitis: a preliminary report. *Curr Ther Res* 1993;53:441–443.
9. Ofek I, Beachey EH. Mannose binding and epithelial cell adherence of Escherichia coli. *Infect Immun* 1978;22(1):247–254.

10. Ruggieri MR, Hanno PM, Levin RM. Mannose inhibition of Escherichia coli adherence to urinary bladder epithelium: comparison with yeast agglutination. *Urol Res* 1985;13(2): 79–84.
11. Michaels EK, Chmiel JS, Plotkin BJ, Schaeffer AJ. Effect of D-mannose and D-glucose on Escherichia coli bacteriuria in rats. *Urol Res* 1983;11(2):97–102.
12. Suvarna R, Pirmohamed M, Henderson L. Possible interaction between warfarin and cranberry juice. *BMJ* 2003;327(7429):1454.
13. Li Z, Seeram NP, Carpenter CL, Thames G, Minutti C, Bowerman S Cranberry does not affect prothrombin time in male subjects on warfarin. *J Am Diet Assoc* 2006;106(12): 2057–2061.
14. Lilja JJ, Backman JT, Neuvonen PJ. Effects of daily ingestion of cranberry juice on the pharmacokinetics of warfarin, tizanidine, and midazolam–probes of CYP2C9, CYP1A2, and CYP3A4. *Clin Pharmacol Ther* 2007;81(6):833–839.
15. Blumenthal M, ed. *The Complete German Commission E Monographs: Therapeutic Guide to Herbal Medicines*. Boston, MA: American Botanical Council; 1998.
16. Newall CA AL, Philpson JD. *Herbal Medicine: A Guide for Healthcare Professionals.* London, UK: The Pharmaceutical Press; 1996.
17. Gruenwald J, BrendlerT, Jaenicke C. *PDR for Herbal Medicines.* 1st ed. Montvale, NJ: Medical Economics Company, Inc; 1998.

IX

Quick Reference Guide

CHAPTER 53

Natural Medicines in Clinical Management—A Quick Reference Guide to Common Conditions

Robert Alan Bonakdar

The following section provides a bottom-line categorization of dietary supplements in common clinical scenarios as provided by the *Natural Medicines Comprehensive Database*. The reader is provided a graphic categorization of several supplements based on safety and efficacy. The supplements listing are a brief sampling of the most typical initial choices based on available level of efficacy and safety, although many others supplements may be appropriate to place on the chart. This chart is followed by specific recommendation as available including supplement formulation, dosing, and brand names utilized in clinical trials. An outline of the format used for the following chapters is noted below. This section is especially pertinent for the busy clinician who is typically presented with a patient with a particular condition in need of additional options.

The question "What else can I take" or the clinician's query "What else can I try here?" can be daunting, especially if the answer is in the dietary supplement realm where the clinician may not have "go-to" answers. This section is meant to provide some initial options when delving into the dietary supplement recommendations. It should not be seen as the question answered but simply as the beginning of the discussion and a few key points should be kept in mind before using these guidelines.

First, these recommendations are meant as a static starting point for the busy clinicians in a rapidly evolving field. Beyond this chart, the reader should refer to regular updates and in-depth information available through the Natural Medicines Comprehensive Database at www.naturaldatabase.com. The charts available on the Web site provide a comprehensive list of supplements including those with less efficacy and safety as well as background references. Next, these recommendation need to be placed into context. For example, although the totality of evidence places a supplement with less than optimal efficacy or safety, there may be specific formulations, both those listed here and others as noted by Marilyn Barrett (chapter 31), which demonstrate better evidence or safety when examined individually.

In all cases, the supplement needs to be individualized for the patient in mind. Two supplements with similar safety profiles in a generic sense may have different safety profiles based on the medical history, medication intake, and supplement regimen utilized by a particular patient. For further elaboration of this point, the clinical case studies are presented as examples. Lastly, as the clinician becomes comfortable with these "go-to" answers, there are often more questions than answers in the area of dosing, regulation, and additional choices among others. This can lead the reader to the introductory chapters of the book as well as other resources reviewed which provide the background needed to confidently practice in this arena.

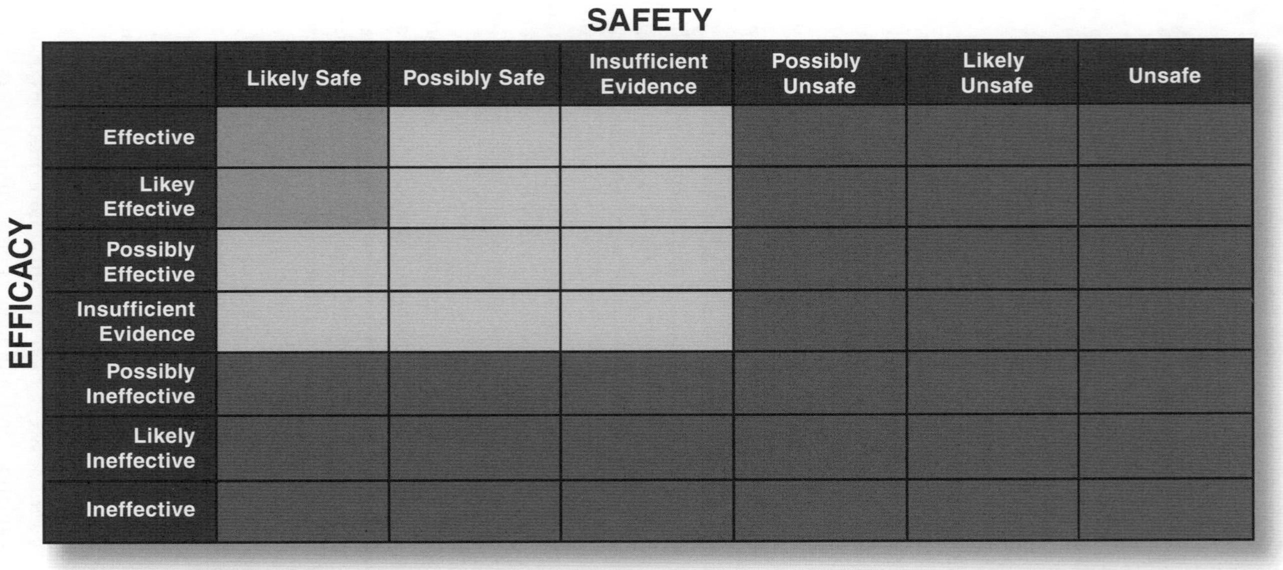

SAFETY

EFFICACY	Likely Safe	Possibly Safe	Insufficient Evidence	Possibly Unsafe	Likely Unsafe	Unsafe
Effective						
Likey Effective						
Possibly Effective						
Insufficient Evidence						
Possibly Ineffective						
Likely Ineffective						
Ineffective						

Figure 53.1 • Recommendation chart for natural medicines.

Notes:

- **Supplement name** (glucosamine sulfate)
  - **Formulation details if applicable** (tablet, extract, standardization, etc.)
  - **Dosing if standardized**: (1,500 mg/d)
  - **Example of specific formulations (maker/distributor) and dosages utilized in clinical trials if different from above:**
    - (Dona Glucosamine (Rotta Pharmaceuticals)
    - **Notes regarding formulation**
- Example:
- Devil's Claw (*Harpagophytum procumbens*)
  - Typically standardized to 50 to 100 mg harpagoside component per day
  - Example:
    - Harpadol (Arkopharma)
      - 2.6 g/d providing 57 mg of the harpagoside constituent and 87 mg of total iridoid glycosides.
    - Doloteffin (Ardeypharm)
      - 2,400 mg/d providing 60 mg/d of harpagoside
- **Combination products (if applicable)**
  - **Formulation name if available and combination ingredients per serving:** Phlogenzym (Mucos Pharma GMBH & Co)
    - Bromelain 90 mg
    - Trypsin 48 mg
    - Rutin (Rutosid Trihydrate) 100 mg
    - **Dosing** 2 to 3 times/d

The following chapters are excerpted from *Natural Medicines Comprehensive Database* with Commentary by Dr. Bonakdar.

CHAPTER 54

Natural Medicines in Attention-Deficit Hyperactivity Disorder (ADHD)

Robert Alan Bonakdar

SAFETY

EFFICACY	Likely Safe	Possibly Safe	Insufficient Evidence
Effective			
Likely Effective			
Possibly Effective		Fish oil Zinc	
Insufficient Evidence	SAMe *St. John's Wort* Magnesium	*Ginkgo biloba* *American ginseng* Flaxseed oil L-carnitine	
Possibly Ineffective			

[a]Ratings courtesy of *Natural Medicines Comprehensive Database*. See full detailed chart and product monograph at www.naturaldatabase.com.

Figure 54.1 • Recommendation chart for natural medicines[a].

Notes:

- Zinc sulfate
  - 150 mg/d
- Combination products
  - Eye Q (Novasel), each 2 capsules contains
    - Fish oils 400 mg, including
      - Eicosapentaenoic acid (EPA) 92 mg
      - Docosahexaenoic acid (DHA) 29 mg
    - Evening primrose oil 100 mg containing
      - Gamma linolenic acid (GLA) 10 mg

    - Dosing: 6 capsules/d
    - Note: Appears to improve cognitive function, hyperactivity, inattentiveness, and behavior
- AD-FX (CV Technologies)
    - American ginseng extract (200 mg)
    - Ginkgo biloba extract (50 mg)
    - Dosing: 2×/d

CHAPTER 55

Natural Medicines in the Clinical Management of Allergic Rhinitis

Robert Alan Bonakdar

SAFETY

EFFICACY	Likely Safe	Possibly Safe	Insufficient Evidence
Effective			
Likely Effective			
Possibly Effective	Vitamin C	Butterbur *Tinospora cordifolia* *Phleum pratense*	
Insufficient Evidence		*Echinacea* (various) MSM Pycnogenol Quercetin Stinging Nettle (*Urtica dioica*)	

[a]Ratings courtesy of *Natural Medicines Comprehensive Database*. See full detailed chart and product monograph at www.naturaldatabase.com.

Figure 55.1 • Recommendation chart for natural medicines[a].

Notes:

- Butterbur (*Petasites hybridus*)
  - Butterbur leaf extract standardized to 8 mg total petasin
    - Tesalin, Ze 339, (Zeller AG)
    - One tablet 3 to 4×/d
  - A whole butterbur root extract
    - Petaforce (Bioforce)
    - 50 mg 2×/d
- *Phleum pratense*
  - SUBLINGUAL:
    - Grazax (Alk Abello)
      - Containing 75,000 SQ-T (standardized quality tablet) units daily, corresponding to 15 mcg
      - Utilized 8 weeks before and continued through pollen season

- **SUBCUTANEOUS:**
  - Alutard SQ (Alk Abello)
    - 100,000 SQ (standardized quality) units, corresponding to 20 mcg
    - 2× weekly starting 8 weeks before and continued through grass pollen season has been used.
- *Tinospora cordifolia*
  - Tinofend (Verdure Sciences) aqueous stem extract
    - 300 mg 3×/d

CHAPTER 56

Natural Medicines in the Clinical Management of Alzheimer's

Robert Alan Bonakdar

SAFETY / EFFICACY

EFFICACY	Likely Safe	Possibly Safe	Insufficient Evidence
Effective			
Likely Effective			
Possibly Effective	*Ginkgo* leaf Vitamin E Lemon balm (*Melissa officinalis*)	Acetyl-L-carnitine Alpha-GPC (Alpha Glycerol Phosphoryl Choline) Huperzine A Citicoline Idebenone Phosphotidyl-serine Vinpocetine Sage (*Salvia officianalis*) Niacin	
Insufficient Evidence		Vitamin B6	

[a]Ratings courtesy of *Natural Medicines Comprehensive Database*. See full detailed chart and product monograph at www.naturaldatabase.com.

Figure 56.1 • Recommendation chart for natural medicines[a].

Notes:

- Carnitine (various formulations)
  - Acetyl-L-carnitine
  - Acetyl levocarnitine hydrochloride
  - 1.5 to 3 g/d
  - Note: Meta-analysis demonstrates benefit on both clinical and psychometric testing starting at 3 months and increasing over time
- Idebenone
  - 90 to 120 mg 3×/d

- Phosphatidylserine
  - 100 mg 3×/d
- Alpha-GPC (Alpha Glycerol Phosphoryl Choline)
  - 1200 mg/d
  - Examples:
    - In Europe, Alpha-GPC is available as a prescription product for Alzheimer's under the name Gliatilin
- Citicoline
  - 1000 mg/d
- Zinc
  - 30 mg/d

CHAPTER 57

Natural Medicines in the Clinical Management of Anxiety

Robert Alan Bonakdar

SAFETY

EFFICACY	Likely Safe	Possibly Safe	Insufficient Evidence
Effective			
Likely Effective			
Possibly Effective		Passionflower (*Passiflora incarnata*) Melatonin (peri-operative anxiety)	Kava (*Piper metysticum*)
Insufficient Evidence	SAMe St. John's Wort (*Hypericum Perforatum*) Roseroot (*Rhodiola rosea*)	Theanine Valerian	Skullcap (*Scutellaria baicalensis*)

[a]Ratings courtesy of *Natural Medicines Comprehensive Database*. See full detailed chart and product monograph at www.naturaldatabase.com.

Figure 57.1 • Recommendation chart for natural medicines[a].

Notes:

- Kava (*Piper metysticum*)
  - 100 mg, 3×/d, standardized to 70% kavalactones
  - Example:
    - WS 1490 (W. Schwabe)
- Melatonin (perioperative anxiety)
  - .05, 0.1, or 0.2 mg/kg
- Passionflower (*Passiflora incarnata*)
  - Various formulations:
    - Liquid extract 45 drops daily
    - Tablets: 90 mg/d

- L-theanine
  - 200 mg/d
- Roseroot (*Rhodiola rosea*)
  - 170 mg 2×/d for 10 weeks
  - Example:
    - Rhodax

CHAPTER 58

Natural Medicines in Athletic Performance

Robert Alan Bonakdar

SAFETY

EFFICACY	Likely Safe	Possibly Safe	Insufficient Evidence
Effective			
Likely Effective			
Possibly Effective	Creatine Caffeine Vitamin C	Pycnogenol Whey protein Deanol Roseroot (*Rhodiola rosea*)	
Insufficient Evidence			

[a]Ratings courtesy of *Natural Medicines Comprehensive Database*. See full detailed chart and product monograph at www.naturaldatabase.com.

Figure 58.1 • Recommendation chart for natural medicines in Athletic Performance[a].

Notes:

- Pycnogenol (French Maritime Pine Bark Extract [*Pinus pinaster*])
  - Treadmill capacity/delayed onset muscle soreness
  - 200 mg daily
  - Note: Pycnogenol is the US registered trademark for the extract
- Creatine
  - Acutely loaded with 20 g/d (or 0.3 g/kg) for 5 days followed by a maintenance dose of 2 or more grams (0.03 g/kg) daily
  - Alternately: 3 g/d for 28 days
  - During creatine supplementation, water intake should be increased to at least 64 ounces per day

- L-carnitine
  - 1–3 g/d
- Roseroot (*Rhodiola rosea*)
  - 200 mg/d
  - Example:
    - Finzelberg (GmbH, Germany) standardized to contain 3% rosavin and 1% salidroside

CHAPTER 59

Natural Medicines in the Clinical Management of Benign Prostatic Hyperplasia (BPH)

Robert Alan Bonakdar

SAFETY

EFFICACY	Likely Safe	Possibly Safe	Insufficient Evidence
Effective			
Likely Effective	Beta-sitosterol Pygum (*Prunus africana*) Saw palmetto (*Serenoa repens*)		
Possibly Effective	Rye grass pollen	Pumpkin seed oil extract (*Cucurbita pepo*) African wild potato	
Insufficient Evidence			

[a]Ratings courtesy of *Natural Medicines Comprehensive Database*. See full detailed chart and product monograph at www.naturaldatabase.com.

Figure 59.1 • Recommendation chart for Natural Medicines in the Clinical Management of Benign Prostatic Hyperplasia (BPH)[a].

Notes:

- Saw palmetto (*Serenoa repens*):
  - 160 mg twice daily or 320 mg once daily of a lipophilic extract containing 80% to 90% fatty acids
  - Examples:
    - ProstActive (Nature's Way)
      - (aka Prostagutt [WS1473], Schwabe Pharm.)
    - Sabalselect (Indena USA, Inc)
      - (aka Prostaserene (Therabel Research)
    - SG 291 (Indena USA, Inc)
      - (aka Talso (Sanofi Synthelabo GmbH)

- Beta-sitosterol/African wild potato/South African Star Grass (*Hypoxis rooperi*)
  - 60 to 130 mg of beta-sitosterol divided into 2 to 3 doses daily
  - Examples:
    - Harzol (Hoyer-Madaus GmbH)
    - Azuprostat (Azupharma)
- Pygum (*Prunus africana*)
  - 75 to 200 mg standardized lipophilic extract (14% triterpenes, 0.5% *n*-docosanol) 1 to 2×/d
- Pumpkin seed oil extract (*Cucurbita pepo*)
  - 480 mg/d in 3 divided doses
- Combination products
  - ProstActive Plus (Nature's Way)
    - (aka Prostagutt Forte, WS1473 (Schwabe Pharm), contains
      - Saw palmetto berry 12:1 extract 160 mg
      - Stinging nettle root 10:1 extract concentrate 120 mg
      - Dose: Typically 2 tabs/d

CHAPTER 60

Natural Medicines in the Clinical Management Breast Cancer (Prevention)

Robert Alan Bonakdar

SAFETY

EFFICACY	Likely Safe	Possibly Safe	Insufficient Evidence
Effective			
Likely Effective			
Possibly Effective	Beta-carotene Folic acid Green tea (*Camellia sinensis*) Fish oil Olive oil (*Olea europaea*) Soy (*Glycine max*) Vitamin A		
Insufficient Evidence	Flaxseed (*Linum usitatissimum*) Shitake mushroom (*Lentinus edodes*)	Beta-glucans Indole-3-carbinol Red clover (*Trifolium pratense*)	Vitamin D

[a]Ratings courtesy of *Natural Medicines Comprehensive Database*. See full detailed chart and product monograph at www.naturaldatabase.com.

Figure 60.1 • Recommendation chart for Natural Medicines in the Clinical Management Breast Cancer (Prevention)[a].

Notes:

- Beta-carotene (prevention)
  - 15 to 50 mg/d
- Folic acid (prevention)
  - Minimum 400 mcg/d
  - Note: In general, premenopausal women with five or more servings of fruits and vegetables per day have modestly lower risk as compared with those consuming less than two servings.
  - This trend appears to be related most significantly to specific nutrients and dietary components including more frequent intake of:
    - Soy
    - Vitamin A
    - Carotenoids
    - Vitamin C
    - Olive oil

CHAPTER 61

Natural Medicines in the Clinical Management of Cataracts

Robert Alan Bonakdar

SAFETY

EFFICACY	Likely Safe	Possibly Safe	Insufficient Evidence
Effective			
Likely Effective	Lutein Niacin Riboflavin		
Possibly Effective	Acetyl-L-carnitine Selenium Vitamin C Vitamin A	Alpha lipoic acid Bilberry (*Vaccinium myrtillus*) Glutathione Lycopene Pyruvate Quercetin	Carnosine Methoxylated flavones
Insufficient Evidence			

[a]Ratings courtesy of *Natural Medicines Comprehensive Database*. See full detailed chart and product monograph at www.naturaldatabase.com.

Figure 61.1 • Recommendation chart for natural medicines[a].

Notes:

- Lutein (dietary intake or supplement)
  - 6 to 12 mg/d
- Niacin (vitamin B_3) (dietary intake)
  - 44 mg/d
- Riboflavin (vitamin B_2) (dietary intake)
  - 2.6 mg/d
- Combination products:
  - Riboflavin 3 mg/d
  - Niacin 40 mg/d
  - Note: The above combination reduced risk of developing nuclear cataracts compared to placebo by up to 44%

CHAPTER 62

Natural Medicines in the Clinical Management of Cold and Flu

Robert Alan Bonakdar

SAFETY

EFFICACY	Likely Safe	Possibly Safe	Insufficient Evidence
Effective			
Likely Effective			
Possibly Effective		American ginseng (*Panax quinquefolium*)	
Insufficient Evidence	Alpha-Linolenic acid Garlic (*Allium sativum*) Lactobacillus GG	Andrographis (*Andrographis paniculata*) Astralagus (Astragalus membranaceus) Linoleic acid (from flax) Panax ginseng (*Panax quinquefolium*)	

[a]Ratings courtesy of *Natural Medicines Comprehensive Database*. See full detailed chart and product monograph at www.naturaldatabase.com.

Figure 62.1 • Recommendation chart for natural medicines for cold and flu (prevention)[a].

Notes:

- Andrographis (*Andrographis paniculata*) (see combination products)
- American ginseng (*Panax quinquefolium*)
  - 200 mg 2 to 3×/d
  - Examples:
    - Cold-FX (CV Technologies, Canada)
    - Prevention: 200 mg 2×/d over a 3- to 4-month period
    - Note: Taking during influenza season might modestly decrease the risk of developing symptoms of an upper respiratory tract infection
    - Treatment: 200 mg 2 to 3/d during symptoms
- Echinacea (*Echinacea purpurea*)
  - Dosing varies
  - Examples:
    - Tablet: Echinaforce, (Bioforce AG)

SAFETY / **EFFICACY**

	Likely Safe	Possibly Safe	Insufficient Evidence
Effective			
Likely Effective			
Possibly Effective	Andrographis (*Andrographis paniculata*) Echinacea (*Echinacea purpurea*) Vitamin C (Extreme conditions)	Elderberry (*Sambucus nigra*)	
Insufficient Evidence	Oscilococcinum	Astralagus (*Astragalus membranaceus*) Goldenseal (*Hydrastis canadensis*) Larch arabino-galactan (*Larch arabinogalactan*) Siberian ginseng (*Eleutherococcus senticosus*)	Zinc lozenges Bee propolis

[a]Ratings courtesy of *Natural Medicines Comprehensive Database.* See full detailed chart and product monograph at www.naturaldatabase.com.

Figure 62.2 • Recommendation chart for natural medicines used for cold and flu (treatment)[a].

- A tablet containing 6.78 mg of *E. purpurea* crude extract based on 95% herb and 5% root is dosed as
- 2 tablets 3×/d
- Tea: Echinacea plus (traditional medicinals)
  - Combination of *E. purpurea* and *E. angustifolia*
  - 5 to 6 cups of tea on day 1 of symptoms
  - Titrating to 1 cup/d over the next 5 days
- Liquid: Echinagard (Nature's Way)
  - 20 drops q 2 hours on day 1 of symptoms
  - 20 drops 3×/d for up to 10 days
- Siberian ginseng (*Eleutherococcus senticosus*) (see combination products)
- Combination products
  - Kan Jang (Swedish Herbal Institute), each tablet contains:
    - Andrographis (*A. paniculata*), 178 to 266 mg, standardized to 4 to 5.6 mg andrographolide
    - Siberian ginseng (*E. senticosus*) 20 to 30 mg
      - Treatment: 1 to 2 tablets 3×/d
      - Prevention: 1 tablet/d 5 d/wk
      - Note: Appears to significantly improve symptoms of the common cold when started within 72 hours of symptom onset.

CHAPTER 63

Natural Medicines in the Clinical Management of Congestive Heart Failure

Robert Alan Bonakdar

SAFETY

EFFICACY	Likely Safe	Possibly Safe	Insufficient Evidence
Effective			
Likely Effective			
Possibly Effective	Coenzyme Q10 L-arginine L-carnitine	Hawthorne (*Crataegus monogyna*) Taurine *Terminalia arjuna*	
Insufficient Evidence			

[a]Ratings courtesy of *Natural Medicines Comprehensive Database*. See full detailed chart and product monograph at www.naturaldatabase.com.

Figure 63.1 • Recommendation chart for natural medicines[a].

Notes:

- Coenzyme Q10
  - 100 mg/d divided
- L-arginine
  - 6 to 20 g/d
- L-carnitine
  - 1 g twice daily
- Hawthorne (*Crataegus monogyna*)
  - Standardized hawthorn leaf with flower extract
  - Example:
    - LI 132 or WS 1442
    - Dose: 160 to 1800 mg/d (3.5 to 39.6 mg of total flavonoids calculated as hyperoside or 30 to 338 mg of proanthocyanidins) in 2 to 3 divided doses daily
- Taurine
  - 2 to 6 g/d in 2 to 3 divided doses
- *Terminalia arjuna*
  - 500 mg every 8 hours has been used

CHAPTER 64

Natural Medicines in the Clinical Management of Depression

Robert Alan Bonakdar

SAFETY

EFFICACY	Likely Safe	Possibly Safe	Insufficient Evidence
Effective			
Likely Effective	SAMe (*S-adenosyl-L-methionine*) St. John's Wort (*Hypericum perforatum*)		
Possibly Effective	Fish oil Folic acid	Saffron (*Crocus sativus*)	5-HTP (*5-hydroxy-tryptophan*)
Insufficient Evidence	Acetyl-L-carnitine	Turmeric (*Curcumae longa*)	

[a]Ratings courtesy of *Natural Medicines Comprehensive Database*. See full detailed chart and product monograph at www.naturaldatabase.com.

Figure 64.1 • Recommendation chart for Natural Medicines in the Clinical Management of Depression[a].

Notes:

- St. John's Wort
  - Varies based on formulation, typically 300 mg 2–4×/day
  - Examples
    - Lichtwer LI 160, containing 0.3% hypericin
      - LI 160 , Kira (Lichtwer Pharma US, Inc.).
    - Lichtwer LI 160 WS is the hyperforin-stabilized version of LI 160.
      - Quanterra Emotional Balance (Warner-Lambert).
    - ZE 117, containing 0.2% hypericin
      - Remotiv (Zeller).
    - WS 5572, containing 5% hyperforin
      - Movana (Pharmaton)
- SAMe (*S-adenosyl-L-methionine*)
  - 400 to 1600 mg/d

- Acetyl L-carnitine
  - 1,500 to 3,000 mg daily
- Eicosapentaenoic acid (EPA)
  - 1 g 2×/daily
- Fish oils (along with antidepressants)
  - up to 6.6 g/d
- Folic acid (along with antidepressants)
  - 200 to 500 mcg/d
- Saffron (*Crocus sativus*)
  - 30 mg/d (Novin Zaferan Co., Iran)

CHAPTER 65

Natural Medicines in the Clinical Management of Diabetes

Robert Alan Bonakdar

SAFETY

EFFICACY	Likely Safe	Possibly Safe	Insufficient Evidence
Effective			
Likely Effective			
Possibly Effective	Blond psyllium (*Plantago ovata*) Guar gum (*Cyamopsis tetragonoloba*) Oat bran (*Avena sativa*) Soy (*Glycine max*) Magnesium	Alpha-lipoic acid *American* ginseng (Panax quinquefolius) Chromium Glucomannan (*Amorphophallus konjac*) *Panax ginseng* Prickly pear cactus (*Opuntia ficus-indica*) Agaricus mushroom (*Agaricus blazei*) Milk thistle (*Silybum marianum*) Niacin	
Insufficient Evidence	Cassia cinnamon (*Cinnamomum aromaticum*)	Banaba (*Lagerstroemia speciosa*) Bitter melon (*Momordica charantia*) Fenugreek (*Trigonella foenum-graecum*) Gymnema (*Gymnema sylvestre*) Stevia (*Stevia rebaudiana*)	

[a]Ratings courtesy of *Natural Medicines Comprehensive Database.* See full detailed chart and product monograph at www.naturaldatabase.com.

Figure 65.1 • Recommendation chart for Natural Medicines in the Clinical Management of Diabetes[a].

Notes:

- Alpha-lipoic acid (ALA)
  - 600 to 1,800 mg orally or 500 to 1,000 mg intravenously
  - Note: Appears to improve insulin sensitivity and glucose disposal in patients with type 2 diabetes after 4 weeks of oral or 1 to 10 days of intravenous treatment
  - Note: ALA also appears to improve neuropathic sensory symptoms and objective measures related to diabetic neuropathy
- American ginseng (*Panax quinquefolius*)
  - 3 g orally, up to 2 hours before a meal
    - Note: Can significantly reduce postprandial glucose levels in patients with type 2 diabetes
- Chromium picolinate
  - 200 to 1,000 mcg daily
  - Example:
    - Chromax (Nutrition 21)
- Blond psyllium seed husk (*Plantago ovata*)
  - 10 to 30 g/d in divided doses advancing based on GI toleralability
  - Note: Psyllium seems to reduce postprandial blood glucose levels in patients with type II diabetes by 14% to 20%, total cholesterol by about 9%, and LDL cholesterol by 13%
  - Note: Blond psyllium's maximum effect on the glucose levels occurs when psyllium is mixed and consumed with foods
- Soy (*Glycine max*)
  - 10 to 30 g/d soy protein, 75 to 150 mg isoflavones
  - Note: In postmenopausal women with type 2 diabetes, 30 g of soy protein (132 mg isoflavones) daily × 12 weeks lowers fasting insulin levels, hemoglobin A1c, insulin resistance, and low-density lipoprotein (LDL) cholesterol
  - Note: Touchi, a fermented soybean product, may acts as an alpha-glucosidase inhibitor.
  - Note: Soy has shown preliminary benefit in the treatment of diabetic nephropathy and reducing urinary albumin excretion
- **Combination products**
  - Diachrome (Nutrition 21)
    - Chromium 600 mcg with biotin

CHAPTER 66

Natural Medicines in the Clinical Management of Fatigue

Robert Alan Bonakdar

SAFETY

EFFICACY	Likely Safe	Possibly Safe	Insufficient Evidence
Effective			
Likely Effective			
Possibly Effective	Magnesium	Alpha-lipoic acid Roseroot (*Rhodiola rosea*) D-Ribose	
Insufficient Evidence	Coenzyme Q10 Carnitine Iron		

[a]Ratings courtesy of *Natural Medicines Comprehensive Database*. See full detailed chart and product monograph at www.naturaldatabase.com.

Figure 66.1 • Recommendation chart for natural medicines in the Clinical Management of Fatigue[a].

Notes:

- Magnesium (In people with low red blood cell magnesium)
  - 1 g magnesium sulfate, intramuscular injections
- Coenzyme Q10 (fatigue related to a physical task)
  - 100 to 300 mg/d
- Carnitine:
- L-carnitine: (Age-related fatigue)
  - 2 g/d × 30 days
  - Above dosing appears to improve physical and mental fatigue, increases muscle mass, and decreases fat mass compared to placebo in elderly patients
- Acetyl-L-carnitine (chronic fatigue syndrome)
- Propionyl-L-carnitine (chronic fatigue syndrome)
  - 2 g/d of either of the above
  - Note: Acetylcarnitine had main effect on mental fatigue and propionylcarnitine on general fatigue in 12-week clinical trial. Less improvement was found with combined treatment.

- Iron (ferrous sulfate)
  - 80 mg/d may improve fatigue primarily in women with borderline or low serum ferritin concentration)
- Roseroot (*Rhodiola rosea*)
  - 100 to 750 mg/d based on formulation
  - Example
    - SHR-5 (ProActive BioProducts, Inc.)
  - 170 mg tabs 1 to 4×/d
- D-Ribose
  - 5 g 3×/d
    - Example:
      - Corvalen (Valen Labs)

CHAPTER 67

Natural Medicines in the Clinical Management of Fibromyalgia

Robert Alan Bonakdar

SAFETY

EFFICACY	Likely Safe	Possibly Safe	Insufficient Evidence
Effective			
Likely Effective			
Possibly Effective	SAMe (S-adenosyl -L-methionine) Capsicum (*Capsicum frutescens*) Magnesium		5-HTP (5-hydroxy-tryptophan)
Insufficient Evidence	St. John's Wort (*Hypericum perforatum*)	*American ginseng* (*Panax quinquefolius*) Ashwaganda (*Withania somnifera*) Astralagus (*Astragalus membranaceus*) German chamomile (*Matricaria recutita*) Malic acid Melatonin *Panax ginseng* Passionflower (*Passiflora incarnata*) Valerian (*Valeriana officinalis*)	

[a]Ratings courtesy of *Natural Medicines Comprehensive Database*. See full detailed chart and product monograph at www.naturaldatabase.com.

Figure 67.1 • Recommendation chart for Natural Medicines in the Clinical Management of Fibromyalgia[a].

Notes:

- SAMe (S-adenosyl-L-methionine)
  - 800 mg/d
- Capsicum topical (*Capsicum frutescens*)
  - 0.025% 4×/d
- 5-HTP (5-hydroxytryptophan)
  - 100 mg 3 times daily
- Combination products
  - Super Malic, containing:
    - Malic acid 200 mg
    - Magnesium 50 mg
    - Dose: 3 tabs 2×/d

CHAPTER 68

Natural Medicines in the Clinical Management of Glaucoma

Robert Alan Bonakdar

SAFETY

EFFICACY	Likely Safe	Possibly Safe	Insufficient Evidence
Effective			
Likely Effective			
Possibly Effective	*Ginkgo biloba*	Marijuana	
Insufficient Evidence	Fish oil Glucosamine sulfate Vitamin C	Forskolin	Citicoline

[a]Ratings courtesy of *Natural Medicines Comprehensive Database*. See full detailed chart and product monograph at www.naturaldatabase.com.

Figure 68.1 • Recommendation chart for natural medicines[a].

Notes:

- *Ginkgo biloba*
    - Ginkgo leaf extract
    - 40 mg 3×/d
    - Note: Use for up to 4 weeks appears to improve preexisting visual field damage in patients with normal tension glaucoma

CHAPTER 69

Natural Medicines in the Clinical Management of Migraine Headache

Robert Alan Bonakdar

SAFETY

EFFICACY

	Likely Safe	Possibly Safe	Insufficient Evidence
Effective	Caffeine		
Likely Effective			
Possibly Effective		Butterbur (*Petasites hybridus*) Feverfew (*Tanacetum parthenium*) Coenzyme Q-10 Magnesium Riboflavin (Vitamin B-2) Melatonin Peppermint (*Mentha x piperita*)	
Insufficient Evidence			

[a]Ratings courtesy of *Natural Medicines Comprehensive Database*. See full detailed chart and product monograph at www.naturaldatabase.com.

Figure 69.1 • Recommendation chart for Natural Medicines in the Clinical Management of Migraine Headache[a].

Notes:

- Butterbur (*Petasites hybridus*)
  - 150 mg/d of rhizome extract standardized to 15% petasin and isopetasin
  - Example:
    - Petadolex (Weber & Weber International)
- Feverfew (*Tanacetum parthenium*)
  - 50 to 100 mg/d of feverfew extract. Most extracts used in clinical studies were standardized to 0.2% to 0.7%, or
  - 6.25 mg 3×/d of a supercritical carbon dioxide feverfew extract (MIG-99)

- Coenzyme Q10
  - 100 to 300 mg/d based on a brand. Bioabsorption varies widely
  - Examples
    - CoQMax, CF(crystal free) (Xymogen)
    - Dose: 100 to 300 mg/d
- Magnesium
  - Various formulations, base on GI tolerability of salts. 200 to 800 mg 1 to 3×/d, advance as tolerated
  - Example:
    - Magnesium citrate (610 mg three times daily), trimagnesium dicitrate (600 mg daily)
- Riboflavin (vitamin B-2)
  - 400 mg/d
- Melatonin
  - 3 mg extended release at bedtime
- **Combination products**
  - Migra-Lieve (Natural Science Corp. of America)
    - Feverfew extract (*T. parthenium*, standardized to 0.7% Parthenolide) 100 mg
    - Magnesium (citrate/oxide 1:1) 300 mg
    - Riboflavin (vitamin B_2) 400 mg.
  - Gelstat Migraine (GelStat Corporation) (sublingual) at onset of migraine as directed
    - Feverfew (*T. parthenium*)
      - Dose: Homeopathic 3×
    - Ginger (*Zingiber officinale*)
      - Dose: Homeopathic 2×

CHAPTER 70

Natural Medicines in the Clinical Management of Hyperlipidemia

Robert Alan Bonakdar

SAFETY

EFFICACY	Likely Safe	Possibly Safe	Insufficient Evidence
Effective	Fish oil Niacin		
Likely Effective	Oat bran (*Avena sativa*) Plant sterols Blond psyllium (*Plantago ovata*)	Red yeast rice (*Monascus purpureus*)	
Possibly Effective	Soy (*Glycine max*)	Artichoke extract (*Cynara cardunculus*) Alfalfa (*Medicago sativa*)	Inositol nicotinate
Insufficient Evidence		Policosanol	

[a]Ratings courtesy of *Natural Medicines Comprehensive Database*. See full detailed chart and product monograph at www.naturaldatabase.com.

Figure 70.1 • Recommendation chart for Natural Medicines in the Clinical Management of Hyperlipidemia[a].

Notes:

- Fish oil (hypertriglyceridemia)
  - 1 to 6 g/d
    - Examples: Multiple over-the-counter brands are available. Look for brand with a high level of eicosapentaenoic acid (EPA)/docosahexaenoic acid (DHA) combination per gram of fish oil
    - Note: An prescription preparation approved for hypertriglyceridemia (Lovaza, formerly known as Omacor, GlaxoSmithKline, contains) 465 mg of EPA and 375 mg of DHA in 1 g capsules
- Niacin (vitamin B_3):
  - HDL increase 1,200 to 1,500 mg/d
  - Low-density lipoprotein (LDL) decrease 2,000 to 3,000 mg/d

Summary of the Lipid Effects of Selected Drugs and Natural Products

	LDL	HDL	TGs
Statins	↓ Upto 55%	↑ 6%–14%	↓ 15%–35%
Bile acid sequestrants	↓ 10%–30%		Variable; sometimes ↑
Ezetimibe	↓ 18%–24%		↓ 10 %
Niacin	↓ 10%–15%	↑ 35%	↓ 20%–50%
Fibrates	Variable	↑ 5%–15%	
Artichoke extract	↓ Upto 23%		
Soy	↓ Upto 10%		
Walnuts	↓ 8%–16%		
Fish Oil			↓ 20%–50%
Plant stanols and sterols	↓ 5%–17%		
Fiber: Blond psyllium, oat bran	↓ 5%–26%		

See full detailed chart and product monograph at www.naturaldatabase.com.

    - Note: Several Food and Drug Administration–approved formulation are available. Monitoring for liver function is recommended with long-term use
    - Note: Flushing can be a common side effect and can be minimized with slow-dose titration, using extended release formulations, pretreating with aspirin, or taking regular-release niacin with meals or the sustained-release product at bedtime
- Plant sterols/stanols
  - 800 mg to 6 g/d divided and typically given before meals.
  - Example: Available in various formulations including tables and butter replacements including Take Control and Benecol
- Red yeast rice (*Monascus purpureus*)
  - 600 to 3,150 mg daily
  - Example:
    - Xuezhikang (Beijing WBLPeking University Biotech Co.)
  - Note: As red yeast rice products contain varying levels of statins (lovastatin), liver function monitoring is recommended

CHAPTER 71

Natural Medicines in the Clinical Management of Hypertension

Robert Alan Bonakdar

SAFETY

EFFICACY	Likely Safe	Possibly Safe	Insufficient Evidence
Effective			
Likely Effective			
Possibly Effective	Alpha-linolenic acid Blond pysllium (*Plantago ovata*) Calcium Cocoa (*Theobroma cacao*) Coenzyme Q10 Fish oil Garlic (*Allium sativum*)	Pycnogenol (Pinus pinaster/ Pinus maritima)	Casein peptide
Insufficient Evidence	Green tea (*Camellia sinensis*) Magnesium Pomegranate (*Punica granatum*) Vitamin D	L-arginine Tomato extract (*Lycopersicon esculentum*)	

[a]Ratings courtesy of *Natural Medicines Comprehensive Database*. See full detailed chart and product monograph at www.naturaldatabase.com.

Figure 71.1 • Recommendation chart for Natural Medicines in the Clinical Management of Hypertension[a].

Notes:

- Fish oil
  - 4 g of fish oils or eicosapentaenoic acid (EPA) 2.04 g and docosahexaenoic acid (DHA) 1.4 g/d used in trials
  - Note: Also used at 4 g/d for hypertension secondary to cyclosporine in heart transplant patients

- Alpha-linolenic acid
  - 1.6g/d as part of a Mediterranean diet
  - A diet high in linolenic acid seems to reduce risk of hypertension by about a third (Djousse L et al. Dietary linolenic acid is associated with a lower prevalence of hypertension in the NHLBI Family Heart Study. *Hypertension* 2005;45:368–373.)
- Cocoa
  - Consuming dark (more so than milk) chocolate 46 to 105 g/d (213 to 500 mg of cocoa polyphenols) lowers systolic blood pressure by 4.7 mm Hg and diastolic blood pressure by 2.8 mm Hg
  - 6.3 g/d (30 mg of polyphenols) decreases systolic blood pressure by 2.9 mm Hg and diastolic blood pressure by 1.9 mm Hg when consumed for 18 weeks by patients with prehypertension or mild hypertension
  - Example:
    - Ritter Sport Halbbitter (Alfred Ritter GmbH & Co.) used in both the above studies
- Garlic
  - Garlic powder 600 to 900 mg/d
  - Example
    - Kwai (Lichtwer Pharma).
  - Note: An aged garlic extract 2,400 mg daily has also been used
  - Note: It has been shown to reduce systolic blood pressure by about 8% and diastolic blood pressure by about 7%
- Combination approaches (dietary)
  - DASH diet
  - In a 2,000-calorie DASH diet, the following are recommended:
    - 7 to 8 servings of grains
    - 4 to 5 servings of fruits
    - 4 to 5 servings of vegetables
    - 2 to 3 servings of low-fat dairy products
    - 2 or less servings of lean meats
    - Snacks and sweets ≤5 per week

CHAPTER 72

Natural Medicines in the Clinical Management of Insomnia

Robert Alan Bonakdar

SAFETY

EFFICACY	Likely Safe	Possibly Safe	Insufficient Evidence
Effective			
Likely Effective	St. John's Wort (*Hypericum Perforatum*) (insomnia related to depression)		
Possibly Effective	Coenzyme Q10 Melatonin	Valerian (*Valeriana officinalis*)	
Insufficient Evidence		Lavender (*Lavandula augustifolia*) German chamomile (*Matricaria recutita*) Lemon balm (*Melissa officinalis*) Passionflower (*Passiflora incarnata*)	Skullcap (*Scutellaria baicalensis*)

[a]Ratings courtesy of *Natural Medicines Comprehensive Database.* See full detailed chart and product monograph at www.naturaldatabase.com.

Figure 72.1 • Recommendation chart for natural medicines[a].

Notes:

- Valerian (*Valeriana officinalis*)
    - 300 to 900 mg valerian extract 30 to 120 minutes before bedtime
    - Examples:
        - See combination products
- Melatonin
    - For insomnia: 0.3 to 5 mg at bedtime
    - For jet lag, 0.5 to 5 mg at bedtime on the arrival day at the eastbound destination, continuing for 2 to 5 days
    - Note: Both immediate-release and sustained-release preparations have been used
    - Note: The controlled-released melatonin, Circadin, is available as a prescription drug in Canada and Europe

- Lavender (*Lavandula augustifolia*)
  - Aromatherapy provided with via an Aromastream device (Tisserand Aromatherapy, Sussex, UK)
- Coenzyme Q10 (insomnia related to heart failure)
  - 100 to 300 mg/d
- St. John's Wort (related to depression)
  - Examples
    - Lichtwer LI 160, containing 0.3% hypericin
      - LI 160 , Kira (Lichtwer Pharma US, Inc.).
    - Lichtwer LI 160 WS is the hyperforin-stabilized version of LI 160.
      - Quanterra Emotional Balance (Warner-Lambert).
    - ZE 117, containing 0.2% hypericin
      - Remotiv (Zeller).
    - WS 5572, containing 5% hyperforin
      - Movana (Pharmaton)
- Combination products
  - Research-based combination (Morin CM. *Sleep* 2005;28(11):1465–1471.):
    - Valerian (187-mg native extracts; 5 to 8:1, methanol 45% m/m)
    - Hops (41.9-mg native extracts; 7 to 10:1, methanol 45% m/m)
    - Dosing: 2 tablets nightly for 28 days
    - Note: This combination demonstrated benefit similar to diphenhydramine in several sleep parameters with residual sedation or rebound insomnia.
  - Euvegal forte (Schwabe Pharmaceuticals)
    - Lemon balm leaf extract 80 mg
    - Valerian root extract 160 mg
    - Dose: 3 times/d
    - Note: Above product appears to improve the quality of sleep in healthy subjects

CHAPTER 73

Natural Medicines in the Clinical Management of Irritable Bowel Syndrome (IBS)

Robert Alan Bonakdar

SAFETY

EFFICACY	Likely Safe	Possibly Safe	Insufficient Evidence
Effective	Blond psyllium seed husk (*Plantago ovata*)	Cascara (*Frangula purshiana*) European buckthorn (*Rhamnus cathartica*)	
Likely Effective	Senna (*Senna alexandrina*)		
Possibly Effective	Bifidobacteria Karaya gum (*Sterculia urens*)	Aloe (*Aloe vera*)	
Insufficient Evidence	Lactobacillus	Artichoke leaf extract (*Cynara cardunculus*) Peppermint oil (*Mentha x piperita*)	

[a]Ratings courtesy of *Natural Medicines Comprehensive Database*. See full detailed chart and product monograph at www.naturaldatabase.com.

Figure 73.1 • Recommendation chart for Natural Medicines in the Clinical Management of Irritable Bowel Syndrome (IBS)[a].

Notes:

- Blond psyllium seed husk (*Plantago ovata*)
  - 10 to 30 g/d in divided doses advancing on the basis of GI tolerability
- Bifidobacteria
  - *Bifidobacterium infantis* 35624 (Bifantis, Proctor & Gamble)
    - 1 billion cells daily
    - Note: 8 weeks of use seems to significantly reduce symptoms of irritable bowel syndrome such as abdominal pain and bloating and bowel movement difficulty. Improvement is seen within 1 week of treatment.

- Lactobacillus
  - *Lactobacillus acidophilus* 10 billion heat-killed *L. acidophilus* units
    - Examples
      - Lacteol Fort (Mirren Pty Ltd)
    - Note: 6 weeks significantly improves abdominal pain, bloating, and number and quality of stools compared to placebo
- Peppermint oil
  - 0.2 to 1 ml 3×/d in an enteric-coated tablet
  - Also available as tincture or tea in combination with other essential oils
- Artichoke leaf extract
  - 320 to 640 mg 1 to 3×/d
  - Example:
    - Hepar-SL forte (Serturner Arzneimittel GmbH)
      - 640 mg 3×/d
    - Cynara SL (Lichtwer Pharma)
      - 320 to 640 mg /d
- Combination products
  - VSL#3 (Sigma-Tau Pharmaceuticals, Inc.)
    - Bacteria 450 billion units, including:
    - *Bifidobacterium breve*
    - *Bifidobacterium longum*
    - *Bifidobacterium infantis*
    - *Lactobacillus acidophilus*
    - *Lactobacillus plantarum*
    - *Lactobacillus paracasei*
    - *Lactobacillus bulgaricus*
    - *Streptococcus thermophilus*
    - Dosing: 3 g 2×/d

CHAPTER 74

Natural Medicines in the Clinical Management of Low Back Pain

Robert Alan Bonakdar

SAFETY

EFFICACY	Likely Safe	Possibly Safe	Insufficient Evidence
Effective			
Likely Effective	Capsaicin (*Capsicum frutescens*)		
Possibly Effective	Devil's claw (*Harpagophytum procumbens*) Willow bark (*Salix alba/Salix purpurea*)		
Insufficient Evidence			

[a]Ratings courtesy of *Natural Medicines Comprehensive Database.* See full detailed chart and product monograph at www.naturaldatabase.com.

Figure 74.1 • Recommendation chart for natural medicines[a].

Notes:

- Capsaicin (topical/plaster) (*Capsicum frutescens*)
  - Topical: 0.025% to 0.075%
  - Capsicum-containing plasters:
    - Example: 11 mg capsaicin/plaster or 22 mcg/cm^2 of plaster applied
    - Dose: Plaster is applied in the morning for 4 to 8 hours
- Devil's claw (*Harpagophytum procumbens*)
  - Typically standardized to 50 to 100 mg harpagoside component per day
  - Example:
    - Doloteffin (Ardeypharm)
      - 2,400 mg/d providing 60 mg/d of harpagoside
    - Harpadol (Arkopharma)
      - 2.6 g/d providing 57 mg of the harpagoside constituent and 87 mg of total iridoid glycosides.
- Willow bark extract (*Salix alba/Salix purpurea*)
  - 120 to 240 mg of the salicin daily typically used in various formulations
  - Other forms:
    - Flexipert (Bionorica)
    - 2 tablets—Willow Barks (*Salicis cortex*) = 789.48 mg
      - Dose: 2 tablets 1 to 2×/d

CHAPTER 75

Natural Medicines in the Clinical Management of Macular Degeneration

Robert Alan Bonakdar

SAFETY

EFFICACY	Likely Safe	Possibly Safe	Insufficient Evidence
Effective			
Likely Effective			
Possibly Effective	Lutein and zeaxanthin Beta-carotene Fish oils Zinc Vitamin E		
Insufficient Evidence		*Ginkgo Biloba* leaf extract	

[a]Ratings courtesy of *Natural Medicines Comprehensive Database*. See full detailed chart and product monograph at www.naturaldatabase.com.

Figure 75.1 • Recommendation chart for natural medicines[a].

Notes:

- Lutein and zeaxanthin
  - 10 to 20 mg/d alone or with an antioxidant/vitamin
- Fish oils, docosahexaenoic acid (DHA)
  - >4 servings of fish/wk was associated with a 35% lower risk of age-related macular degeneration (AMD) compared with 3 or less servings/mo
- Combination products:
  - Elemental zinc 80 mg
  - Vitamin C 500 mg
  - Vitamin E 400 IU
  - Beta-carotene 15 mg daily
  - Note: In patients with advanced AMD, above supplement combination caused risk reduction of 27% for visual acuity loss and a 24% for progression of AMD

CHAPTER 76

Natural Medicines in the Clinical Management of Menopause

Robert Alan Bonakdar

SAFETY

EFFICACY	Likely Safe	Possibly Safe	Insufficient Evidence
Effective			
Likely Effective			
Possibly Effective	Flaxseed (*Linum usitatissimum*) Soy (*Glycine max*) EPA St. John's Wort (*Hypericum perforatum*)	Black cohosh (*Cimicifuga racemosa*) Progesterone	
Insufficient Evidence	Chasteberry (*Vitex agnus-castus*)	Hops (*Humulus lupulus*) Kudzu (*Pueraria lobata*) Valerian (*Valeriana officinalis*)	

[a]Ratings courtesy of *Natural Medicines Comprehensive Database*. See full detailed chart and product monograph at www.naturaldatabase.com.

Figure 76.1 • Recommendation chart for Natural Medicines in the Clinical Management of Menopause[a].

Notes:

- Black cohosh (*Cimicifuga racemosa*) root and rhizome extract
  - 20 to 160 mg/d, providing 2 to 16 mg triterpenes
  - Example:
    - Remifemin (Phytopharmica/Enzymatic Therapy).
      - 20 mg tablet standardized to contain 1 mg triterpene glycosides, calculated as 27-deoxyactein,
      - Dose: 20 to 80 mg 2×/d
    - Klimadynon/Menofem/CR BNO 1055 (Bionorica AG)
      - 40 mg/d
- St. John's Wort extract (*Hypericum perforatum*)
  - Standardized to contain hypericin 250 mcg.
  - Dose: 2–4 times/day (see combinations below)

- Flaxseed (*Linum usitatissimum*)
  - 40 g/d significantly reduces symptoms of hot flashes by about 35% and night sweats by about 44% compared to baseline in women with mild menopausal symptoms (Lemay A et al. *Obstet Gynecol* 2002;100:495–504.)
- Soy (*Glycine max*)
  - Diet: Consuming soy protein 20 to 60 g providing 34 to 76 mg of isoflavones daily seems to modestly decrease the frequency and severity of hot flashes in some menopausal women.
  - Supplements: Taking concentrated soy isoflavone extracts, providing 35 to 120 mg of isoflavones per day appears beneficial in trials.
- Combination products:
  - Remifemin plus (Enzymatic Therapy, Germany)
    - Isopropanolic black cohosh extract
      - 20 mg tablets, standardized for triterpene glycosides content, calculated as 27-deoxyactein
    - St. John's Wort extract standardized to contain hypericin 250 mcg.
    - Dose: 1 to 2 tables 2×/d
  - Gynoplus (Jin-Yang Pharm)
    - Black cohosh extract
    - St. John's Wort 48 mg
    - Dose: Per 264 mg tablet:
      - 0.0364 ml of extract from Cimicifugae racemosa rhizome, equivalent to 1 mg terpene glycosides
      - 84 mg of dried extract from *Hypericum perforatum*, equivalent to 0.25 mg hypericin.

CHAPTER 77

Natural Medicines in the Clinical Management of Obesity

Robert Alan Bonakdar

SAFETY

EFFICACY	Likely Safe	Possibly Safe	Insufficient Evidence
Effective			
Likely Effective			
Possibly Effective	Calcium Psyllium (*Plantago ovata*) Vitamin D	Conjugated linoleic acid Fish oil	
Insufficient Evidence	Chromium St. John's Wort (*Hypericum perforatum*)	Glucomannan (*Amorphophallus konjac*) Guggul (*Commiphora wightii*) Pyruvate	

[a]Ratings courtesy of *Natural Medicines Comprehensive Database*. See full detailed chart and product monograph at www.naturaldatabase.com.

Figure 77.1 • Recommendation chart for Natural Medicines in the Clinical Management of Obesity[a].

Notes:

- Calcium/vitamin D (preventing weight gain)
  - 900 to 1,200 mg/d with vitamin D 400 to 800 IU/d
    - Note: Most evidence appears to indicate that calcium may help reduce the chance of gaining weight. In one 3-year study, 1,000 mg plus vitamin D (cholecalciferol) 400 IU daily was associated with less weight gain over time compared to placebo. The inverse effect seems most pronounced in those with inadequate intake

- Conjugated linoleic acid (CLA) (improving body composition)
  - 1.8 to 4.5 g/d
  - Note: CLA appears to improve body fat mass and lean body mass in some patients but does not seem to reduce total body weight or body mass index. CLA may also reduce hunger and improve satiety
  - 300 to 600 mg/d
- Fish oil
  - 6 g daily providing 260 mg DHA/gram and 60 mg EPA/g eicosapentaenoic acid (EPA) and docosahexaenoic acid (DHA)
  - Examples
    - Hi-DHA, (NuMega)
    - Note: Above formulation significantly decreases body fat when combined with exercise

CHAPTER 78

Natural Medicines in the Clinical Management of Osteoarthritis

Robert Alan Bonakdar

SAFETY

EFFICACY	Likely Safe	Possibly Safe	Insufficient Evidence
Effective			
Likely Effective	Glucosamine sulfate S-Adenosyl Methionine-endogenous (SAMe) Capsaicin (topical) (*Capsicum frutescens*)		
Possibly Effective	Chondroitin 4, 6 Sulfate	Avocado soybean unsaponofiables (ASUs) Devil's claw (*Harpagophytum procumbens*) Cetylated fatty acids (oral or topical in combination with menthol) Niacinamide Methylsulfonylmethane (MSM) Bromelain/rutin/trypsin Beta-carotene Cetylated fatty acids	
Insufficient Evidence	Ginger (*Zingiber officinale*)		

[a]Ratings courtesy of *Natural Medicines Comprehensive Database*. See full detailed chart and product monograph at www.naturaldatabase.com.

Figure 78.1 • Recommendation chart for natural medicines[a].

Notes:

- Glucosamine sulfate
  - 1500 mg/d
  - Examples:
    - Dona Glucosamine (Rotta Pharmaceuticals)

- SAMe (S-Adenosyl Methionine - endogenous)
  - 600 to 1,600 mg/d
  - Example:
    - Manufacturer: NOW
- Capsaicin (topical) (*Capsicum frutescens*)
  - 0.025% to 0.075%
- Avocado soybean unsaponifiables (ASUs)
  - 300 to 600 mg/d
- Devil's claw (*Harpagophytum procumbens*)
  - Typically standardized to 50 to 100 mg harpagoside component per day
  - Example:
    - Harpadol (Arkopharma)
      - 2.6 g/d providing 57 mg of the harpagoside constituent and 87 mg of total iridoid glycosides.
    - Doloteffin (Ardeypharm)
      - 2,400 mg/d providing 60 mg/d of harpagoside
- Cetylated fatty acids (oral or topical in combination with menthol)
  - Example:
    - Celadrin (Proprietary Nutritionals, Inc.)
    - 350 mg combined with 50 mg soy lecithin and 75 mg fish oil
    - Topically it has been combined with menthol
- Antioxidants
  - Moderate to high intake of vitamin C > Beta-carotene > vitamin E appears to decrease progression of knee arthritis and pain
- Niacinamide
  - 3 g daily in divided doses
- Methylsulfonylmethane (MSM)
  - 1.5 to 6 g/d
- Ginger (*Zingiber officinale*)
  - Example
    - EV ext-33 (Eurovita)
    - 170 mg three times daily
- Combination products
  - Phlogenzym (Mucos Pharma GMBH & Co)
    - Bromelain 90 mg
    - Trypsin 48 mg
    - Rutin (rutosid trihydrate) 100 mg
    - Dosing 2 to 3 times per day

CHAPTER 79

Natural Medicines in the Clinical Management of Osteoporosis

Robert Alan Bonakdar

SAFETY

EFFICACY	Likely Safe	Possibly Safe	Insufficient Evidence
Effective			
Likely Effective	Calcium Vitamin D Ipriflavone		
Possibly Effective	Magnesium Soy (*Glycine max*) Manganese Strontium ranelate Vitamin K Zinc Fish oil Copper Evening primrose oil (*Oenothera biennis*)	DHEA Silicon	
Insufficient Evidence	Alfalfa (*Medicago sativa*) Green and black tea (*Camellia sinensis*) Boron	Red clover (*Trifolium pratense*) Panax ginseng	

[a]Ratings courtesy of *Natural Medicines Comprehensive Database*. See full detailed chart and product monograph at www.naturaldatabase.com.

Figure 79.1 • Recommendation chart for Natural Medicines in the Clinical Management of Osteoporosis[a].

Notes:

- Vitamin D
  - 800 to 1,000 IU per day, higher based on baseline level
- Calcium
  - Prevention, in postmenopausal women
    - 1 to 1.6 g/d
  - Prevention, in premenopausal women
    - 1 to 1.2 g

- Men
  - 1 g/d has been used in most research
- Note: Absorption of calcium from supplements is greatest when taken with food in doses of 500 mg or less since the active transport system for calcium in the small bowel is easily saturated

- Ipriflavone (isoflavone derived from soy)
  - 1,000 mg daily, typically with calcium
- Strontium ranelate
  - 2 g/d strontium ranelate, providing 680 mg elemental strontium
  - Note: Appears to reduce the risk of vertebral fractures by 40% in postmenopausal women with osteoporosis and a history of vertebral fracture. Some evidence that it may increase bone mineral density in these patients by 14% at the lumbar spine and 8% at the femoral neck

CHAPTER 80

Natural Medicines in the Clinical Management of Premenstrual Syndrome

Robert Alan Bonakdar

SAFETY

EFFICACY	Likely Safe	Possibly Safe	Insufficient Evidence
Effective			
Likely Effective	Calcium		
Possibly Effective	Chasteberry (*Vitex agnus-castus*) Ginkgo (*Ginkgo biloba*) Magnesium Pyridoxine (vitamin B_6) Vitamin E		
Insufficient Evidence	Manganese St. John's Wort SAMe Soy (*Glycine max*) Vitamin D	Black cohosh (*Actaea racemosa*) Dong quai (*Angelica sinensis*) Red clover (*Trifolium pratense*)	

[a]Ratings courtesy of *Natural Medicines Comprehensive Database*. See full detailed chart and product monograph at www.naturaldatabase.com.

Figure 80.1 • Recommendation chart for Natural Medicines in the Clinical Management of Premenstrual Syndrome[a].

Notes:

- Calcium
  - 1,000 to 1,300 mg/d
  - Note: In one trial, women consuming an average of 1,283 mg/d from foods seem to have about a 30% lower risk of developing PMS compared with women consuming an average of 529 mg/d

- Chasteberry (*Vitex agnus-castus*)
    - Examples:
        - Agnolyt (Madaus GmbH)
            - 4 mg daily
        - Ze 440 (Prefemin, Zeller AG)
            - 20 mg/d
        - BNO 1095/Agnucaston/Cyclodynon (Bionorica AG)
            - 20 mg/d
- Pyridoxine (vitamin B_6)
    - 50 to 200 mg/d
- Magnesium (various salts)
    - 200 to 360 mg/d
- Combination products
    - (De Souza MC. *J Womens Health Gend Based Med* 2000;9(2):131–139.)
        - Magnesium 200 mg
        - Vitamin B_6 50 mg
        - Dosing: Once per day
        - Note: Combination demonstrated modest benefit for anxiety-related premenstrual symptoms

CHAPTER 81

Natural Medicines in the Clinical Management of Urinary Tract Infection (UTI)

Robert Alan Bonakdar

SAFETY

EFFICACY	Likely Safe	Possibly Safe	Insufficient Evidence
Effective			
Likely Effective			
Possibly Effective	Cranberry (*Vaccinium macrocarpon*)		
Insufficient Evidence	Echinacea Garlic (*Allium sativum*) Lactobacillus	Asparagus (*Asparagus officinalis*) Bifidobacteria Dandelion (*Taraxacum officinale*)	

[a]Ratings courtesy of *Natural Medicines Comprehensive Database*. See full detailed chart and product monograph at www.naturaldatabase.com.

Figure 81.1 • Recommendation chart for Natural Medicines in the Clinical Management of Urinary Tract Infection[a].

Notes:

- Cranberry
  - Drink:
    - Asymptomatic bacteriuria and urinary tract infections (UTIs) in pregnant women
      - Cranberry juice cocktail 16 oz daily
    - Recurrent UTIs in elderly women
      - Cranberry juice cocktail 26% cranberry juice (Ocean Spray) 300 ml daily
  - Encapsulated: 400 to 500 mg/d
    - Example:
      - Cran-Max (Buckton Scott Health Products)

- Lactobacillus (recurrent UTIs)
  - Vaginal suppositories with L. casei var rhamnosus and *L. fermentum*:
    - 0.5 g (1.6 billion organisms) 2/wk × 2 wk, then monthly
- Combination products
  - 50 ml of cranberry–lingonberry juice concentrate daily for 6 months
    - Dosing: 5 times/wk × 1 y
    - Note: Above combination provided a 20% reduction in absolute risk recurrent UTI compared with the control group with a number needed to treat of 5, oral Lactobacillus did not seem to reduce the recurrence of urinary tract infection.

INDEX